Core Curriculum for Specializing in Intellectual and Developmental Disability

A Resource for Nurses and Other Health Care Professionals

Edited by

Wendy M. Nehring
RN, PhD, FAAN, FAAMR

JONES AND BARTLETT PUBLISHERS
Sudbury, Massachusetts
BOSTON   TORONTO   LONDON   SINGAPORE

World Headquarters

Jones and Bartlett Publishers
40 Tall Pine Drive
Sudbury, MA 01776
978-443-5000
info@jbpub.com
www.jbpub.com

Jones and Bartlett Publishers
Canada
2406 Nikanna Road
Mississauga, ON L5C 2W6
CANADA

Jones and Bartlett Publishers
International
Barb House, Barb Mews
London W6 7PA
UK

Library of Congress Cataloging-in-Publication Data

Core curriculum for specializing in intellectual and developmental disability : a resource for nurses and other health care professionals / [edited by] Wendy M. Nehring.
    p. ; cm.
  Includes bibliographical references and index.
  ISBN 0-7637-4765-3 (pbk. : alk. paper)
  1. People with mental disabilities—Care. 2. Developmentally disabled—Care. 3. Mental retardation—Nursing. 4. Developmental disabilities—Nursing.
  [DNLM: 1. Mental Retardation—nursing. 2. Developmental Disabilities—nursing. 3. Nurse's Role. 4. Quality of Life. WY 160 C797 2005] I. Nehring, Wendy M., 1957–
  RC570.C67 2005
  362.2'0425—dc22

2004021974

Production Credits
Acquisitions Editor: Kevin Sullivan
Production Director: Amy Rose
Production Editor: Jeff Freeland
Editorial Assistant: Amy Sibley
Marketing Manager: Ed McKenna
Associate Marketing Manager: Emily Ekle
Manufacturing and Inventory Coordinator: Amy Bacus
Design and Composition: Paw Print Media
Cover Design: Timothy Dziewit
Printing and Binding: Courier Stoughton

Printed in the United States of America
09 08 07 06 05   10 9 8 7 6 5 4 3 2 1

To Sid, Adam, and Kaitlyn, I love you all very much!

Contents

Section V: Family Perspectives   379

Section VI: Health Care Policy Issues   395

Foreword

The last half of the twentieth century saw a sea of change in our knowledge, attitudes, and beliefs related to individuals with intellectual and development disabilities (I/DD). We have moved through a period of de-institutionalization to full inclusion of those individuals in every aspects of our daily living. These new approaches to a previously disenfranchised population were codified in federal legislation including the Americans with Disabilities Act in 1990, Part H of the Individuals with Disabilities Education Act, (now Part C), and the Early Intervention Program for Infants and Toddlers, and are reflected in the New Freedom Initiative, under which the Office of Disability was established in the Department of Health and Human Services in 2001.

There were likely multiple circumstances that led to those changes, but clearly one key factor was the discovery in the late 1950s that the severe mental retardation associated with phenylketonuria (PKU) could be prevented with a special diet for affected infants and the subsequent establishment of newborn screening programs for that disorder. Today, infants can be screened at birth for many disorders that will result in disability or death if untreated early. These programs are undergoing massive growth as a result of scientific and technologic advances as this manuscript goes to press. The tenets of early detection and intervention are also applied broadly in routine health care at all ages.

The editor has gathered here a comprehensive text on current concepts in I/DD affecting individuals across the lifespan, placed in historical context. The section on basic concepts is particularly important because our terminology has changed so much over the years. The contribution of genetics and the relatively new genomics cannot be underestimated. Although we have seen an explosive growth in our knowledge in recent years, we can only imagine what is yet to be learned. Section IV of the book contains an enormous amount of information that is both informative and practical. Attention to the pivotal role and contribution of families as equal partners in the care of individuals with I/DD cannot be understated. The final section on health care policy reminds us of the importance of attendance to the contribution of culture and ethnicity in an increasingly multicultural society. As our knowledge, attitudes, and beliefs about I/DD continue to evolve, so too, will the ethical and legal issues as well as economic and policy change. The notion of putting computer technology to work in providing additional resources is especially helpful because it can be easily updated.

The contributing authors, many of whom are nurses, are noted in their fields. This is a useful book for students and professionals alike in any and all of the disciplines working with infants, children, and adults with I/DD. I applaud the editor for undertaking the challenge of this comprehensive and very useful volume.

Irene Forsman, RN, MS

Preface

There is a disparity in health care for persons with intellectual and developmental disabilities (I/DD) of all ages in the United States. Part of this problem is due to a lack of knowledge by health care professionals about the specific conditions that cause I/DD, health care management for this population (including secondary conditions), and available financial options and community referrals. It is often the case that educational curriculums at both the undergraduate and graduate levels for all health care disciplines are unable to fit in enough information about and practical experiences with this population.

This is one of only a few books available in which interdisciplinary authors have written on salient topics related to the health care of persons, of all ages, with I/DD. The information presented by the authors is evidence-based. This book is intended to be informational, as well as for use in academic, continuing education, and professional inservice programs. The chapters are presented in outline format so that the user can learn about the major issues on the topic and/or adapt the material for presentation. The book is divided into six sections: history of health professionals' involvement in the care of persons with I/DD, basic concepts, the influence of genetics, nursing and health professionals' roles in the field of I/DD, family perspectives, and health care policy issues. Accompanying links to resources (including books, media, organizations, and web sites), a genetic glossary, and study questions for each chapter are available on the publisher's web site.

The first section provides an overview of the history of health care professionals' involvement in and care of persons with I/DD. Most of the available published literature covers medical and nursing care.

In the second section on basic concepts, the reader is introduced to a discussion of the definitions of mental retardation and similar terms, such as developmental disabilities. Terminology in this field has changed over the years to reflect societal attitudes and, more recently, the perspectives of persons with I/DD. Other chapters cover the etiology and epidemiology of I/DD.

The third section is devoted to genetics. This is an area of science that will have tremendous impact on persons with I/DD in the coming years. Health care professionals will need to be knowledgeable of the many genetic advances, changes in technology to detect I/DD, and accompanying medical advances that will possibly ameliorate future conditions that cause I/DD, but which will also hopefully improve the lives of persons with I/DD.

The fourth section is the longest and covers the roles of nurses and other health care professionals in the field of I/DD as they interact with and care for persons of all ages with I/DD. The reader will note that there is information in many of these chapters that is repeated in other chapters, reflecting the interdisciplinary and multisystem nature of caring for persons with I/DD.

The fifth section focuses on family perspectives. Information is provided on family reactions to initial diagnosis through parental planning for the lifelong care of their child with I/DD. Siblings and grandparents are also discussed.

The sixth and final section is devoted to health care policy issues. The chapters in this section focus on cultural and ethnic, legal and ethical, and economic and health policy issues.

Due to a scarcity of books on these health care topics, it is hoped that the reader will find the information useful and will be able to locate additional resources to supplement the information found in this book. For the reader who is not employed in an academic or health care setting where resources are available on these topics, the public library in any community is an excellent resource. For materials that are not available at that library, inter-library loans can be obtained from other libraries.

Many people who assisted in the completion of this book need to be thanked. These individuals include the members of the Nursing Division and the Health Promotions Coordinating Council of the American Association on Mental Retardation, of which most are authors of the chapters in this book. Special thanks are also extended to Kevin Sullivan, Amy Sibley, and Jeff Freeland of Jones and Bartlett Publishers, whose gentle prodding kept this book on track.

Wendy H. Nehring, RN, PhD, FAAN, FAAMR
Editor

List of Authors/ Contributors to Core Curriculum

Wendy M. Nehring, RN, PhD, FAAN, FAAMR **Editor**
College of Nursing
Rutgers, The State University of New Jersey
180 University Ave., Ackerson Hall, Rm. 102A
Newark, NJ 07102
973/353-5293, x606 (w), 973/353-1277 (f)
nehring@nightingale.rutgers.edu
(Chapter 1, Chapter 2, Chapter 4, Chapter 7, Chapter 10,
    Chapter 12, and Chapter 25)

Sarah Ailey, RN, PhD
Assistant Professor
Rush University College of Nursing
Department of Community and Mental Health Nursing
Armour Academic Center
600 South Paulina Street, Rm. 1080
Chicago, IL 60623
312/942-3383 (w); 312/942-2549 (f)
Sarah_H_Ailey@rush.edu
(Chapter 18)

Judith Amundson, RD, MS, FAAMR
Health Services Consultant
Employment Policy Group
Center for Disabilities and Development
University of Iowa Health Care
100 Hawkins Drive
Iowa City, IA 52242-1011
319/356-1455 (w), 319/356-8284 (f)
judith-amundson@uiowa.edu
(Chapter 16)

Lee S. Barks, RN, ARNP, PhD(c), CDDN, FAAMR
Consulting Nurse Clinical Specialist
1 Village Green
Longwood, FL 32779-9752
407/741-4023 (h), 407/333-2133 (f)
LeeBarks@cfl.rr.com
(Chapter 17)

Cecily A. Betz, RN, PhD, FAAN
Associate Professor
USC University Affiliated Program
Children's Hospital Los Angeles
4650 Sunset Boulevard, Mailstop #53
Los Angeles, CA 90027
323-669-2300 (w), 323/913-1003 (f)
cbetz@usc.edu
(Chapter 11)

Mary Beth Bruder, PhD
Professor of Pediatrics and Educational Psychology
Director, University of Connecticut A. J. Pappanikou
    Center for Excellence in Developmental Disabilities
    Education, Research, and Service
University of Connecticut Health Center
263 Farmington Avenue, Suite 260, MC 6222
Farmington, CT 06030-6222
860/679-1500 (w), 860/679-1588 (f)
bruder@nso1.uchc.edu
(Chapter 8)

Steven Corbin, DDS, MPH
Dean, Special Olympics University
Special Olympics Inc.
Special Olympics University—Health and Research
1325 G Street, NW, Suite 500
Washington, DC 20005
scorbin@specialolympics.org
(Chapter 23)

Jean Nelson Farley, RN, MSN, PNP-C, CRRN
Clinical Instructor
Georgetown University
School of Nursing & Health Studies
3700 Reservoir Road NW
Washington, DC 20007
202/687-7334 (w), 202/687-5553 (f)
farleyj@georgetown.edu
(Chapter 15)

Melissa Spezia Faulkner, RN, DSN
Associate Professor
Department of Maternal Child Nursing
University of Illinois at Chicago
845 S. Damen Ave., Rm. 810
Chicago, IL 60612-7350
312/996-2193 (w), 312/996-8871 (f)
melissaf@uic.edu
(Chapter 7)

Sandra A. Faux, RN, PhD
Associate Professor
Rush University College of Nursing
Armour Academic Building
600 S. Paulina, #1064K
Chicago, IL 60612
312/942-2760 (w), 312/942-2549 (f)
sandra_a_faux@rush.edu
(Chapter 24)

Stanford Fenton, DDS, MDS, FDS RCSEd, FAAPD
Professor and Chair
Department of Pediatric Dentistry & Community Oral
    Health
University of Tennessee College of Dentistry
875 Union Avenue
Memphis, TN 38163
and
Director of Dental Services
Crittenden Memorial Hospital
200 Tyler Avenue
West Memphis, AR 72303
901/448-6206 (w), 901/448-6249 (f)
sfenton@utmem.edu
(Chapter 23)

Irene Forsman, RN, MS
Nurse Consultant
Division of Services for Special Health Needs
Health Resources and Services Administration
18A-18 PKLN
Rockville, MD 20857
301/443-9023 (w)
Iforsman@hrsa.gov
(Foreword)

Carolyn Graff, RNC, PhD
Chief of Nursing

University of Tennessee, Boling Center for Developmental
    Disabilities
711 Jefferson Ave.
Memphis, TN 38105
901/448-6544 (w), 901/448-4121 (f)
cgraff@utmem.edu
(Chapter 6)

Joan Earle Hahn, RN, DNSc, CDDN, CS
Assistant Adjunct Professor
University of California, Los Angeles
School of Nursing
Factor Building Room 5-145
700 Tiverton, Box 956919
Los Angeles, CA 90095-6919
310/206-3339 (w), 310/206-3241 (f)
jhahn@sonnet.ucla.edu
(Chapter 14)

Stanley D. Handmaker, MD, DPhil, FAAMR
Professor of Pediatrics and Psychiatry
Department of Pediatrics
University of New Mexico Health Sciences Center
ACC-3012
Albuquerque, NM 87131-0001
505/272-0344 (w), 505/272-6845 (f)
shandmaker@salud.unm.edu
(Chapter 3)

Barbara Hanley, MSW, MPH, PhD, FAAMR
Director of Social Work and Associate Professor of
    Pediatrics
Cincinnati Children's Hospital Medical Center
460 B, Building E
3333 Burnet Ave.
Cincinnati, OH 45229
513/636-8364 (w), 513/636-3962 (f)
Barbara.Hanley@cchmc.org
(Chapter 20)

Dalice L. Hertzberg, RN, MSN, FNP-C, CRRN
Instructor
JFK Partners
University of Colorado Health Sciences Center at
    Fitzsimmons
1784 Racine St.
Building 401, Room 105
Aurora, CO 80045

303/724-0652 (w), 303/724-0960 (f)
dalice.hertzberg@uchsc.edu
(Chapter 9 and Chapter 13)

Ted Kastner, MD
President
Developmental Disabilities Health Alliance, Inc.
1285 Broad Street
Bloomfield, NJ 07003
973/338-4200 (w), 973/338-4440 (f)
tkastner@ddha.com
(Chapter 27)

Marilyn Krajicek, RN, EdD, FAAN
Professor
University of Colorado Health Sciences Center
School of Nursing
4200 E. 9th Ave., C-288
Denver, CO 80262
303/315-8662 (w), 303/315-5215 (f)
marilyn.krajicek@uchsc.edu
(Chapter 9 and Chapter 13)

Felissa R. Lashley, RN, PhD, ACRN, FACMG, FAAN
Dean and Professor
College of Nursing
Rutgers, The State University of New Jersey
180 University Ave., Ackerson Hall, Rm. 102C
Newark, NJ 07102
973/353-5293, ext. 647 (w), 973/353-1277 (f)
lashley@nightingale.rutgers.edu
(Chapter 21)

Susan McFadden, OTR, MEd, FAOTA
Chief of Occupational Therapy
University of Tennessee, Boling Center for Developmental
    Disabilities
711 Jefferson Ave.
Memphis, TN 38105
901/448-6566 (w), 901/448-7097 (f)
smcfadden@utmem.edu
(Chapter 6)

Laura Murphy, EdD, NCSP
Chief of Psychology, Associate Professor of Psychiatry
University of Tennessee, Boling Center for Developmental
    Disabilities
711 Jefferson Ave.

Memphis, TN 38105
901/448-6511 (w), 901/448-3844 (f)
lmurphy@utmem.edu
(Chapter 6)

Deborah A. Natvig, RN, PhD
Associate Professor of Health Care Management
Lander University
320 Stanley Ave.
Greenwood, SC 29649
864/388-8246 (w), 864/388-8020 (f)
dnatvig@lander.edu
(Chapter 5)

Laura Pickler, MD, MPH
Instructor/Fellow Child Development
1056 East 19th Ave., B140
Denver, CO 80218
303/461-6441 (w), 303/764-8086 (f)
Pickler.Laura@tchden.org
(Chapter 12)

Ann Poindexter, MD, FAAP, FAAMR
1024 Clifton St.
Conway, AR 72034
501/329-8488 (h), 501/336-9831 (f)
dapoin@cyberback.com
(Chapter 2 and Chapter 4)

Leslie Rubin, MD, FAAMR
Director, Division of Developmental Pediatrics
Associate Professor Pediatrics
Emory University School of Medicine
776 Windsor Parkway
Atlanta, GA 30342
404/303-7247 (w), 404/303-7837 (f)
lrubi01@emory.edu
(Chapter 19)

Roy Q. Sanders, MD
Marcus Institute
1920 Briarcliff Road
Atlanta, GA 30329
Director of Psychiatric Services
404/419-5300 (w), 404/419–5410 (f)
(Chapter 19)

Teresa Savage, RN, PhD
Assistant Professor, Research
Maternal-Child Nursing
University of Illinois at Chicago
College of Nursing
845 S. Damen Ave., Room 841
Chicago, IL 60612
and
Associate Director
Center for the Study of Disability Ethics
Rehabilitation Institute of Chicago
345 E. Superior St.
Chicago, IL 60614
312/942-4036 (w), 312/996-8871 (f)
tsavag2@uic.edu
(Chapter 26)

Bob Schalock, PhD
President
Bob Schalock & Associates
113 North Park, P.O. Box 285
Chewelah, WA 99109-0285
509/935-8176 (w), 509/935-6101 (f)
rschalock@ultraplix.com
(Chapter 22)

Kathy Pekala Service, RN, MS, RNC/NP, CDDN
Nurse Practitioner
Franklin-Hampshire Area Office
Department of Mental Retardation
One Roundhouse Plaza
Northampton, MA 01060-4401
413/586-4948, x109 (w); 413/584-0611 (f)
Kathy.Service@state.ma.us
(Chapter 14)

Justine Joan Sheppard, CCC-SLP, PhD, BRS-S
Adjunct Associate Professor
Teachers College, Columbia University
and
Nutritional Management Associates
111 Chincopee Rd.
Lake Hopatcong, NJ 07849-1552
973/663-3630 (w), 973/663-4108 (f)
jjsheppard@worldnet.att.net
(Chapter 17)

David Thomas, MA
Disabilities Consultant
JFK Partners, Department of Pediatrics
University of Colorado Health Sciences Center
4200 E. Ninth Ave., C221
Denver, CO 80262
303/864-5262 (w), 303/864-5270 (f)
Thomas.David@tchden.org
(Chapter 13)

Kevin Walsh, PhD
Director of Quality Management and Research
Developmental Disabilities Health Alliance, Inc.
223 Gibbsboro Road
Clementon, NJ 08021-4135
856/782-8989 (w), 856/782-4976 (f)
kwalsh@ddha.com
(Chapter 27)

Toni M. Whitaker, MD
Assistant Professor of Pediatrics
University of Tennessee, Boling Center for Developmental
    Disabilities
711 Jefferson Ave.
Memphis, TN 38105
901/448-3043 (w), 901/448-7097 (f)
twhitaker@utmem.edu
(Chapter 6)

Sheryl White-Scott, MD, FACP
Director, St. Charles Developmental Disabilities Program,
    SVCMC
Assistant Professor of Medicine, NYMC
Sister Thea Bowman
1205 Sutter Ave.
Brooklyn, NY 11208
718/647-2600, ext. 127 (w), 718/348-0308 (f)
swhite@svcmcny.org
(Chapter 26)

History of Health Professionals' Involvement in the Care of Persons with Intellectual and Developmental Disabilities

I

History of Nursing and Health Professionals in Intellectual and Developmental Disabilities

Wendy M. Nehring, RN, PhD, FAAN, FAAMR

1

Objectives

At the completion of this chapter, the learner will be able to:

1. Identify early attitudes in health care and society regarding persons with intellectual and developmental disabilities (I/DD).
2. Discuss the historical issues across time that are pivotal in the field of I/DD.
3. Describe how nursing and medical care for persons with I/DD evolved over time.
4. Describe nursing and medical education in I/DD across time.

Key Points

- Nurses and physicians have specialized in the care of persons with I/DD since organized nursing and medicine began.
- Nursing and medical care for persons with I/DD has evolved with advances in medical and genetic knowledge, technology, and legislation.
- Education in I/DD has been present since the onset of nursing and medical education, but remains an undervalued area for theoretical and clinical teaching.
- Nursing and medical leaders in I/DD have impacted education, research, clinical practice, and health policy in the United States over the years.
- Across time, nurses have been at the forefront in developing practice guidelines in the field of I/DD.

I.   Background

Prior to the beginning of nursing and medicine as professional careers in this country, nurses and physicians in Europe and other parts of the world were known to care for persons with I/DD.

A. Ancient Civilizations (7000 BC–AD 399)

1. Persons with mental retardation were ostracized and persecuted, as they were thought to be possessed with evil spirits.

2. Women in the family cared for the sick at home.

3. No record is found regarding the care or teaching of persons with mental retardation (Kanner, 1964).

4. After the initiation of healing temples in ancient Egypt and Greece, humane care and remediation of persons with mental illness and epilepsy is described (Bullough & Bullough, 1969).

5. Infanticide was practiced by ancient Greeks, Romans, and Spartans.

6. Persons with mental retardation and epilepsy were often used as "fools" or "jesters" for entertainment (Kanner, 1964).

7. Hebraic and Christian tradition emphasized protection and empathy of persons with mental retardation.

8. Women and clergy from religious orders provided care to persons with mental retardation (Scheerenberger, 1983).

B. Middle Ages (400–1499)

1. Persons with mental retardation were once again used as "jesters" or "fools."

2. Persons with mental retardation were thought to be possessed by evil spirits and were often tortured as a result. Burning at the stake was one method.

3. Exceptions were the care given by the Sisters of Charity at Bicetre, the hospital and asylum in Paris, and by the villagers near the shrine at St. Dymphna at Gheel in Belgium (Bullough & Bullough, 1969).

4. Wine in which the bones of saints were soaked or washed was given as a tonic for persons with mental retardation and felt to be beneficial (Ingram, 1942).

5. Mental retardation was first legally defined in 1324 (Scheerenberger, 1983).

6. Persons with mental retardation lived in hospitals, prisons, almshouses, monasteries, warehouses, work houses, charitable facilities, and pest houses (Scheerenberger, 1983).

C. Reformation (1517–1648)

1. Martin Luther regarded persons with mental retardation as "godless" creatures. Both Luther and John Calvin felt persons with mental retardation should be euthanized as they were possessed by the Devil (Kanner, 1964).

2. Persons with mental retardation continued to be persecuted.

    3. Many hospitals in which many early nurses and physicians cared for persons with mental retardation were closed by the religious wars.

    4. These hospitals re-appeared later during the reign of Henry VIII.

D. Europe in the 18th Century

    1. Opening of England's Bethlehem Royal Hospital or "Bedlam," an early asylum converted from a hospital. Treatment was cruel and often neglectful. No hygiene was practiced. Visitors could pay a few pennies to visit the wards for "entertainment."

    2. Persons with mental retardation were similarly starved, put in stocks, chained, and maltreated at the monastery of Charenton near Paris.

    3. First effective reforms by Philippe Pinel (1745–1826) in France and William Tuke (1732–1822, a friend of Dorthea Dix) in England.

        a. Pinel was the physician director at the Bicetre Asylum and later at the Salpetriere Asylum.

            i. He removed all chains.

            ii. He wrote about the humane and scientific care and treatment of persons with mental illness and mental retardation, including a classification of brain disorders.

                a. Mania

                b. Melancholia

                c. Dementia

                d. Abolition of thought or idiocy

            iii. He was greatly aided by Jean-Baptiste Pussin and his wife, who provided nursing care (Bullough & Bullough, 1969).

        b. Tuke was a businessman who helped establish an asylum referred to as a "retreat" in York in 1796 after the death of a friend.

            i. Emphasized gentleness and sympathy

            ii. Used nurse attendants

II. Issues in Mental Retardation

Across time, health care professionals in the field of I/DD have been concerned with a number of issues affecting the persons they care for.

A. Terminology and Systems of Classification

    1. 19th century

        a. "Idiot" and "feeble-minded" used to describe people with mental retardation at start of 19th century.

        b. Several classifications published:

        i.   Ireland's (1877) *On Idiocy and Imbecility* introduced medical model of mental retardation as a disease.

       ii.   Kerlin (1877)

     iii.   Tuke (1892)

2.   Early decades of 20th century

    a.   Mental enfeeblement seen as one of three divisions of insanity. Further divided into idiocy and imbecility (Laird, 1902).

    b.   Additional classifications were published during this time:

        i.   Barr (1904) classified persons with mental retardation according to their educational potential.

       ii.   Goddard (1912) discussed the Kallikak family.

     iii.   Association of Medical Officers of American Institutions for Idiots and Feeble-Minded Persons (later the American Association on Mental Retardation) formed in 1921, with three levels of mental retardation based solely on intellectual functioning (IQ).

      iv.   Sands (1928)

3.   Next classification system published by American Association on Mental Deficiency in 1934.

    a.   Divided into three categories: idiot, imbecile, and moron.

    b.   Physical defects, neurological status, adaptive behavior, and family history were to be considered in addition to IQ.

    c.   IQ as dynamic rather than static quantity accepted.

    d.   Beginning understanding that intelligence is affected by environment.

4.   Doll (1941) first introduced concept of adaptive behavior in determining mental retardation.

5.   American Psychiatric Association (APA) introduces first *Diagnostic and Statistical Manual of Mental Disorders (DSM-I)* in 1952 and adopts term "mental deficiency" with three levels:

    a.   Mild deficiency (IQ: 70–85); uses highest cutoff to date

    b.   Moderate deficiency (IQ: 50–69)

    c.   Severe deficiency (IQ: 0–49)

6.   Other conditions such as physical handicaps, neurological impairment, behavioral and emotional problems, and learning disabilities were discussed in addition to mental retardation in the 1960s.

7.   Heber revised the next edition of the *Manual on Terminology and Classification in Mental Retardation* in 1961.

    a.   Three components of the definition arise: IQ, adaptive behavior, and origin in the developmental period.

    b. Five levels of mental retardation in 1961:

       i. Borderline (IQ: 83–67) (category eliminated in 1973 edition). May be problem of comorbidity between mild mental retardation and learning disabilities.

       ii. Mild (IQ: 66–50)

       iii. Moderate (IQ: 49–33)

       iv. Severe (IQ: 32–16)

       v. Profound (IQ: 16 or less) (Scheerenberger, 1987).

    c. Attempted to develop definition that would satisfy all disciplines with interest in mental retardation.

    d. Range of IQ scores for each level heavily discussed in 1973 and 1983 editions. In 1983, upper IQ cutoff for diagnosis was 75 (Grossman, 1983; Grossman, 1973).

8. Major changes occurred in the ninth edition of the American Association on Mental Retardation's book on the definition and classification on mental retardation (Luckasson et al., 1992) (see Chapter 2).

    a. Each individual is assessed along four dimensions:

       i. Intellectual functioning and adaptive skills

       ii. Psychological/emotional considerations

       iii. Physical/health/etiology considerations

       iv. Environmental considerations (Luckasson et al., 1992)

    b. Elimination of tiered-system of levels of mental retardation.

9. American Psychological Association (Editorial Board, 1996) published own manual on definition and classification of mental retardation, maintaining levels of mental retardation (i.e., mild, moderate, severe, and profound).

10. The term "developmental disabilities" coined in 1978 with the Developmental Disabilities Act. Originally meant for funding purposes, but has become a diagnostic label. Last defined in 2000 (see Chapter 2).

    a. Developmental disabilities as a category and label broadened in the 1990s to include attention deficit hyperactivity disorder (ADHD), autism, pervasive developmental disorder (PDD), emotional disorders (Craft & Wolraich, 1997), dual diagnosis, learning disabilities, and pediatric HIV infection.

11. Mental retardation as condition divided by biological and social definitions.

    a. Zigler and associates (1984) posited theory of mental retardation based on organic and familial or environmental etiologies. Prevalence rates differ when examining by different models. In 1986, Zigler and Hodapp added a third group: "undifferentiated."

    b. Mercer's (1973) discussion of the 3% prevalence of mental retardation as determined by the standard deviations on standardized IQ tests. Led to discussion of "six-hour child" as a child with established cognitive limitations based on IQ testing in school, and no obvious limitations in adaptive functioning while outside the school or after graduation.

B. Educational to Custodial Care

1. Educational instruction was given to children with mental retardation, epilepsy, and hearing impairment in Connecticut, New York, Ohio, and Massachusetts during the 19th century.

2. Edward Sequin (1812–1880) gains national attention with physiological education program. Believes in proper hygiene, exercise, and nutrition (Deutsch, 1949).

3. Methods to reverse cognitive impairment through sensory stimulation.

4. Worcester State Hospital in Massachusetts becomes first mental hospital in 1833 to deliver therapeutic care. Philosophy is that mental retardation is caused by disease rather than evil spirits or immorality.

5. By the end of the 19th century, care in almshouses, jails, and asylums became more custodial. Large numbers of patients admitted and treated with cages, abuse, chains, and neglect.

6. Large institutions built to house these increasingly large numbers of persons with mental retardation and mental illness away from the cities.

7. Custodial care influenced by the eugenics movement and works of Darwin and Galton. Belief in the etiology of mental retardation due to immorality and alcoholism greatly increased.

C. Segregation

1. Segregation of persons with mental retardation in institutions rose from the end of the the 19th century until 1967, when the population of persons with mental retardation reached its highest level.

2. Persons with mental retardation were not felt to be valuable and contributing members of society.

D. Sterilization

1. First sterilization law passed in 1907 in Indiana.

2. *Buck v. Bell* in 1927 resulted in decision to control numbers of persons with mental retardation through sterilization.

3. Many sterilization laws remained in place until the 1950s (Devine, 1983).

4. The effort to control and reduce the numbers of persons with mental retardation, which was unsuccessful, did not occur as a result of sterilization (Deutsch, 1949).

E. Mental Testing

1. Introduction of intelligence or IQ testing through the Binet-Simon test during the early 20th century.

    2. Alpha and Beta Army Scales during World War I resulted in large percentage (40%) of White soldiers found to be mentally retarded as determined by scoring of test (Haskell, 1944).

F. Mental Hygiene Movement and Child Guidance Clinics

    1. Mental hygiene movement and child guidance clinics began in an effort to prevent mental illness (Kassin & Veo, 1930–1931).

    2. Distinction began to be made between mental retardation and mental illness.

    3. Special education classes, vocational training, or placement in institutions was recommended when children with mental retardation were seen in the child guidance clinics (Kanner, 1967).

    4. Fernald opened outpatient diagnostic clinic in 1920 for children with mental retardation.

    5. Regional and community centers were established after World War II for the purposes of case finding, diagnosis, treatment, and rehabilitation (Wallace, 1958).

        a. Psychiatrists, psychologists, nutritionists, social workers, and public health and school nurses took part in these clinics.

G. Medical and Health Care Advances

    1. Throughout the 20th century, increased understanding of environmental influences on intelligence (e.g., adverse effects of drugs, alcohol, and caffeine on the fetus; lead; toxic chemicals; infections; child abuse; and malnutrition) and genetic inheritance patterns (e.g., inborn errors of metabolism, X-linked disorders, and mitochondrial disorders) occurred (Scheerenberger, 1983, 1987).

    2. Identification and description of phenylketonuria (PKU) by Folling in 1934 and the double-helix model of DNA by Watson and Crick in 1953 were significant discoveries.

    3. Advancements in prenatal and postnatal care, birth delivery techniques, immunizations, penicillin and sulfa drugs, treatment for subdural hematomas and neurological congenital defects, Rh incompatibility, and TB and birth defect prevention in the 1940s (Gittens, 1994; "Retrospect and Prospect in Mental Deficiency," 1945; Whitney, 1950).

    4. Knowledge and treatment of prematurity, newborn screening programs, and new understanding of parent–infant bonding.

    5. Human Genome Project has identified and described all genes located on the human genome. Proteomics and pharmacogenetics will be household words and standard treatment in a few years.

    6. Primary prevention and treatment involving prenatal care, newborn screening and treatment, genetic counseling, dietary supplements, and immunizations are widely practiced in developed countries.

H. Federal and Legislative Influences

1. The development of the Children's Bureau in 1912.

2. The Social Security Act of 1935 and later amendments.

3. Presidency of John F. Kennedy (1960–1963). Included among many recommendations, policies, and programs initiated by Kennedy was the institution of the University Affiliated Facilities and Programs (Kennedy, 1963; Scheerenberger, 1987) and the President's Panel (later Committee) on Mental Retardation.

4. *Wyatt v. Stickney* (1972) was a class action suit that determined that persons with mental retardation living in institutional settings had the right to refuse participation in research studies and must receive informed consent. Institutional Review Board approval of all research studies conducted in institutional settings must also be obtained.

5. *Pennsylvania Association for Retarded Children v. Commonwealth of Pennsylvania* (1971) and *Mills v. Board of Education* (1972) were landmark court cases that preceded Public Law 94-142 and found that no child could be denied public education in the state of Pennsylvania and Washington, D.C. respectively.

6. Section 504 of the Rehabilitation Act in 1973.

7. Public Law 94-142, the "Education for All Handicapped Children Act," passed in 1975, mandated educational services for all children between the ages of 3 and 21 years. Provided for individualized education plans (IEPs), placement in the least restrictive environment, protection from incorrect placement and classification, and due process.

8. *Pennhurst State School v. Halderman* (1981), a court case that supported deinstitutionalization and advocated for appropriate community supports. Was not upheld by the Supreme Court in 1981.

9. Public Law 99-457, which mandated educational services for all children between the ages of 3 and 5 years (Part B), with optional funding for the establishment of early intervention services for children from birth to 3 years of age (Part H). The two educational laws were combined into the "Individuals with Disabilities Educational Act" (IDEA) in 1990. IDEA was last amended and reauthorized in 2000 (P.L. 106-402).

10. "Americans with Disabilities Act of 1990" (ADA) (P.L. 101-336) was the largest civil rights legislation since the 1960s. The ADA addresses discrimination due to disability by public entities; employment; public accommodations; and architectural, communications, and transportation barriers (Gittler, 1997).

I. Deinstitutionalization

1. Blatt and Kaplan's (1966) book, *Christmas in Purgatory* and Geraldo Rivera's expose of Willowbrook in 1972 alarmed the public about conditions in institutions.

2. Edgerton's (1967) book, *The Cloak of Competence*, about the lives of persons with mild mental retardation after dismissal from an institution also influenced policy regarding decreasing the numbers of persons with mental retardation in institutions.

3. As states began the process of deinstitutionalization in the 1970s, foster care living arrangements, semi-independent living arrangements, group homes, developmental centers, and intermediate care facilities were established in the communities.

   a. All persons with mental retardation are currently living in the community in many states. Institutional enrollment is greatly reduced in all other states.

J. Normalization

1. Introduced by Bank-Mikkelsen and Nirje of Sweden in 1969.

2. Normalization means "making it possible for the mentally subnormal to experience the normal rhythm of the day, the weeks, the seasons and the year, supporting the normal development of the life circle, encouraging normal personal considerations, giving opportunity for bisexual contacts, confronting them with economical problems and providing for them normal living facilities, all with due consideration to the specific handicap of the individual" (Nirje, 1973, p. 29).

3. In 1983, Wolfensberger renamed normalization as "social role valorization" in an effort to focus on the individual's personhood and strengths.

K. Self-Advocacy

1. Acting as individuals, small groups, or organizations, persons with mental retardation and developmental disabilities are acting as their own advocates to obtain needed services, lifestyle choices, and self-respect. This has occurred more frequently over the past 20 years.

III. Nursing Care for Persons with I/DD

Nursing care was first provided to persons with I/DD by female members of the family, and later by religious nursing orders, "better" patients, and concerned individuals, prior to the onset of organized nursing. Nursing care in this country, beginning in the 19th century, was often crude and unsophisticated, but evolved to a specialized area of nursing where evidence-based care is the norm.

A. The 19th Century in America

1. In the early 19th century, "nursing care" was delivered by former or higher-functioning patients in the institutions across the country. In some institutions, nursing care was provided by slaves.

2. An early description of the nursing role in 1840 included the responsibilities of delivering personal hygiene and comfort to the patients, providing amusements, ambulating the patients, preventing their escape, and protecting the patients' safety.

3. No set standards of care were in place in institutions in most places until the late 19th century. Linda Richards was instrumental in influencing this change beginning in 1899.

4. In 1896, Howe described the nursing role as treating the patient with electricity and massage, and assisting with personal hygiene and exercise. The nurse also assisted the physician by charting.

B. 1900 to 1929

1. In the early years of the 20th century, nurses caring for persons with mental retardation were viewed as a "servant" of the physician and a housekeeper.

   a. Nutrition, skin integrity, and personal hygiene were important aspects of the nursing role.

   b. Nurses worked 14 hours for the day shift and 10 hours if they worked the night shift for 6.5 days per week (Santos & Stainbrook, 1949).

   c. Male nurses received an average of $34.33 per month and female nurses received an average of $28.13 per month (Barrus, 1908).

2. During the eugenic period in the early decades of the 20th century, Bradley (1914) suggested that nurses act as role models by their example and teaching. This meant that nurses must abstain from alcohol and uphold the highest moral values in their behavior.

   a. The nursing role consisted of giving verbal and written reports, physical assessment, feeding, toileting, hydrotherapy, bathing, care of epileptics and bedridden patients, exercise, entertainment, and the admission of new patients (Mabon, 1910; Purcell, 1911).

   b. Salaries averaged between $75 and $100 per month (Tucker, 1916).

C. 1930 to 1959

1. In the 1930s, the nursing literature first distinguished between nurses caring for persons with mental retardation and those caring for persons with mental illness.

2. Nurses cared for persons with mental retardation in a variety of settings, and working conditions improved for some nurses.

   a. Public health nurses were working with children with mental retardation and their families in homes and clinics. Advised parents on issues of communicable diseases, child welfare, health, and morality (Sloan & Stevens, 1976).

   b. Pediatric nurses were advised to recommend institutionalization for many cases (Jeans & Rand, 1936).

    c. Black American nurses received less pay than White nurses (Noll, 1995).

    d. The work day was decreased from 10 hours per day to 8 hours per day in 1935 (Wallace, 1948).

    e. In the 1940s, monthly salaries averaged from $150 to $220 for the staff nurse position (Nursing Documentation, Lincoln Developmental Center, March 1994).

  3. The high number of men serving in World War II brought about changes in the nursing care of persons with mental retardation.

    a. With many physicians called away from the institutions, nurses had to be responsible for a majority of the care. Many nurses were not experienced or well-qualified (Corcoran, 1947).

    b. Nurses' daily responsibilities in the institution included nursing reports, housekeeping, baths, dressing, feeding, checking patients' clothing, linen count, occupational therapy, admission of new patients, and care of the patients in the treatment ward (Dick, 1941). No medical records were found on the wards even in the 1950s (Devine, 1983).

    c. Nurses in the institutions were also beginning to provide continuing education to nurses in the community and to attendants in the institution regarding the care of children with mental retardation (Julian & Mischke, 1980).

    d. Nurses were now being mentioned as being a part of the interdisciplinary team (Julian & Mischke, 1980).

    e. Public health and school nurses were actively involved in casefinding and providing referrals for evaluation and diagnosis of mental retardation. These nurses taught parenting skills and counseled parents as needed, but often helped parents to complete the application for the institution (Corcoran, 1947; Julian & Mischke, 1980).

    f. Nurses wishing to work in this field were encouraged to have knowledge of normal and abnormal growth and development, psychiatry, psychology, sociology, and home economics (Clarke, 1942).

  4. By the 1950s, nurses in the community were helping families raise their children with mental retardation in the home (Flory, 1957).

D. Nursing care during the 1960s was directly influenced by the Kennedy administration.

  1. The nurse specializing in this field was now encouraged to be knowledgeable in human development, embryology, genetics, microbiology, prevention screening, nutrition, psychology, and health care (Murray & Barnard, 1966).

  2. The institutional environment continued to be unsafe and unsanitary until changes were made after the exposés by Blatt and Rivera in 1972 (Devine, 1983).

a. In some institutions, the ratio of nurses to patients was 1 to 55 (Miller, 1979).

b. Medications were used in abundance. For example, one nurse remembered giving 22,000 doses of medications to 162 patients in one month in 1960 (Ellibee, 1960).

3. Standing medical orders were present for every patient.

4. The 1960s, in many institutions, heralded the initiation of nursing documentation in the patient's charts. Nurses recorded the patient's vital signs, intake and output, height and weight, medications, restraint and isolation care, range of motion exercises, and provided brief nurse's notes and a weekly summary report.

5. Surgeries were often performed at the institutions until the 1970s and 1980s. In fact, it is reported that some of the employees also partook of this opportunity to have their surgeries done in the institution.

6. Programming by nurses for the patients was documented in the 1960s. These programs involved, for example:

a. Operant therapy (Barnard, 1968).

b. Aversive therapy (Slamar & Kachoyeanos, 1969).

c. Sensory-motor training (Pothier, 1968).

d. Self-care skills (Devine, 1983).

7. Nurses began to be involved in research. In 1965, Patricia McNelly, the Director of Nursing at the Central Wisconsin Colony and Training School, headed a research project to examine team nursing with a small group of four children (Miller, 1979).

8. In the community, public health nurses wrote important guides that were often found in every nurse's public health bag:

a. *A Guide for Public Health Nurses Working with Mentally Retarded Children* (Holtgrewe, 1964).

b. *Guide for Public Health Nurses Working with Children from the Developmental Point of View* (Borlick, 1961).

c. *A Developmental Approach to Casefinding Among Infants and Young Children* (Haynes, 1967).

9. A number of programs were also initiated by the nurses caring for children with mental retardation in the community. These programs included topics on:

a. Case management (Belfint & Sylvester, 1962).

b. Developmental assessment (Paulus, 1966).

c. Home training (Dittman, 1961; Steele, 1966).

d. Feeding and positioning (Haynes, 1968).

e. Parent support (Fackler, 1966) and education (McCarty & Chisholm, 1966) groups.

E. The 1970s heralded the onset of the modern era of nursing care for persons with mental retardation and developmental disabilities.

1. The developmental model of delivery of care replaced the medical model in 1976 (Miller, 1979).

2. Programming continued for the residents in the institutions on such topics as:

    a. Behavioral modification (Knapp, O'Neil, & Allen, 1974) and behavioral therapy (Etters, 1975).

    b. Therapeutic handling (Pothier, 1971).

    c. Elimination of rumination (Libby & Phillips, 1978).

3. Nursing care in the community during the 1970s took on these roles and functions concerning persons with mental retardation:

    a. Casefinding.

    b. Prevention of mental retardation.

    c. Developing infant programs.

    d. Working in interdisciplinary clinics.

    e. Offering genetic counseling.

    f. Working in neonatal intensive care units.

    g. Counseling individuals and/or groups.

    h. Providing community follow-up.

    i. Using screening tools.

    j. Offering specific programs in behavior modification and sex education (Krajicek & Roberts, 1976).

4. Nurses were now working in a variety of community settings caring for persons with mental retardation:

    a. The institution.

    b. The community.

    c. Hospital nursing units.

    d. University-affiliated facilities or programs.

    e. Health maintenance organizations.

    f. Colleges and schools of nursing.

    g. Federal agencies.

    h. Schools.

    i. Group homes (Worthy, 1975; see Chapter 6).

5. Additional nursing specialties arose around the care of children and adults with mental retardation and developmental disabilities including:

    a. The nurse in early intervention (Godfrey, 1975).

    b. The nurse in genetics (Scanlon & Fibison, 1995).

F. During the 1980s on into the current year, deinstitutionalization and scientific and technological advances have influenced nursing care.

   1. Residents remaining in institutional settings currently have more complex and multiple diagnoses and are older. They may be nonambulatory, have uncontrollable seizure disorders, have behavioral problems, and/or be diagnosed with many comorbidities.

   2. Important national nursing conferences were held during the past 25 years in the areas of early intervention, mental retardation and developmental disabilities, genetics, and implementing the Individuals with Disabilities Education Act (IDEA) in regards to invasive procedures.

      a. Specifically, six national workshops for nurses in mental retardation took place from 1958 to 1974.

IV. Medical Care for Persons with I/DD Across Time

Medical care has been provided in some measure to persons with I/DD since the middle ages. Early care was crude and reflected societal attitudes and the treatments of the time. Today, medical practice in the care of persons with I/DD continues to evolve and utilizes evidence-based care.

A. Middle Ages

   1. Avicenna (980–1037) first described levels of intelligence and felt that variances in a person's "vital energy" affected intelligence. His textbook, *Canon of Medicine* (n.d.) continued to be used in the 16th century (Scheerenberger, 1983).

   2. Paulus Bagellandes first described epilepsy in a textbook on children's diseases in 1472 (Redfield, 1947).

   3. Paracelsus (1493–1541) first described cretinism and discussed mental retardation and mental illness (Scheerenberger, 1983).

B. 17th and 18th Centuries

   1. Walter Harris (1647–1732), a pediatrician, first considered heredity as a cause of disease (Scheerenberger, 1983).

   2. Thomas Willis wrote about "stupidity" and "foolishness" in the 17th century. He felt that "stupidity" was related to blood and nervous problems. Willis further felt that in some cases "stupidity" could be erased, but if it was due to heredity, it probably could not. Medical care consisted of such treatments as evacuations, chocolate, coffee, and moderate sleep. "Foolishness" was Willis's term for epilepsy; he felt this condition was due to blockages in the brain. He believed that if evacuations did not work, then there was nothing that could be done (Andrews, 1998).

3. Benjamin Rush (1745–1813) was the first American physician to write about medical care for persons with mental retardation. He invented a spinning chair and a mechanical contraption that would cool a person down when their behaviors were too erratic (Scheerenberger, 1983).

C. 19th and 20th Centuries

1. Guggenbuhl (1816–1863) built an institution in Switzerland to care for persons with cretinism. He advocated for good diet, baths, exercise, medications, and training to develop the senses (Miller, 1996).

2. By the last half of the 19th century, greater than 50% of persons residing in institutions were epileptic. Treatments included exercise, chloroform, caffeine, arsenic, bleeding, and digitalis (Scheerenberger, 1983).

3. Tranquilizers became popular medical "restraints" during the 1940s through the 1970s.

4. A lack of access to mental health professionals and services was identified in the 1980s.

5. Dental care is another current area of need for persons of all ages with I/DD.

D. 21st Century

1. Discoveries, as a result of the Human Genome Project, have greatly affected medical care. New genetic findings and patterns of inheritance will lead to the advent of new methods of medical care in this century.

V. Nursing Training and Education in I/DD

Up until the middle of the 20th century, nursing training and education often took place in segregated settings, namely the institution, away from the hospitals where general nursing was taught. Today, the nursing curriculum generally has little to no content on I/DD. If taught, information on the care of persons with I/DD is often not presented across the lifespan. With the current daily advances in genetic knowledge, it is important to discuss mental retardation and developmental disabilities in this context.

A. Early training schools for nurse instruction in mental retardation took place in asylums by physicians. Most of these schools in the late 19th century were in the New England states.

1. The training of nurses and attendants was often indistinguishable.

2. The first training school for nurses in an asylum was conducted by Dr. Cowles at the McLean Asylum in Somerville, Massachusetts, in 1882 (Cowles, 1887).

   a. In the first year, nursing students learned about illness and injury, as well as basic nursing skills.

b. In the second year, nursing students learned about the philosophy and theory of "mental" nursing.

c. Each year of study consisted of 30 lectures over eight months (Cowles, 1887).

3. Physicians were hesitant to conduct training courses for nurses in case "She would want to be a doctor herself" (Cowles, 1887, p. 178).

4. Applicants to the early nursing training programs had to meet similar criteria as did those applying to general nursing programs (i.e., between 20 and 35 years of age, of good moral character, and unmarried) (Russell, 1945).

B. Nursing Education During the First Three Decades of the 20th Century

1. From 1900 to 1930, nurses received training in the care of persons with mental retardation in general hospitals, asylums, mental hospitals, and institutions.

2. The first general hospital program to affiliate with a mental hospital was The Presbyterian Hospital in Chicago, Illinois, in 1909 (Goodnow, 1949).

3. The nursing curriculum in institutional-based programs was similar to nursing curricula today, with the exception of instruction in hydrotherapy (from *Lectures from the Training School at the Lincoln State School & Colony, 1912–1918*, 1996).

4. Students on average received a stipend ranging from $15 to $35 per month. Students were also on duty between 12 and 15.5 hours a day with one-half day off per week (Tucker, 1916).

5. By the end of the 1920s, most nursing training took place in the general hospital (Haydon, 1928).

6. In the 1926 National League for Nursing Practice's revised curriculum guide, lectures in psychology were to include problems of the mental deviate, theories of intelligence, IQ, mental age, and mental testing. Lectures in psychiatry were to include feeblemindedness and idiocy, diagnoses, etiology, mental testing, grades and types, care, education, legal and state responsibilities, and colonies and institutions (*Revision of the Standard Curriculum: Psychology*, 1926).

7. Unfortunately, in some institutions, physicians were teaching the high functioning patients to be nurses. Interestingly, some of these "nurses" obtained positions as nurses in other institutions and as private-duty nurses (Trent, 1994).

C. Nursing education in mental retardation content changed little between 1930 and 1959.

D. Beginning in 1960, nursing education in mental retardation took place most often in collegiate schools of nursing.

1. Many nurse educators wrote about nursing content and clinical experiences provided for student nurses during the 1960s and 1970s (Lange & Whitney, 1966; Pennington, 1968)

2. A post-graduate program was developed for the study of children with handicaps at the University of Washington in Seattle in 1965 by Kathryn Barnard.

E. Several nurses provided in-services for other nurses in the institutions and in the community regarding mental retardation.

1. Most noteworthy were the in-services provided by Una Haynes on the physical and developmental assessment of infants, which were delivered across the country. Live babies were used for hands-on practice by the nurses in attendance. When these seminars ended in the late 1970s, over 17,000 nurses had attended.

2. From a working group of nursing leaders in the field came the publication *Guidelines for Continuing Education in Developmental Disabilities* (Haynes, Bumbalo, Cook, Haar, Krajicek, & Slamar, 1978). This publication was updated in 1996 as a booklet, *Continuing Education Needs for Nurses Caring for Children with Special Health Care Needs* (Austin & Donohoe, 1996).

F. In 1989, Brandt and Magyary developed a graduate nursing program for the clinical nurse specialist in early intervention.

G. Since the 1990s, the Maternal Child Health Bureau has provided funding to university nursing schools to prepare pediatric nurse practitioners for leadership roles in the management of children with special health care needs, including developmental disabilities.

VI. Training and Education in I/DD in Other Health Care Disciplines

Less is known about the history of education of other health care disciplines that specialize in I/DD.

A. Medical education would have involved some instruction through the early years in mental retardation as a subset of mental illness or insanity.

1. As in nursing, this emphasis would have been differentiated more specifically in the 20th century.

B. In both nursing and medicine, the content on and clinical experiences with persons with I/DD is most often found in pediatric courses, followed by psychiatric and community or public health courses.

C. Emphasis on the care of persons with I/DD in the disciplines of social work, nutrition, and psychology most likely appeared at the turn of the 20th century and was more recent in physical, occupational, and speech therapy.

VII. Standards of Care and Practice

Currently, health insurance companies through managed care require professionals to provide standards of practice by which to legally guide practice in a responsible manner. Nurses specializing in mental retardation and

developmental disabilities should be aware of the following standards of care and practice:

A. *Statement on the Scope and Standards for the Nurse Who Specializes in Developmental Disabilities and/or Mental Retardation* (Nehring, Roth, Natvig, Morse, & Krajicek, 1998; second edition in press).

B. *Standards of Nursing Practice in Mental Retardation/Developmental Disabilities* (Aggen et al., 1995).

C. *Standards of Nursing Practice for the Care of Children and Adolescents with Special Health and Developmental Needs* (Consensus Committee, 1994).

D. *Statement on the Scope and Standards of Genetics Clinical Nursing Practice* (International Society of Nurses in Genetics, 1998).

VIII. Summary

The history of care given by nurses and other health care professionals and their education in this specialization has evolved across time (Nehring, 1999). Many issues and societal attitudes have influenced this care and education. Today, health care for this population is evidence-based, and many organizations exist for professionals specializing in this field.

References

Aggen, R. L., DeGenaro, M. D., Fox, L., Hahn, J. E., Logan, B. A., & VonFumetti, L. (1995). *Standards of nursing practice in mental retardation/developmental disabilities.* Eugene, OR: Developmental Disabilities Nurses Association.

American Psychiatric Association. (1952). *Diagnostic and statistical manual of mental disorders: DSM-I.* Washington, DC: Author.

Americans with Disabilities Act of 1990, Pub. L. No. 101–133, 104 Stat. 328 (1991).

Andrews, J. (1998). Begging the question of idiocy: The definition and socio-cultural meaning of idiocy in early Britain: Part 2. *History of Psychiatry, 9,* 179–200.

Austin, J. R. D., & Donohoe, M. L. (1996). *Continuing education needs for nurses caring for children with special health care needs.* MCH Grant #MCU115042, Washington, DC: Health Resources and Services Administration, Maternal and Child Health Bureau and Georgetown University Child Development Center.

Barnard, K. (1968). Teaching the retarded child is a family affair. *American Journal of Nursing, 68,* 305–311.

Barr, M. W. (1904). *Mental defectives: Their history, treatment and training.* Philadelphia: P. Blakiston Son & Co.

Barrus, C. (1908). *Nursing the insane.* New York: The Macmillan Company.

Belfint, E. K., & Sylvester, L. W. (1962). Delaware's program for mentally retarded children. *Nursing Outlook, 10,* 442–444.

Blatt, B., & Kaplan, F. (1966). *Christmas in purgatory.* Boston: Allyn & Bacon.

Borlick, M. M. (1961). *Guide for public health nurses working with children from the developmental point of view.* Washington, DC: U.S. Department of Health, Education, and Welfare, Children's Bureau, Publ. No. 392-1961.

Bradley, E. B. (1914). The problem of the feeble-minded. *American Journal of Nursing, 14*, 628–631.

Buck v. Bell, 274 U.S. 200 (1927).

Bullough, V. L., & Bullough, B. (1969). *The emergence of modern nursing* (2nd ed.). London: Macmillan.

Clarke, E. K. (1942). *Mental hygiene for community nursing*. Minneapolis, MN: University of Minnesota Press.

Consensus Committee. (1994). *Standards of nursing practice for the care of children and adolescents with special health and developmental needs*. Vienna, VA: National Maternal and Child Health Clearinghouse.

Corcoran, M. E. (1947). Observations and suggestions for improving the care of mental defectives. *American Journal of Mental Deficiency, 51*, 599–605.

Cowles, E. (1887). Nursing-reform for the insane. *Journal of Insanity, 44*, 176–191.

Craft, L. T., & Wolraich, M. L. (1997). Conditions. In H. M. Wallace, J. C. MacQueen, R. F. Biehl, & J. A. Blackman (Eds.). *Mosby's resource guide to children with disabilities and chronic illness* (pp. 441–467). St. Louis, MO: Mosby.

Deutsch, A. (1949). *The mentally ill in America*. New York: Columbia University Press.

Developmental Disabilities Assistance and Bill of Rights Act of 2000, Pub. L. No. 102-402, 114 Stat. 1677 (2000).

Devine, P. (1983). Mental retardation: An early subspecialty in psychiatric nursing. *Journal of Psychiatric Nursing and Mental Health Services, 21*, 21–30.

Dick, K. R. (1941). Nursing in a state hospital. *American Journal of Nursing, 41*, 401–407.

Dittmann, L. L. (1961). *The nurse in home training programs for the retarded child*. Washington, DC: U.S. Department of Health, Education, and Welfare, Children's Bureau and Social Security Administration, U.S. Government Printing Office.

Doll, E. A. (1941). The essentials of an inclusive concept of mental deficiency. *American Journal of Mental Deficiency, 46*, 214–219.

Edgerton, R. (1967). *The cloak of competence*. Berkeley, CA: University of California Press.

Editorial Board. (1996). Definition of mental retardation. In J. W. Jacobsen & J. A. Mulick (Eds.). *Manual of diagnosis and professional practice in mental retardation* (pp. 13–41). Washington, DC: American Psychological Association.

Education for All Handicapped Children Act of 1975, Pub. L. No. 94-142, 89 Stat. 773 (1975).

Education of the Handicapped Act Amendments of 1986, Pub. L. No. 99-457, 100 Stat. 1145(1986).

Ellibee, E. (1960). *Annual report 1959–1960*. Unpublished document, Madison, WI: Central Wisconsin Colony and Training School.

Etters, L. E. (1975). Adolescent retardates in a therapy group. *American Journal of Nursing, 75*, 1174–1175.

Fackler, E. (1966). Community organization in culturally deprived areas. *Mental Retardation, 4*, 12–14.

Flory, M. C. (1957). Training the mentally retarded child. *Nursing Outlook, 5*, 344–347.

Gittens, J. (1994). *Poor relations: The child of the State of Illinois, 1818–1990*. Chicago, IL: University of Illinois Press.

Gittler, J. (1997). Legal rights of children with disabilities. In H. M. Wallace, J. C. McQueen, R. F. Biehl, & J. A. Blackman (Eds.). *Mosby's resource guide to children with disabilities and chronic illness* (pp. 97–105). St. Louis, MO: Mosby.

Goddard, H. (1912). *The Kallikak family: A study in the heredity of feeble-mindedness*. New York: Macmillan.

Godfrey, A. B. (1975). Sensory-motor stimulation: A specialized program. *American Journal of Nursing, 75,* 56-62.

Goodnow, M. (1949). *Nursing history* (8th ed.). Philadelphia: W. B. Saunders.

Grossman, H. (Ed.). (1983). *Classification in mental retardation.* Washington, DC: American Association in Mental Deficiency.

Grossman, H. (Ed.). (1973). *Manual on terminology and classification in mental retardation.* Washington, DC: American Association on Mental Deficiency.

Haskell, R. H. (1944). Mental deficiency over a hundred years: A brief historical sketch of trends in this field. *American Journal of Psychiatry, 100,* 107–118.

Haydon, E. M. (1928). Teaching and supervision of mental nursing. *American Journal of Nursing, 28,* 499–501.

Haynes, U. (1967). *A developmental approach to casefinding among infants and young children.* Washington, DC: U.S. Department of Health, Education and Welfare, Children's Bureau.

Haynes, U. (1968). *An ad hoc committee project–Sub-committee on nursing, American Association for Mental Deficiency guidelines for nursing standards in residential centers for the mentally retarded.* Washington, DC: United Cerebral Palsy Associations, Inc.

Haynes, U., Bumbalo, J., Cook, C., Haar, D., Krajicek, M., & Slamar, C. F. (1978). *Guidelines for continuing education in developmental disabilities.* Kansas City, MO: American Nurses Association, NP-58.

Heber, R. (1961). *A manual on terminology and classification in mental retardation* (2nd ed.). *American Journal on Mental Deficiency* (Mongraph suppl.).

Holtgrewe, M. M. (1964). *A guide for public health nurses working with mentally retarded children.* Washington, DC: Superintendent of Documents, U.S. Government Printing Office, #422-1964.

Individuals with Disabilities Education Act (IDEA) of 1990, Pub. L. No. 101-476, S 101, 104 Stat. 1103 (1990).

Individuals with Disabilities Education Act, Pub. L. No. 105-17, 111 Stat. 37 (1997).

International Society of Nurses in Genetics. (1998). *Statement on the scope and standards of genetics clinical nursing practice.* Washington, DC: American Nurses Publishing and author.

Ireland, W. W. (1877). *On idiocy and imbecility.* London: J. & A. Churchill.

Jeans, P. C., & Rand, W. (1936). *Essentials of pediatrics* (3rd ed.). Philadelphia: J. B. Lippincott.

Julian, D., & Mischke, K. (1980). Nursing and mental retardation: An Oregon perspective 1900–1979. *Oregon Nurse, 12,* 10–15.

Kanner, L. (1964). *A history of the care and study of the mentally retarded.* Springfield, IL: Charles C. Thomas.

Kanner, L. (1967). Medicine in the history of mental retardation 1800–1965. *American Journal of Mental Deficiency, 72,* 165–189.

Kassin, J., & Veo, L. (1930–31). The early recognition of mental diseases in children. *American Journal of Orthopsychiatry, 1,* 406–429.

Kennedy, J. F. (1963). *Message from the President of the United States relative to mental illness and mental retardation.* Document #58, 88th Congress, 1st Session, House of Representatives, Washington, DC: U. S. Government Printing Office.

Kerlin, I. N. (1877). *The organization of establishments for idiotic and imbecile classes.* Proceedings of the Association of Medical Officers of American Institutions for Idiotic and Feeble-Minded Persons, 19–28.

Knapp, M. E., O'Neil, S. M., & Allen, K. E. (1974). Teaching Suzi to walk by behavior modification of motor skills. *Nursing Forum, 13,* 158–183.

Krajicek, M. J., & Roberts, P. (1976). Nursing. In R. B. Johnston & P. R. Magrab (Eds.), *Developmental disorders: Assessment, treatment, education* (pp. 363–374). Baltimore: University Park Press.

Laird, S. L. (1902). Nursing of the insane. *American Journal of Nursing, 2,* 170–180.

Lange, S., & Whitney, L. (1966). Teaching mental retardation nursing: The faculty learn. *Nursing Outlook, 14,* 58–63.

Lectures from the Training School at the Lincoln State School & Colony, 1912–1918. (1996). Lincoln State School & Colony, Record Series 254.55, Illinois State Archives.

Libby, D. G., & Phillips, E. (1978). Eliminating rumination behavior in a profoundly retarded adolescent: An exploratory study. *Mental Retardation, 16,* 57.

Lincoln Developmental Center (March 1994). Nursing documentation. Unpublished documents. Lincoln, Illinois.

Luckasson, R., Coulter, D. L., Polloway, E. A., Reiss, S., Schalock, R. L., & Snell, M. E. (1992). *Mental retardation: Definition, classification, and systems of support* (9th ed.). Washington, DC: American Association on Mental Retardation.

Mabon, W. (1910). The nursing care of the insane. *American Journal of Nursing, 10,* 887–896.

McCarty, K. A., & Chisholm, M. M. (1966). Group education with mothers of retarded children. *Nursing Clinics of North America, 1,* 703–713.

Mercer, J. (1973). The myth of the 3% prevalence. In R. K. Eyman, C. E. Meyers, & G. Tarjan (Eds.). *Sociobehavioral studies in mental retardation* (pp. 1–18), Monograph #1, Washington, DC: American Association on Mental Deficiency.

Miller, E. (1996). Idiocy in the nineteenth century. *History of Psychiatry, 7,* 361–373.

Miller, J. A. (1979). A history of nursing at Central Wisconsin Center for the developmentally disabled. Unpublished manuscript. University of Illinois at Chicago, Chicago, IL.

Mills v. Board of Education, 348 F. Supp. 868 (D.D.C. 1972).

Murray, B. L., & Barnard, K. E. (1966). The nursing specialist in mental retardation. *Nursing Clinics of North America, 1,* 631–640.

Nehring, W. M. (1999). *A history of nursing in the field of mental retardation and developmental disabilities.* Washington, DC: American Association on Mental Retardation.

Nehring, W. M., Roth, S. P., Natvig, D. M., Morse, J. S., & Krajicek, M. (1998). *Statement on the scope and standards for the nurse who specializes in developmental disabilities and/or mental retardation.* Washington, DC: American Nurses Publishing and the Nursing Division of the American Association on Mental Retardation.

Nirje, B. (1973). The normalization principle—Implications and comments. In H. C. Gunzburg (Ed.). *Advances in the care of the mentally handicapped* (pp. 29–38). Baltimore: Williams & Wilkins.

Noll, S. (1995). *Feeble-minded in our midst: Institutions for the mentally retarded in the South, 1900-1940s.* Chapel Hill, NC: University of North Carolina Press.

Nursing documentation. (1994). Lincoln, IL: Lincoln Developmental Center.

Paulus, A. C. (1966). A tool for the assessment of the retarded child. *Nursing Clinics of North America, 1,* 659–668.

Pennhurst State School v. Halderman, Civil Action Nos. 79-1404, 79-1408, 79-1414, 79-1415, 79-1489, U.S. Third Circuit Court of Appeals (1981).

Pennington, M. (1968). Nursing students work with the mentally retarded. *Nursing Outlook, 16,* 38–39.

Pennsylvania Association for Retarded Children v. Commonwealth of Pennsylvania, 343 F. Supp. 279 (D.Pa. 1972).

Pothier, P. C. (1968). Implementing a training program with a severely retarded young child in a home setting. *ANA Clinical Sessions* (pp. 332–337). New York: Appleton-Century-Crofts.

Pothier, P. C. (1971). Therapeutic handling of the severely handicapped child. *American Journal of Nursing, 71,* 321–324.

Purcell, M. (1911). Nursing care of the insane. *American Journal of Nursing, 11,* 430–433.

Redfield, R. (1947). The folk society. *American Journal of Sociology, 52*, 293–308.

Rehabilitation Act of 1973, Pub. L. No. 93-112, 87 Stat. 355 (1973).

Retrospect and prospect in mental deficiency. (1945). *American Journal of Mental Deficiency, 49*, 8–18.

Revision of the standard curriculum: Psychology. (1926). *American Journal of Nursing, 26*, 140–146.

Russell, W. L. (1945). *The New York Hospital: A history of the psychiatric service 1771–1936.* New York: Columbia University Press.

Sands, I. J. (1928). *Nervous and mental diseases for nurses.* Philadelphia: W. B. Saunders.

Santos, E. H., & Stainbrook, E. (1949). A history of psychiatric nursing in the nineteenth century. Part I. *Journal of the History of Medicine, 4*, 48–60.

Scanlon, C., & Fibison, W. (1995). *Managing genetic information: Implications for nursing practice.* Washington, DC: American Nurses Association.

Scheerenberger, R. C. (1983). *A history of mental retardation.* Baltimore: Paul H. Brookes.

Scheerenberger, R. C. (1987). *A history of mental retardation: A quarter century of promise.* Baltimore: Paul H. Brookes.

Slamar, C. F., & Kachoyeanos, M. K. (1969). Nursing therapy in a combined treatment approach to rumination. *ANA Clinical Sessions* (pp. 185–195). New York: Appleton-Century-Crofts.

Sloan, W., & Stevens, H. A. (1976). *A century of concern: A history of the American Association on Mental Deficiency 1876–1976.* Washington, DC: American Association on Mental Deficiency.

Steele, S. (1966). The role of the public health nurse in the discharge of the handicapped child in the community. *Nursing Clinics of North America, 1*, 153–162.

Trent, J. W. (1994). *Inventing the feeble mind: A history of mental retardation in the United States.* Los Angeles: University of California Press.

Tucker, K. (1916). Nursing care of the insane in the United States. *American Journal of Nursing, 16*, 198–202.

Tuke, D. H. (Ed.). (1892). *A dictionary of psychological medicine* (Vol. 1). Philadelphia: P. Blakiston, Son & Co.

Wallace, A. M. (1948). *History of the Walter E. Fernald State School.* Unpublished document, Waverley, MA: Walter E. Fernald State School.

Wallace, H. M. (1958). Progress and problems in maternal and child health. *Nursing Outlook, 6*, 278–281.

Whitney, E. A. (1950). Mental deficiency in the 1880's and 1940's: A brief review of sixty year's progress. *American Journal of Mental Deficiency, 54*, 151–154.

Wolfensberger, W. (1983). Social role valorization: A proposed new term for the principle of normalization. *Mental Retardation, 21*, 234–239.

Worthy, E. J. (1975). Symposium on the child with developmental disabilities. *Nursing Clinics of North America, 10*, 307–308.

Wyatt v. Stickney, 344 F. Supp 373 (N.D. Ala. 1972).

Zigler, E., Balla, D., & Hodapp, R. (1984). On the definition and classification of mental retardation. *American Journal of Mental Deficiency, 89*, 215–230.

Zigler, E., & Hodapp, R. M. (1986). *Understanding mental retardation.* New York: Cambridge University Press.

Basic Concepts

II

Definition of Mental Retardation/Developmental Disabilities

2

Ann R. Poindexter, MD, FAAMR, and
Wendy M. Nehring, RN, PhD, FAAN, FAAMR

Objectives

At the completion of this chapter, the learner will be able to:

1. Identify different definitions of mental retardation.
2. List the three essential elements that must be present to make a diagnosis of mental retardation.
3. Describe the particular importance of adaptive behavior as related to the individual's age, community, and culture.
4. Understand the purpose(s) of determining limitations for a particular individual.
5. Identify definitions of developmental disability and special health care needs.

Key Points

- Three criteria must be present to diagnose mental retardation: significant limitations in intellectual functioning, significant limitations in adaptive behavior, and manifestation before the age of 18 years.

- Limitations in functioning must be assessed within the current context of the typical environment of a person of similar age and culture.

- Health professionals must consider a variety of factors—including diversity and differences in the developmental domains of communication, sensori-motor, and behavior—when assessing for mental retardation.

- For every individual, strengths and limitations co-exist.

- Describing a person's limitations is done in order to identify a list of necessary supports which may be prioritized according to immediate need and/or economic status.

- It is assumed that a person with intellectual and developmental disabilities will have a higher quality of life with appropriate supports across their lifespan.

- A number of terms exist that describe persons with intellectual and developmental disabilities.

I.   Definitions of Mental Retardation

Several definitions of mental retardation have been written over the last century. Similar elements in these definitions include IQ, adaptive functioning, and age of onset. Historically, these definitions were first written by physicians and by the 1900s were written by organizations, such as the American Association on Mental Retardation (AAMR) and the American Psychological Association (APA). The *Diagnostic and Statistical Manual-IV-TR* (American Psychiatric Association, 2000) also includes a definition of mental retardation. Each state further identifies its own definition of mental retardation, which may be one of the above organizational definitions (see Schroeder, Gerry, Gertz, & Velazquez, 2002). The latest definitions are provided below.

A. According to the AAMR (Luckasson et al., 2002), mental retardation is "a disability (not a diagnosis) characterized by significant limitations both in intellectual functioning and in adaptive behavior as expressed in conceptual, social, and practical adaptive skills. This disability originates before age 18" (Luckasson et al., 2002, p. 19).

   1. Definition of mental retardation as a disability does not consider a long-term prognosis as the definition of mental retardation, and is based upon the individual's level of functioning when assessed (Editorial Board, 1996).

   2. The theoretical model behind the 2002 definition involves the dimensions of intelligence, adaptive behavior, interactions and roles in world, health, and environment and culture.

   3. Any limitations identified in an individual's present level of functioning must be assessed within the environments typical of the individual's age and ethnicity. Examples of an individual's environments include homes, neighborhoods, places of worship, schools, workplaces, social settings, and other settings where individuals of similar age spend their time.

   4. Cultural and linguistic diversity are essential in the consideration of a definition of mental retardation, as well as differences in other developmental domains: motor, language and communication, behavior, and sensory (Jones & Menchetti, 2001; Luckasson et al., 2002).

   5. It is essential in assessing a person for mental retardation to identify a list of strengths and limitations.

   6. From the list of limitations, a number of supports, of varying intensity, can be identified to assist in improving the person's quality of life and functioning. *Supports Intensity Scale* (Thompson et al., 2004), a new instrument to quantify needed supports, is available from AAMR.

   7. Such supports and their effectiveness should be evaluated periodically (Luckasson et al., 2002).

   8. Significant intellectual limitations are usually defined as scoring two standard deviations (S.D.s) below the mean on a standardized tool for measuring intelligence.

9. Significant limitations in adaptive behavior may also be measured by standardized tools, such as the AAMR *Adaptive Behavior Scales* (Lambert, Nihira, & Leland, 1993; Nihira, Leland, & Lambert, 1993).

10. Whereas the current AAMR definition of mental retardation focuses on supports, the authors recognize that levels of IQ performance may be used to provide services. Other variables that can be used to categorize people include the etiology of mental retardation (e.g., organic versus nonorganic), adaptive behavior limitations, and mental health diagnoses (Luckasson et. al., 2002).

B. The APA (Jacobson & Mulick, 1996) defines mental retardation as "(a) significant limitations in general intellectual functioning; (b) significant limitations in adaptive functioning, which exist concurrently; and (c) onset of intellectual and adaptive limitations before the age of 22 years" (Editorial Board, 1996, p. 13).

1. All three criteria must be present for a diagnosis of mental retardation.

2. The APA defines four categories of severity: mild (IQ of 55–70), moderate (IQ of 35–54), severe (IQ of 20–34), and profound (IQ of below 20). These IQ scores correspond to 2 S.D. below the mean and lower.

3. Adaptive behavior limitations for the mild and moderate categories are in two or more domains. For the remaining two categories, adaptive behavior limitations are found in all domains.

4. Socioeconomic status, language and communication, ethnicity, and the person's environment as compared to the environment of a person of similar age and ethnicity must also be considered when assessing for mental retardation.

5. The age for onset was increased to 22 years to take into consideration the delay of onset of adulthood, as evidenced by economic and social independence, until typically after a person's 22nd birthday (Editorial Board, 1996).

C. The American Psychiatric Association publishes the *Diagnostic and Statistical Manual of Mental Disorders: DSM-IV-TR* (2000). The definition of mental retardation varies slightly here from the other definitions:

(a) Significantly subaverage intellectual functioning: an IQ score of approximately 70 or below on an individually administered IQ test (for infants, a clinical judgment of significantly subaverage intellectual functioning). (b) Concurrent deficits or impairments in present adaptive functioning (i.e., the person's effectiveness in meeting the standards expected for his or her age by his or her cultural group) in at least two of the following areas: communication, self-care, home living, social/interpersonal skills, use of community resources, self-direction, functional academic skills, work, leisure, health, and safety. (c) The onset is before age 18 years. (p. 46)

1. ICD-10 codes are given for each degree of severity based on IQ, and for a fifth category of severity unspecified when a person's IQ is untestable (APA, 2000).

2. Some professionals argue to decrease the categories of severity to two: mild (50 to approximately 70) and severe (below 50) due to the organic versus

nonorganic argument (Batshaw, 2002). This argument focuses on the fact that most individuals identified in the mild category have been diagnosed with mental retardation as a result of social and environmental deficits, whereas persons in the most severe categories are mentally retarded due to biological causes.

II.   Definitions of Disability

A. The World Health Organization publishes the *International Classification of Functioning, Disability, and Health (ICIDH-2)* (2001). This classification is divided into two parts and emphasizes the person's interaction with their environment: functioning and disability and contextual factors. Functioning and disability is further divided into body functions and structures and activities and participation. Contextual factors also has two parts: environmental and personal. In this classification system, disability refers to activity limitations, impairments, and/or restrictions in full participation. An aspect of this classification are the ICD-10 codes.

1. The term *mental retardation* is defined as "significantly subaverage general intellectual functioning with deficits in adaptive functioning" (p. 42 of Appendix 1 to Subpart P of Part 404). Diagnosis is made by age, IQ, and adaptive functioning.

B. Developmental disability is defined as:

A severe, chronic disability of an individual that (a) is attributable to mental or physical impairment or combination of mental and physical impairments; (b) is manifested before the individual attains the age of 22; (c) is likely to continue indefinitely; (d) results in substantial functional limitations in three or more of the following areas of major life activity: self-care, receptive and expressive language, learning, mobility, self-direction, capacity for independent living, and economic self-sufficiency; and (e) reflects the individual's need for a combination and sequence of special, interdisciplinary, or generic services; individualized supports; or other forms of assistance that are of lifelong or extended duration and are individually planned and coordinated. (Developmental Disabilities Assistance and Bill of Rights Act of 2000, Public Law 106-402)

1. Special compensation is given to children from birth to 9 years of age who have a specific acquired or congenital condition or a substantial developmental delay, in that they do not need to meet three or more of the areas listed above, if it is felt that a high probability exists for them to meet those criteria later in life.

C. The authors of *Healthy People 2010* (Healthy People 2010, 2000) call for a definition of disability, rather than just qualifying this condition as levels of limitation to activities of daily living.

III. Children with Special Health Care Needs

A. Pediatric health care professionals often refer to the term "children with special health care needs." The Maternal and Child Health Bureau's Division of Services for Children with Special Health Care Needs established the following definition: "children with special health care needs are those who have or are at increased risk for a chronic physical, developmental, behavioral, or emotional condition and who also require health and related services of a type or amount beyond that required by children generally" (McPherson et al., 1998).

B. A similar definition is not available for adults.

IV. Future Considerations for Terms and Definitions

A. Current terminology is similar in the three criteria: age, intelligence, and adaptive behavior. Emphasis on current levels of functioning and needed supports separates the AAMR definition from the rest.

B. There is a public and self-advocate demand for less negative terms to replace mental retardation and developmental disabilities, for example. Further discoveries in genetics, neurological functioning, and environmental effects may alter our knowledge so that more specific terminology can arise and umbrella terms, such as disability, will not undermine the specific supports and health needs that are present for this population.

C. Schalock (2002) suggests that technological advances will also impact the functional abilities of persons with intellectual and developmental disabilities in the future, and that the measure of and interventions for persons with intellectual and developmental disabilities will be based on the quality and level of interaction that an individual has with his or her environment.

V. Summary

Terminology has evolved across time to describe persons with and conditions resulting in intellectual and developmental disabilities. It is important to understand this history and influence future terminology that is more positive and less stigmatized.

References

American Psychiatric Association. (2000). *Diagnostic and statistical manual of mental disorders* (4th ed., text rev.). Washington, DC: Author.

Batshaw, M. L. (Ed.). (2002). *Children with disabilities* (5th ed.). Washington, DC: Paul H. Brookes.

Developmental Disabilities Assistance and Bill of Rights Act Amendments of 2000, Pub. L. No. 106-402, 114 Stat. 1677 (2000).

Editorial Board. (1996). Definition of mental retardation. In J. W. Jacobson & J. A. Mulick (Eds.), *Manual of diagnosis and professional practice in mental retardation* (pp. 13–41). Washington, DC: American Psychological Association.

Healthy People 2010. (2000). Retrieved January 20, 2002, from http://www.health.gov/healthypeople/document/

Jacobson, J. W., & Mulick, J. A. (Eds.). (1996). *The manual of diagnosis and professional practice in mental retardation.* Washington, DC: American Psychological Association.

Jones, L., & Menchetti, B. M. (2001). Identification of variables contributing to definitions of mild and moderate mental retardation in Florida. *Journal of Black Studies, 31,* 619–634.

Lambert, N., Nihira, K., & Leland, H. (1993). *AAMR adaptive behavior scale—School and community.* Austin, TX: Pro-Ed.

Luckasson, R., Borthwick-Duffy, S., Buntinx, W. H. E., Coulter, D. L., Craig, E. M., Reeve, A., et al. (2002). *Mental retardation: Definition, classification, and systems of support.* Washington, DC: American Association on Mental Retardation.

McPherson, M., Arango, P., Fox, H., Lauver, C., McManus, M., & Newachek, P. W. (1998). A new definition of children with special health care needs. *Pediatrics, 102,* 137–140.

Nihira, K., Leland, H., & Lambert, N. (1993). *AAMR adaptive behavior scale—Residential and community version* (2nd ed.). Austin, TX: Pro-Ed.

Schalock, R. L. (2002). Definitional issues. In R. L. Schalock, P. C. Baker, & M. D. Croser (Eds.). *Embarking on a new century: Mental retardation at the end of the 20th century* (pp. 45–66). Washington, DC: American Association on Mental Retardation.

Schroeder, S. R., Gerry, M., Gertz, G., & Velazquez, F. (2002). *Use of the term "mental retardation": Language, image and public education.* Retrieved May 25, 2004, from http://www.ssa.gov/disability/MentalRetardationReport.pdf.

Thompson, J. R., Bryant, B. R., Campbell, E. M., Craig, E. M., Hughes, C. M., & Rotholz, D. A., et al. (2004). *Supports intensity scale.* Washington, DC: American Association on Mental Retardation.

World Health Organization. (2001). *International classification of functioning, disability, and health (ICIDH-2).* Retrieved September 25, 2002, from http://www.who.int/icidh/intro.htm

Etiology of Intellectual and Developmental Disabilities

3

Stanley D. Handmaker, MD, PhD, FAAMR

Objectives

At the completion of this chapter, the learner will be able to:

1. Identify the major known causes of intellectual and developmental disabilities (I/DD).

2. Understand how the etiologies of I/DD are determined.

3. Describe the importance of recognizing specific etiologies in the prevention of I/DD.

4. Discuss some important clinical characteristics associated with the most common specific etiologies of I/DD.

5. Describe the four categories of risk factors for I/DD.

6. List interventions that have proven helpful for all levels of prevention.

Key Points

- I/DDs are often due to brain dysfunction resulting from malformation of or damage to the developing brain.

- Most of the identified etiologies, i.e., known causes of I/DD, are prenatal in origin.

- Of these known causes, genetic causes are the most common etiologies of I/DD.

- Identifying specific etiologies often facilitates prevention and therapeutic intervention and affects ultimate prognosis of persons with I/DD.

I.   Overview

A. Approximately 85% of all individuals with mental retardation have mild mental retardation.

B. The likelihood of identifying a specific etiology in any given individual depends on the level of severity of the I/DD.

C. The more severe the level of I/DD, the greater the likelihood that the underlying cause is biomedical in nature, and, therefore, the greater the likelihood of identifying a specific cause. In approximately 75% of cases of severe mental retardation, a biological cause can be determined.

D. Mild mental retardation has also been shown to have substantial heritability.

E. Specific etiologies are determined by obtaining thorough medical histories, including multiple generations; performing complete physical examinations, including dysmorphological and neurological assessments; and laboratory tests, such as chromosome examinations, including high-resolution banding; DNA testing, e.g., fluorescent in-situ hybridization (FISH); metabolic screening, e.g., using tandem mass spectrometry; infectious disease identifications, e.g., using cultures, antibody levels, etc.; heavy metal (e.g., lead and mercury) determinations; and brain imaging techniques, including computerized tomographic (CT) scans, magnetic resonance imaging (MRI), proton emission tomographic (PET) scans, etc.

F. Prenatal causes account for the largest proportion (from 64% to 80%) of etiologies identified in individuals with moderate–severe I/DD.

G. It is estimated that about 10% of all cases of I/DD have perinatal etiologies.

H. Less than 15% of all cases of I/DD have a postnatal cause.

I. It is estimated that as many as 50% of all cases of I/DD have more than one cause.

J. For example, advanced maternal age is associated with increased risk of having autosomal trisomy, e.g., Down syndrome, and of having a neural tube defect, e.g., spina bifida.

K. Neural tube defects, e.g., spina bifida, result from both polygenic causes and folate deficiency in the pregnant mother.

L. Another example of multiple etiologies is prenatal alcohol exposure, e.g., Fetal Alcohol Syndrome, which is due to increased exposure to toxic amounts of alcohol during the pregnancy and also genetic causes of alcoholism as well as genetic causes of fetal susceptibility.

M. Making a specific diagnosis is helpful in counseling the parents of a child with I/DD.

N. Identifying a specific etiology also is sometimes helpful in identifying a targeted intervention to benefit the affected child.

O. In addition, identifying a specific etiology can enable prevention of subsequent individuals with that disorder in the family.

P. There is an increased risk of recurrence in families having a previously affected child with mental retardation.

Q. The risk of having an affected child is also greater when parents have mental retardation.

R. The risk of having an affected child is 20% when one parent has mental retardation and 40% when both parents have mental retardation.

S. A significant proportion of individuals with mental retardation also have comorbidities, e.g., cerebral palsy, epilepsy, autism, attention deficit hyperactivity disorder (ADHD), etc.

T. It is estimated that 25% to 33% of individuals with moderate–severe I/DD also have serious psychiatric/emotional problems as well (Aicardi, 1998; Curry et al., 1997; Hunter, 2000; Luckasson et al., 2002; McLaren & Bryson, 1987; Stromme & Hagberg, 2000).

II. Classification of Known Etiologies of I/DD

A. Prenatal Causes of I/DD

  1. Prenatal causes include genetic abnormalities, congenital infections, alcohol and other drug exposure, other teratogens, and disorders in the pregnant woman.

  2. Genetic abnormalities are the most common identified causes of moderate to severe mental retardation.

  3. However, twin studies have shown that even mild mental retardation has substantial heritability.

  4. Prenatal alcohol exposure is believed to be the most common single known cause of all I/DD (Aicardi, 1998; Knight et al., 1999; McLaren & Bryson, 1987).

B. Perinatal Causes of I/DD

  1. Perinatal causes include placental complications, pre-eclampsia and eclampsia, birth trauma (disturbances in the delivery), metabolic abnormalities, e.g., hypoglycemia and hypocalcemia, and complications of prematurity, including intracerebral bleeding causing hypoxia/ischemia (Aicardi, 1998; Luckasson et al., 2002).

C. Postnatal Causes of I/DD

  1. Postnatal causes include meningitis/encephalitis, accidental or nonaccidental trauma, environmental pollutants (e.g., lead poisoning), and environmental deprivation, including malnutrition.

2. The two most common postnatal causes are nonaccidental trauma (e.g., shaken baby syndrome), and bacterial meningitis (Aicardi, 1998; Luckasson et al., 2002).

III. Categories of Genetic Causes of I/DD

A. There are at least 500 and as many as 750 different genetic disorders which have been identified as I/DD.

B. The genetic disorders include chromosomal abnormalities, single gene disorders, and polygenic/multifactorial conditions.

C. Chromosomal abnormalities are believed to be the most common genetic abnormalities.

D. Chromosomal abnormalities are found in about 40% of all individuals with moderate to severe mental retardation (IQ < 50) (Hodapp & DesJardin, 2002; Knight et al., 1999; Shaffer & Lupski, 2000; Skellern, Lennox, & Glass, 2000).

E. Chromosomal (see Chapter 5)

    1. Autosomal trisomy

    2. X-chromosomal

    3. Structural rearrangements

        a. Deletions (e.g., microdeletions)

            i. Interstitial

            ii. Terminal (telomeric) or subtelomeric

        b. Translocations

        c. Inversions

        d. Duplications

    4. Recent studies of individuals without a previously known cause of mental retardation have found as many as 5–10% with subtelomeric rearrangements (deletions, duplications, etc. at the ends of chromosomes) (DeVries, Winter, Schinzel, & van Ravenswaaij-Arts, 2003; Slavotinek et al., 1999).

F. Single gene (Mendelian) abnormalities

    1. X-linked recessive

    2. Autosomal recessive

    3. Autosomal dominant

G. Polygenic/multifactorial

IV. Specific Genetic Causes of I/DD

A. Chromosomal (Knight et al., 1999; Rosenberg et al., 2000)

    1. Autosomal trisomy

     a. Down syndrome (Trisomy 21)

        i. Down syndrome is the most common genetic disorder causing mental retardation, accounting for as much as one third of all cases.

     b. Edwards syndrome (Trisomy 18)

     c. Patau syndrome (Trisomy 13)

2. X-chromosomal

     a. Klinefelter syndrome (XXY)

     b. Turner syndrome (XO)

     c. XXX syndrome

     d. Others (e.g., XXXY, XXXXY)

        i. In individuals having more than two sex chromosomes, the greater the number of X chromosomes (three or more), the greater the probability of having associated mental retardation.

3. Microdeletions

     a. Prader-Willi syndrome is the most common microdeletion syndrome.

     b. Angelman syndrome

        i. Prader-Willi syndrome and Angelman syndrome are due to the same deletion on chromosome 15 and are examples of genetic imprinting.

       ii. If the deletion is transmitted through the father, the result is Prader-Willi syndrome; if the same deletion is maternally derived, the result is Angelman syndrome.

     c. Williams syndrome is due to a microdeletion on chromosome 7.

     d. Smith-Magenis syndrome is caused by a microdeletion on chromosome 17.

4. Subtelomeric rearrangements (deletions, duplications, etc. at the ends of chromosomes.

B. Single gene (Mendelian) abnormalities

  1. X-linked recessive (Zechner, Wilda, Kehrer-Sawatzki, Vogel, & Fundele, 2001)

     a. Fragile X syndrome (Hunter, 2000; Plomin, DeFries, McClearn, & McGuffin, 2001)

        i. Fragile X syndrome is the most common single gene disorder (1/3000 males) causing mental retardation.

       ii. The disorder is due a tandem repeating trinucleotide (CGG) sequence of >200 resulting in deficient expression of the FMR 1 gene on the long arm of the X chromosome.

      iii. Males with <200 copies of the CGG triplet are phenotypically normal but pass this premutation on to their daughters.

        iv. During oogenesis, this premutation with <200 copies of the CGG triplet then often expands to >200 copies in their offspring, with males being more severely affected than females.

    b. Duchenne Muscular Dystrophy

        i. Duchenne Muscular Dystophy (DMD) is the most common of the muscular dystrophies.

        ii. A milder variant of DMD is known as Becker Muscular Dystrophy (BMD).

    c. Lesch-Nyhan syndrome

        i. Lesch-Nyhan syndrome is characterized by self-mutilating behaviors, including chewing on lips and fingers and head banging.

2. Autosomal recessive (Wilcken, Wiley, Hammond, & Carpenter, 2003)

    a. The autosomal recessive disorders include metabolic conditions (e.g., the inborn errors of metabolism, such as congenital hypothyroidism, phenylketonuria, galactosemia, and Maple Syrup Urine Disease) and neurodegenerative disorders, such as Tay-Sachs disease and metachromatic leukodystrophy.

    b. Phenylketonuria (PKU)

        i. Phenylketonuria (PKU) was the first condition that was detected by newborn screening and in which the mental retardation was prevented by treatment of the affected individual with a selected diet (see Table 3.1).

    c. Congenital hypothyroidism

        i. Congenital hypothyroidism is the most common disorder that is detected by newborn screening programs in which treatment can prevent mental retardation (see Table 3.1).

Table 3.1 Prevention of Mental Retardation in Specific Etiologies	
ETIOLOGY	**PREVENTION**
Genetic disorders	Genetic counseling and prenatal diagnosis
Phenylketonuria (PKU)	Newborn screening and diet with low phenylalanine and added tyrosine
Galactosemia	Newborn screening and diet without galactose
Hypothyroidism	Newborn screening and thyroid hormone replacement
Prenatal alcohol exposure	Abstaining from alcohol during pregnancy
Spina bifida (meningomyelocele)	Increased folic acid in the diet

3. Autosomal dominant

   a. Neurofibromatosis, Type 1 (NF 1)

      i. The most common autosomal dominant disorder causing developmental disabilities is Neurofibromatosis, Type 1 (NF 1).

   b. Tuberous sclerosis

      i. The other prominent autosomal dominant neurocutaneous disorder causing mental retardation is tuberous sclerosis, which also often causes severe epilepsy.

4. Polygenic/multifactorial

   a. Spina bifida (myelomeningocele)

      i. Spina bifida is the most common specific condition with a polygenic/multifactorial etiology.

      ii. Spina bifida is also the most common cause of severe physical disability in children.

      iii. This is a neural tube defect which is often detectable prenatally by elevated alphafetoprotein (AFP) levels or by ultrasound examination.

      iv. A significant proportion of cases are preventable by folic acid (folate) supplementation prior to conception.

   b. Mild mental retardation

      i. A significant proportion of cases of mild mental retardation are believed to have a polygenic/multifactorial etiology. (Spinath, Harlaar, Ronald, & Plomin, 2004; Stromme & Hagberg, 2000)

V. Specific Nongenetic Prenatal Causes of I/DD

A. Toxic

   1. Alcohol

      a. Prenatal alcohol exposure (PAE) is believed to be one of the major, if not *the* major, single known cause of I/DD, including mild mental retardation.

         i. Infants with PAE, including fetal alcohol syndrome (FAS), may be recognized by their prenatal growth deficiency, CNS problems (e.g., increased irritability as a newborn), and facial dysmorphology.

         ii. Characteristic facies of FAS include midfacial hypoplasia with narrow palpebral fissures; epicanthal folds; small, upturned nose; simple philtrum; and thin upper lip.

         iii. Individuals with PAE typically are very social, but they have poor judgment and often have features of ADHD.

   2. Phenytoin (Hydantoin, Dilantin)

   3. Other drugs

B. Infectious (TORCH)

1. Toxoplasmosis

2. Other, including syphilus

3. Rubella

4. Cytomegalovirus (CMV) is the most common TORCH infection to cause mental retardation.

5. Herpes

VI.   Specific Nongenetic Perinatal Causes of I/DD

A. Anoxia/ischemia

1. Premature babies are at greater risk of intracerebral bleeding causing hypoxic-ischemic encephalopathy (HIE).

B. Infectious

1. The most significant perinatal infectious cause of mental retardation is bacterial meningitis.

C. Trauma

1. Trauma due to complications (e.g., cephalopelvic disproportion) at birth can result in brain damage.

VII.   Specific Nongenetic Postnatal Causes of I/DD

A. Meningitis/encephalitis

1. *Haemophilus influenzae* type b (Hib) has previously been identified as causing nearly half (47%) of all meningitis cases causing I/DD.

2. With the use of the Hib vaccine, we are now able to prevent Hib meningitis.

3. *Streptococcus pneumoniae (Pneumococcus)* is now the leading cause of bacterial meningitis causing I/DD.

B. Trauma

1. Accidental

a. Falls

b. Motor vehicle accidents

c. Near-drowning

2. Non-accidental (child abuse, shaken baby syndrome)

C. Malnutrition

D. Environmental pollutants

1. Lead poisoning

2. Methylmercury

3. Others

E. Environmental deprivation

1. Mild mental retardation is frequently believed to be caused by environmental deprivation, in addition to the genetic causes.

VIII. Clinical Features Associated with Common and/or Well-Known Etiologies of I/DD

A number of etiologies of I/DD are often identified initially based on their clinical characteristics that make up the phenotype. It is also important to be aware of behavioral phenotypes (see e.g., Dykens & Hodapp, 2001; Dykens, Hodapp, & Finucane, 2000; Luckasson et al., 2002).

A. Down syndrome

1. Down syndrome is most often diagnosed at birth.

2. Newborn babies with Down syndrome are almost always very hypotonic with a poor suck.

3. Characteristic appearance includes flattened facies with epicanthal folds and upslanted eyes; small mouth with protruding tongue; flattened occiput; short neck; small hands with short, incurved fifth fingers; and, about half the time, a transverse palmar crease.

B. Fragile X syndrome

1. Fragile X syndrome is most often recognized by there being multiple males in the family with mental retardation.

2. Characteristic appearance is elongated facies with prominent ears.

3. Another characteristic physical feature in older males is enlarged testes.

4. Behavioral characteristics sometimes include ADHD and autism.

C. Prader-Willi syndrome

1. Prader-Willi syndrome (PWS) is characterized by decreased fetal activity, obesity, muscular hypotonia, mental retardation, short stature, hypogonadotropic hypogonadism, and small hands and feet.

2. In early childhood, patients with Prader-Willi syndrome often have feeding problems and poor weight gain associated with their hypotonia.

3. Typically, between one and six years of age, these children develop hyperphagia and obesity.

D. Angelman Syndrome

1. Angelman syndrome is characterized by a happy individual with little or no speech, unsteady gait, and movement disorders.

2. Developmental delay is usually obvious by 6–12 months of age and is severe.

3. Seizures are frequent, with onset usually before three years of age.

E. Williams Syndrome

1. Williams syndrome is characterized by elfin facies; low birth weight; feeding difficulties; cardiovascular abnormalities, most typically supravalvular aortic stenosis; hypercalcemia; and small, wide-spaced teeth.

2. Behavioral features include increased irritability as infants and later multiple fears and anxieties.

3. Language skills are typically better developed, and they have poor visual-spatial skills (see Table 3.2).

Table 3.2 Comparison of Language Skills vs. Visual-Spatial Skills in Different Etiologies	
ETIOLOGY	RELATIVE STRENGTH
Down syndrome	Visual-spatial > language skills
Fragile X syndrome	Language > visual-spatial skills
Williams syndrome	Language > visual-spatial skills

F. Smith-Magenis Syndrome

1. Smith-Magenis syndrome is characterized by brachycephaly; broad, flat facies; and short fingers.

2. Behavioral abnormalities include self-mutilation (e.g., pulling out fingernails and toenails) and antisocial behavior.

G. Lesch-Nyhan syndrome

1. Lesch-Nyhan syndrome also has an associated very characteristic pattern of self-mutilation; individuals with this disorder will chew away portions of their lips and fingers if not properly treated.

2. Onset of symptoms is usually between three and six months of age.

3. The initial symptom is often orange colored (uric acid) crystals in the diaper.

H. Duchenne Muscular Dystrophy

1. Duchenne Muscular Dystophy (DMD) is characterized by progressive muscle wasting and weakness, beginning in the extremities and the trunk.

2. Onset of symptoms is usually around two to six years of age.

3. Early symptoms noted are muscle weakness and swelling of the calves.

4. DMD is also known as pseudohypertrophic muscular dystrophy because of the swelling of the calves.

I. Rett Syndrome

1. Rett syndrome is typically seen in girls and is characterized by normal development initially with progressive loss of previously acquired skills in motor function, cognition, and speech.

2. The most characteristic finding is stereotypical hand movements (e.g., wringing and squeezing, sometimes flapping).

3. Also, patients with Rett syndrome tend to have decreasing head circumference after birth.

J. Neurofibromatosis

1. Neurofibromatosis, Type 1 (NF 1) is most often diagnosed initially by the café-au-lait spots characteristic of this condition.

2. NF also can result in multiple tumors along the nerves (neurofibromas) anywhere in the body.

3. NF also can have midbrain (diencephalic) tumors.

K. Tuberous sclerosis

1. Tuberous sclerosis (TS) is often recognized by the facial condition of adenoma sebaceum or depigmented skin lesions in the shape of a mountain ash leaf.

2. TS also often includes severe epilepsy.

IX. Categories of Risk Factors and Interventions Towards Levels of Prevention

A. Categories of Risk Factors—each of the four categories must be assessed individually and also for interactions between two or more categories, which may hasten the need for appropriate interventions (Luckasson et al., 2002).

1. Biomedical risk factors

a. Prenatal—chromosomal disorders, metabolic disorders, parental age, maternal illnesses, syndromes, and single-gene disorders

b. Perinatal—prematurity, birth injury, and neonatal disorders

c. Postnatal—malnutrition, degenerative disorders, seizure disorders, meningoencephalitis, and traumatic brain injury

2. Social risk factors

a. Prenatal—maternal malnutrition, lack of availability or access to quality prenatal care, domestic violence, and poverty

b. Perinatal—lack of birth care, lack of access to birth care, or lack of quality birth care

c. Postnatal—institutionalization, family poverty, inadequate or inappropriate child caregiver, and lack of appropriate stimulation to child

3. Behavioral risk factors

a. Prenatal—parental use of drugs, alcohol, and/or nicotine; and other unsafe behavior

b. Perinatal—parental abandonment or neglect of child

      c. Postnatal—domestic and/or child abuse, inappropriate safety precautions taken, difficult child temperament, and social deprivation

   4. Educational risk factors

      a. Prenatal—cognitive impairment in one or both parents without existing supports, and inadequate preparation for pregnancy, labor, delivery, and parenthood

      b. Perinatal—lack of appropriate assessment of parenting limitations leading to a lack of referral for appropriate services (e.g., parenting classes, foster grandparents, referral to a pediatrician, etc.)

      c. Postnatal—delayed diagnosis, inadequate formal and informal supports, impaired parenting, and inadequate referrals for supports

  B. Primary Prevention Activities

   1. Biomedical—e.g., lead screening, nutrition classes, and appropriate prenatal care

   2. Social—e.g., assisting in providing appropriate informal and formal emotional support, domestic violence programs, and anger management programs

   3. Behavioral—e.g., avoiding alcohol, drugs, and nicotine; adapting a healthy lifestyle; and courses that prepare one emotionally to be a parent

   4. Educational—e.g., education programs that focus on infant care, parenting, healthy lifestyles, sexuality, and environmental hazards

  C. Secondary Prevention

   1. Biomedical—e.g., lead screening, metabolic screening, condition-specific screening, and developmental screening

   2. Social—e.g., family and environmental assessments, promotion of parent–child bonding and interactions, and assisting in enhancing family support

   3. Behavioral—e.g., promoting safety in the environment, including the home, workplace, and community where residing; and promoting appropriate behavior with child

   4. Educational—e.g., referral to appropriate formal and informal support networks, such as early intervention programs, condition-specific parent support groups, therapies, parenting groups, and daycare

  D. Tertiary Prevention

   1. Biomedical—e.g., maintaining a healthy lifestyle

   2. Social—e.g., maintaining an informal and formal support network that brings happiness and contentment

   3. Behavioral—e.g., exercise, leisure, and pleasurable experiences on a regular basis

   4. Educational—e.g., lifelong learning activities to enhance current strengths and limitations

X. Summary

Accurate information based on up-to-date biochemical, genetic, and psychosocial testing is necessary for individual and family well-being, current and future health care planning and interventions, prevention planning, and the ultimate prognosis for the individual with I/DD.

XI. References

Aicardi, J. (1998). The etiology of developmental delay. *Seminars in Pediatric Neurology, 5,* 15–20.

Curry, C. J., Aughton, D., Byrne, J., Carey, J. C., Cassidy, S., Cuniff, C., et al. (1997). Evaluation of mental retardation: Recommendations of a consensus conference. *American Journal of Medical Genetics, 72,* 468–477.

De Vries, R. B., Winter, R., Schinzel, A., & van Ravenswaaij-Arts, C. (2003). Telomeres: A diagnosis at the end of the chromosomes. *Journal of Medical Genetics, 40,* 385–398.

Dykens, E. M., & Hodapp, R. M. (2001). Research in mental retardation: Toward an etiologic approach. *Journal of Child Psychology and Psychiatry, 42,* 49–71.

Dykens, E. M., Hodapp, R. M., & Finucane, B. M. (2000). *Genetics and mental retardation syndromes: A new look at behavior and interventions.* Baltimore: Paul H. Brookes.

Hodapp, R. M., & DesJardin, J. L. (2002). Genetic etiologies of mental retardation: Issues for interventions and interventionists. *Journal of Developmental and Physical Disabilities, 14,* 323–338.

Hunter, A. G. (2000). Outcome of the routine assessment of patients with mental retardation in a genetics clinic. *American Journal of Medical Genetics, 90,* 60–68.

Knight, S. J., Regan, R., Nicod, A., Horsley, S. W., Kearney, L., Homfray, T., et al. (1999). Subtle chromosomal rearrangements in children with unexplained mental retardation. *Lancet, 354,* 1676–1681.

Luckasson, R., Borthwick-Duffy, S., Buntinx, W. H. E., Coulter, D. L., Craig, E. M., Reeve, A., et al. (2002). *Mental retardation: Definition, classification, and systems of supports* (10th ed.). Washington, DC: American Association on Mental Retardation.

McLaren, J., & Bryson, S.E. (1987). Review of recent epidemiological studies of mental retardation: Prevalence, associated disorders, and etiology. *American Journal on Mental Retardation, 92,* 243–254.

Plomin, R., DeFries, J. C., McClearn, G. E., & McGuffin, P. (2001). *Behavioral Genetics* (4th ed.). New York: Worth.

Rosenberg, M. J., Vaske, P., Killoran, C. E., Ning, Y., Wargowski, D., Hudgins, L., et al. (2000). Detection of chromosomal aberrations by a whole-genome microsatellite screen. *American Journal of Human Genetics, 66,* 419–427.

Shaffer, L. G., & Lupski, J. R. (2000). Molecular mechanisms for constitutional chromosomal rearrangements in humans. *Annual Reviews of Genetics, 34,* 297–329.

Skellern, C., Lennox, N., & Glass, I. (2000). New insights into the genetic basis of intellectual disabilities. *Australian Family Physician, 29,* 41–45.

Slavotinek, A., Rosenberg, M., Knight, S., Gaunt, L., Ferguson, W., Killoran, C., et al. (1999). Screening for submicroscopic chromosome rearrangements in children with idiopathic mental retardation using microsatellite markers for the chromosome telomeres. *Journal of Medical Genetics, 36,* 405–411.

Spinath, F. M., Harlaar, N., Ronald, A., & Plomin, R. (2004). Substantial genetic influence on mild mental impairment in early childhood. *American Journal on Mental Retardation, 109,* 34–43.

Stromme, P., & Hagberg, G. (2000). Aetiology in severe and mild mental retardation: A population-based study of Norwegian children. *Developmental Medicine & Child Neurology, 42,* 76–86.

Wilcken, B., Wiley, V., Hammond, J., & Carpenter, K. (2003). Screening newborns for inborn errors of metabolism by tandem mass spectrometry. *New England Journal of Medicine, 348,* 2304–2312.

Zechner, U., Wilda, M., Kehrer-Sawatzki, H., Vogel, W., & Fundele, R. (2001). A high density of X-linked genes for general cognitive ability: A run-away process for shaping human evolution? *Trends in Genetics, 17,* 697–701.

Epidemiology of Intellectual and Developmental Disabilities

Wendy M. Nehring, RN, PhD, FAAN, FAAMR
and Ann R. Poindexter, MD, FAAMR

4

Objectives

At the completion of this chapter, the learner will be able to:

1. Define epidemiology and describe its importance to the field of intellectual and developmental disabilities (I/DD).

2. List the factors that may cause variation in noted rates of mental retardation.

3. Describe the possible reasons for variation in rates of mental retardation in various groups, such as gender, socioeconomic status, and ethnicity.

4. Discuss prevalence rates and findings regarding special health care needs and disability from recent national surveys involving children.

Key Points

• Epidemiology is defined as the study of the relationships of the various factors determining the frequency and distribution of diseases in human communities.

• Studying the epidemiology of I/DD helps to examine how common these conditions are in the community, whether the incidence or prevalence has changed over time, and whether certain population subgroups are more or less likely to be affected.

• Researchers have found considerable variation in estimates of prevalence across countries and regions.

• Variation in prevalence rates may be due to a variety of factors.

• Variation in prevalence rates should be studied carefully to determine factors which can be modified to decrease the prevalence of I/DD and to improve health care and related services.

I.   Definition of Epidemiology

Epidemiology is defined as the study of the relationships of the various factors that determine the frequency and distribution of diseases in a given human community (or communities). An epidemiological study can indicate:

A.   How common the condition or disease is in the area of interest.

B.   Whether the incidence or prevalence of the condition or disease has changed across time.

C.   If certain groups are more susceptible than others in acquiring the condition or disease. Categories of groups may include ethnicity, gender, place of residence, or socioeconomic status (Leonard & Wen, 2002).

II.   Prevalence of Mental Retardation

Researchers have found extreme variation in the estimated prevalence of mental retardation across the world, ranging from 2 to 85 per 1000 (Roeleveld, Ziethuis, & Gabreels, 1997). This is most likely due to the wide range of definitions and classification systems available, as well as the use of different methodologies available to estimate this number in a given population, including differences in measures of intelligence and factors related to the test administrators (Durkin, 2002; Leonard & Wen, 2002; Roeleveld, Ziethuis, & Gabreels, 1997).

A.   The prevalence of severe mental retardation in both developed and developing countries is ~3–4 per 1000 in both children (Roeleveld, Ziethuis & Gabreels, 1997; Starza-Smith, 1989) and adults (Kiely, 1987; Reschly, 1992), although Durkin (2002) stressed in developing countries this figure varies more widely from 2.9 per 1000 in Beijing to 22 per 1000 in slum regions in Pakistan (Durkin, Hasan, & Hasan, 1998; Zuo et al., 1986). An identified cause is twice as likely to be determined for severe mental retardation as for mild mental retardation (Crow & Tolmie, 1998). Batshaw and Shapiro (2002) attribute this to a combination of improved health care and emerging diseases.

B.   The prevalence of mild mental retardation is higher at 10.6 per 1000 (Leonard & Wen, 2002). In the school-age population, Roeleveld, Ziethuis, and Gabreels (1997) estimate a true prevalence rate at 29.8 per 1000, although they caution that this number has questionable validity due to methodological problems in the studies analyzed to reach this figure. In developing countries, this prevalence rate is strongly associated with socioeconomic status (Islam, Durkin, & Zaman, 1993). Christianson et al. (2002) estimate a prevalence of 29.1 per 1000 in South Africa.

C.   According to Social Security Administration data from 1993, in the United States the estimated prevalence of persons age 6 to 64 years with mental retardation of any degree was 7.6 per 1000. The lowest rate was in Alaska and the highest in West Virginia. For children 6 to 17 years of age, the prevalence rate was estimated at 11.4 per 1000, with the lowest rate in New Jersey and the highest in Alabama. For adults, 18 to 64 years, the prevalence rate was estimated at 6.6 per 1000, with the lowest rate in Alaska and the highest in West Virginia. Factors contributing to these findings were identified as socioeconomic status, births to adolescents, and low maternal education (Massey & McDermott, 1995).

D. Many factors influence prevalence numbers, such as:

1. Age—The prevalence of mental retardation is higher during the school years due to the ability to obtain better estimates of true numbers of children with mental retardation based on standardized intelligence testing. The highest prevalence rates have been reported during the period from 10 to 14 years of age (Batshaw & Shapiro, 2002; Wen, 1997). Boyle et al. (1996) reported a prevalence rate of 5.2 per 1000 in children 3 to 4 years, 8.7 per 1000 in children 3 to 10 years, and 12.3 per 1000 in children 9 to 10 years in a sample of metropolitan Atlanta, Georgia, children in 1991. They reported that the increase in numbers was largely due to increasing numbers of children identified with mild mental retardation. The numbers decline in adulthood due probably to the ability of persons with mild mental retardation to adapt in society and the lack of opportunities to assess intelligence. The criteria of limitations in adaptive behavior helped to identify more people outside of the school system. In addition, lack of sufficient information on death certificates may limit the ability to obtain accurate prevalence estimates based on mortality (Leonard & Wen, 2002).

2. Gender—Males are approximately 1.65 times more likely to be identified with mental retardation than are females (Drews, Yeargin-Allsopp, Decoufle, & Murphy, 1995). Factors influencing this gender difference include X-linked genetic conditions (Chelly & Mandel, 2001), neonatal mortality (Stevenson et al., 2000), maternal smoking (Zaren, Lindmark, & Bakketeig, 2000), and low birthweight (Zubrick et al., 2000). Boys are also enrolled in special education more often. Gissler, Jarvelin, Louhiala, and Hemminki (1999) question whether there are social as well as biological determinants for this gender difference.

3. Socioeconomic status—Mild mental retardation has been found to be more prevalent in lower socioeconomic settings than in other socioeconomic strata. The metropolitan Atlanta study (Drews et al., 1995) found support for two forms of mental retardation: biologically based with more often lower intelligence, and socially and economically based with mild mental retardation predominant, discussed originally by Zigler, Balla, and Hodapp (1984). In developing countries, prevention of mental retardation can occur if nutritional changes are made, such as in iodine deficiency (Delange, de Benoist, Pretell, & Dunn, 2001).

4. Maternal factors—IQ scores below 70, low maternal education, pregnancy weight gain less than 10 pounds, and multiple births accounted for higher rates of children with mental retardation (Camp, Broman, Nichols, & Leff, 1998; Decoufle & Boyle, 1995). Older maternal age affected prevalence of severe mental retardation (Drews et al., 1995).

5. Ethnicity—Higher incidence of mental retardation in African-American children, especially mild mental retardation, even after controlling for maternal education, maternal age, gender, and economic status (Boyle et al., 1996; Yeargin-Allsopp, Drews, Decoufle, & Murphy, 1995). Similar findings are present for Australian indigenous groups in Australia (Leonard, Petterson, Bower, & Sanders, 2002). Researchers have speculated that the higher incidences of hypertension, anemia in pregnancy, diabetes, and chronic renal disease in adults from African-American and Australian indigenous groups, as well as higher lead levels and anemia in children, may contribute to this outcome (Camp et al., 1998; Leonard & Wen, 2002; McLennan & Madden, 1999; Yeargin-Allsopp et al., 1995). Urinary tract infection during pregnancy was found to be a risk factor in mental retardation in whites, accounting for 6% of the cases of mental retardation studied (Camp et al., 1998). Breslau et al. (2001) emphasized that disadvantaged environments do influence IQ scores in children. Overall, it is important to carefully consider the operational definitions, sampling, research, and analytical measures used in individual studies in making conclusions about the prevalence of mental retardation in any group (Leonard & Wen, 2002).

6. Low-income countries—Specific factors attributing to higher incidences of mental retardation include increased numbers of births to mothers older than 35 years, genetic diseases, nutritional deficiencies (e.g., vitamin A deficiency, iodine deficiency, and iron deficiency anemia), trauma, infections (in pregnant mothers and in children), toxic exposures, and consanguinity. In these countries, prenatal care and availability of contraception is limited, access to genetic counseling and screening is rare, a higher birth and childhood mortality rate exists, services for children with mental retardation are not widely available, and such children often do not attend school. There exists a crucial need for effective prevention programs in these countries (Durkin, 2002).

E. Recurrence rates for severe mental retardation vary between 3.5% and 14% according to present research studies. Advances in genetic screening should derive more accurate rates in the future (Crow & Tolmie, 1998). Recurrence rates for conditions of mental retardation with known causes, for example, Down syndrome, have specific recurrence rates (Batshaw & Shapiro, 2002).

III. **Prevalence of Special Health Care Needs in Children in the United States**

    A. In 1994, 12.6 million children under the age of 18 years were diagnosed with a chronic developmental, behavioral, physical, or emotional condition that required health or other related services, according to the 1994 National Health Interview Survey on Disability. This survey was completed on 30,032 children.

    B. Prevalence was greater for boys, children from low income families, African-American children, older children, and children from single-parent families.

    C. Eleven percent of these children were not insured.

    D. Six percent did not have an identified source of health care.

    E. Thirteen percent had health needs that were not addressed by a health care professional, such as prescription medications, mental health care, or dental care.

    F. There is a need to develop research methodologies in order to identify children at risk for special health care needs. (Newachek et al., 1998)

IV. **Prevalence of Childhood Disability in U.S. Children**

    A. Newacheck and Halfon (1998) defined disability as "a long-term reduction in ability to conduct social role activities, such as school or play, because of a chronic physical or mental condition" (p. 610).

    B. According to the 1992–1994 National Health Interview Survey of 99,513 children younger than 18 years, 6.5% of all children experience some form of disability. Impairment of speech, special sense, or intelligence was found in 1,696 per 100,000 children. An additional 246 children per 100,000 were considered to have a disability if you included these conditions as a secondary cause.

    C. Prevalence rates increased after the age of 5 years. This may be due to increased social demands while in school.

    D. As in the National Health Interview Survey on Disabilities, the results of The National Health Interview survey also found higher prevalences in boys, low income families, single-parent families, and African-American children. Region of the country and family size only had slight variances in prevalence.

    E. Daily activities were restricted on average for about 2 weeks per year in children with disabilities.

    F. Children with impairments of speech, special sense, and intelligence were:

        1. The least likely to report poor or fair health (8.8%).

        2. Missed one or less school day annually on average (mean = 0.5).

        3. Did not have school attendance problems (2.5% were limited in or unable to attend school).

4. Had the lowest rates of physician visits among the children with disabilities (mean = 4.7 visits). In fact, the rates were similar to children without disabilities (mean = 2.9 visits).

5. Were hospitalized for fewer days (246 hospital days per 1000 in past year) than other categories of children with activity-limiting chronic conditions. (Newacheck & Halfon, 1998)

V. Secondary Conditions

Conditions resulting in mental retardation often have secondary conditions, such as cerebral palsy, seizure disorders, mental health and behavioral problems, and sensorimotor impairments. This prevalence is correlated to the severity of the mental retardation. Greater than half of the children with severe mental retardation have sensory impairments (55%), followed by mental health and behavioral problems (50%) and seizure disorders (21%). Children with mild mental retardation have secondary conditions less often, but when they do, they are most likely mental health and behavioral problems (25%) and sensory impairments (24%). The prevalence of secondary conditions is also specific to individual conditions causing mental retardation, such as Down syndrome, and literature is available for these conditions (Batshaw & Shapiro, 2002; Kiely, 1987).

VI. Implications for Nurses and Other Health Care Professionals in Understanding Epidemiological Information

A. Developing and planning for services, including health care, social, vocational, residential, and educational programs. Could more services be available for adults with I/DD if prevalence numbers were more accurate and valid?

B. Developing and planning for more successful transition programs between infant and preschool services, adolescent and adult services, and adult to older adult services.

C. Education regarding secondary conditions and risk factors.

D. Developing and planning for better public health prevention programs and/or evaluation of existing programs.

E. Focused research on prevalence rates due to specific causes, including environmental influences and emerging disabling conditions, such as shaken baby syndrome, mitochondrial conditions, and long-term effects of childhood cancer survivors, HIV-infected children, and persons affected by lead in childhood.

F. Working to get more children and adults insured for health care. (Ireys & Katz, 1997)

VII. Summary

This is not just a pediatric problem or issue. There is a need to determine and identify prevalence rates of mental retardation in general and specifically for a variety of I/DD as they are identified and understood. Calls for registries by leaders in the field (e.g., Gershon Berkson) have been made for this population, and maybe now is the time to do this. Registries are available for such conditions as Rett syndrome, and they can be instituted for others. Services in all systems of care—educational, health, vocational, social, and residential—can be developed and successfully implemented when there is a justified need.

References

Batshaw, M. L., & Shapiro, B. (2002). Mental retardation. In M. L. Batshaw (Ed.). *Children with disabilities* (5th ed., pp. 287–305). Baltimore: Paul H. Brookes.

Boyle, C. A., Yeargin-Allsopp, M., Doernberg, N. S., Holmgreen, P., Murphy, C. C., & Schendel, D. E. (1996). Prevalence of selected developmental disabilities in children 3–10 years of age: The metropolitan Atlanta developmental disabilities surveillance program, 1991. *Mortality and Morbidity Weekly Report, 45*(SS-2), 1–14.

Breslau, N., Chilcoat, H. D. Susser, E. S., Matte, T., Liang, K. Y., & Peterson, C. L. (2001). Stability and change in children's intelligence quotient scores: A comparison of two socioeconomically disparate communities. *American Journal of Epidemiology, 154,* 711–717.

Camp, B. W., Broman, S. H., Nichols, P. L., & Leff, M. (1998). Maternal and neonatal risk factors for mental retardation: Defining the "at-risk" child. *Early Human Development, 50,* 159–173.

Chelly, J., & Mandel, J. L. (2001). Monogenic causes of X-linked mental retardation. *National Review of Genetics, 2,* 669–680.

Christianson, A. L., Zwane, M. E., Manga, P., Rosen, E., Venter, A., & Downs, D. (2002). Children with intellectual disability in rural South Africa: Prevalence and associated disability. *Journal of Intellectual Disability Research, 46* (Part 2), 179–186.

Crow, Y. J., & Tolmie, J. L. (1998). Recurrence risks in mental retardation. *Journal of Medical Genetics, 35,* 177–182.

Decoufle, P., & Boyle, C. A. (1995). The relationship between maternal education and mental retardation in 10-year-old children. *Annals of Epidemiology, 5,* 347–353.

Delange, F., de Benoist, B., Pretell, E., & Dunn, J. T. (2001). Iodine deficiency in the world: Where do we stand at the turn of the century? *Thyroid, 11,* 437–447.

Drews, C. D., Yeargin-Allsopp, M., Decoufle, P., & Murphy, C. C. (1995). Variation in the influence of selected sociodemographic risk factors for mental retardation. *American Journal of Public Health, 85,* 329–334.

Durkin, M. (2002). The epidemiology of developmental disabilities in low-income countries. *Mental Retardation and Developmental Disabilities Research Reviews, 8,* 206–211.

Durkin, M. S., Hasan, Z. M., & Hasan, K. Z. (1998). Prevalence and correlates of mental retardation among children in Karachi, Pakistan. *American Journal of Epidemiology, 147,* 281–288.

Gissler, M., Jarvelin, M. R., Louhiala, P., & Hemminki, E. (1999). Boys have more health problems in childhood than girls: Follow-up of the 1987 Finnish birth cohort. *Acta Paediatrica, 88,* 310–314.

Ireys, H. T., & Katz, S. (1997). The demography of disability and chronic illness among children. In H. M. Wallace, R. F. Biehl, J. C. MacQueen, & J. A. Blackman (Eds.). *Mosby's resource guide to children with disabilities and chronic illness* (pp. 3–12). St. Louis, MO: Mosby.

Islam, S., Durkin, M. S., & Zaman, S. S. (1993). Socioeconomic status and the prevalence of mental retardation in Bangladesh. *Mental Retardation, 31*, 412–417.

Kiely, M. (1987). The prevalence of mental retardation. *Epidemiological Reviews, 9*, 194–218.

Leonard, H., Petterson, B., Bower, C., & Sanders, R. (2002). Prevalence of infants born with Down's syndrome: 1980–96. *Paediatrics Perinatalogy and Epidemiology, 14*, 163–171.

Leonard, H., & Wen, X. (2002). The epidemiology of mental retardation: Challenges and opportunities in the new millennium. *Mental Retardation & Developmental Disabilities Research Reviews, 8*, 117–134.

Massey, P. S., & McDermott, S. (1995). State-specific rates of mental retardation—United States, 1993. *Morbidity & Mortality Weekly Report, 45*(3), 61–65.

McLennan, W., & Madden, R. (1999). *The health and welfare of Australia's Aboriginal and Torres Strait Islander peoples*. Canberra: Australian Bureau of Statistics, Australian Institute of Health and Welfare.

Newacheck, P. W., & Halfon, N. (1998). Prevalence and impact of disabling chronic conditions in childhood. *American Journal of Public Health, 88*, 610–617.

Newacheck, P. W., Strickland, B., Shonkoff, J. P., Perrin, J. M., McPherson, M., & McManus, M. (1998). An epidemiologic profile of children with special health care needs. *Pediatrics, 102*, 117–123.

Reschly, D. (1992). Mental retardation: Conceptual foundations, definitional criteria, and diagnostic operations. In S. Hooper, G. Hynd, & R. Mattison (Eds.). *Developmental disorders: Diagnostic criteria and clinical assessment*. Hillsdale, NJ: Lawrence Erlbaum Associates.

Roeleveld, N., Ziethuis, G. A., & Gabreels, F. (1997). The prevalence of mental retardation: A critical review of recent literature. *Developmental Medicine & Child Neurology, 39*, 194–218.

Starza-Smith, A. (1989). Recent trends in prevalence studies of children with severe mental retardation. *Disability, Handicap & Society, 4*, 177–195.

Stevenson, D. K., Verter, J., Fanaroff, A. A., Oh, W., Ehrenkranz, R. A., & Shankaran, S. (2000). Sex differences in outcomes of very low birthweight infants: The newborn male disadvantage. *Archives of Diseases in Childhood Fetal Neonatal Edition, 83*, F182–185.

Wen, X. (1997). *The definition and prevalence of intellectual disability in Australia*. Canberra: Australian Institute of Health and Welfare.

Yeargin-Allsopp, M., Drews, C. D., Decoufle, P., & Murphy, C. C. (1995). Mild mental retardation in black and white children in metropolitan Atlanta: A case-control study. *American Journal of Public Health, 85*, 324–328.

Zaren, B., Lindmark, G., & Bakketeig, L. (2000). Maternal smoking affects fetal growth more in the male fetus. *Paediatric Perinatal Epidemiology, 14*, 118–126.

Zigler, E., Balla, D., & Hodapp, R. (1984). On the definition and classification of mental retardation. *American Journal of Mental Deficiency, 89*, 215–230.

Zubrick, S. R., Kurinczuk, J. J., McDermott, B. M. C., McKelvey, R. S., Silburn, S. R., & Davies, L. C. (2000). Fetal growth and subsequent mental health problems in children aged 4 to 13 years. *Developmental Medicine & Child Neurology, 42*, 14–20.

Zuo, Q. H., Zhang, X. Z., Li, Z., Qian, Y. P., Wu, X. R., & Lin, Q. (1986). An epidemiological study on mental retardation among children in Chang-Qiao area of Beijing. *Chinese Medical Journal, 99*, 9–14.

The Influence of Genetics

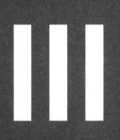

Genetic Concepts

Deborah A. Natvig, RN, PhD

5

Objectives

At the completion of this chapter, the learner will be able to:

1. Discuss the importance of the Human Genome Project.
2. Discuss concepts of basic human genetics.
3. Describe advances in genetic information and technology.
4. Identify ethical dilemmas and societal issues related to advances in genetic information and technology.
5. Discuss how concepts of genetics impact on practice for nurses and other health care professionals in I/DD.
6. Use and understand terminology related to genetics.

Key Points

- Knowledge and understanding of the Human Genome Project will help nurses and other health professionals apply the latest genetic information to clinical practice.

- There are many diseases and disorders that are the result of genetic abnormalities, environmental factors, or a combination of both.

- There are four main types of genetic disorders: (a) chromosomal disorders, (b) single-gene disorders, (c) multifactorial disorders, and (d) nontraditional disorders.

- The etiology of mental retardation is unknown for approximately 50% of affected individuals.

- The purpose of genetic screening, evaluation, diagnosis and counseling is to (a) assist families to have healthy babies, (b) help children born with disabilities reach their highest potential, and (c) help affected families stay healthy as they adjust to their child's special needs.

Key Points *(continued)*

- The major components of genetic screening, evaluation, diagnosis, and counseling include: (a) development of a three-generation pedigree, (b) pre-, peri-, and post-natal history, (c) complete physical evaluation that focuses on presence of minor anomalies, (d) a neurological examination, and (e) assessment of how the individual responds to and interacts with others and the environment.

- Longitudinal follow-up is very important, as it allows for individuals to be evaluated over time for physical and behavioral changes that may be significant in diagnosing many conditions.

- The ethical, legal, and societal issues become more complex as the knowledge of genetics increases.

I. **Human Genome Project** (National Human Genome Research Institute (n.d.); Human Genome Program, 2003).

The U.S. Human Genome Project was an international collaborative research project that began in 1990 and was completed in 2003. The purpose of the project was to (a) identify all of the genes in human DNA, (b) determine the sequence of the 3 billion DNA building blocks that account for life's diversity, (c) store this information in databases, (d) develop tools for data analysis, and (e) address the ethical, legal, and social issues (ELSI) that may arise from the project. The National Institutes of Health and the U.S. Department of Energy coordinated the project, which was completed two years ahead of the original schedule. To achieve these goals, the project also included the study of the genetic make-up of nonhuman organisms including (a) *escherichia coli*, (b) the fruit fly, and (c) the laboratory mouse.

A. What is a genome and why is it important?

1. A genome is all the DNA in an organism, including its genes.

2. DNA is made up of four similar chemicals called bases. They are adenine (A), thymine (T), cytosine (C), and guanine (G). They are repeated millions of times throughout the genome. The human genome has 3 billion pairs of bases.

3. The particular order of the As, Ts, Cs, and Gs is very important and determines if an organism is human or another species. It also determines the diversity or differences among individuals in the human species.

4. All organisms are related through similarities in DNA sequences. Because of this, knowledge gained from nonhuman genomes often leads to new knowledge about human biology.

5. There are 46 chromosomes in the human somatic cell and in the zygote. This total number is composed of 22 pairs of autosomes and 1 pair of sex chromosomes.

6. Each chromosome contains many genes that are the basic physical and functional units of heredity. It is estimated that the human genome contains 30,000 genes.

B. Practical benefits to learning about DNA include new ways to assess, diagnose, treat, and prevent thousands of disorders that affect us.

II. Overview

A large number of diseases and disorders are the result of genetic abnormalities, environmental factors, or a combination of both. The etiology of mental retardation is unknown for approximately 50% of affected individuals, however (Curry et al., 1997). Currently 282 genes have been identified as molecularly related to mental retardation (Inlow & Restifo, 2004). It is important to distinguish among those disorders in which defects in the genetic information are of prime importance, those in which environmental hazards (including hazards of the intrauterine environment) are chiefly to blame, and those in which a combination of genetic and environmental factors are responsible. A family history is essential as the initial step in delineating the genetic diagnosis. There are four main types of genetic disorders: (a) chromosome disorders, (b) single-gene disorders, (c) multifactorial disorders, and (d) nontraditional.

A. Family History

1. An adequate family history is an essential part of the assessment of a patient with a genetic disorder.

2. Family history may be helpful in determining if a condition has a genetic basis.

3. A pedigree or family tree is a schematic drawing of a person's family history.

    a. Can help distinguish among chromosomal disorders, single-gene disorders, and multifactorial disorders.

    b. Universal symbols are used in drawing pedigrees (see Figure 5.1).

B. Chromosome Disorders—Chromosome abnormalities are reported in 4% to 28% of individuals with mental retardation. As the severity of mental retardation and presence of congenital anomalies increases, the presence of chromosomal abnormality also increases (Curry et al., 1997).

1. Chromosomes are the nuclear structures that carry the basic units of inheritance, the genes.

Figure 5.1 Pedigree Symbols

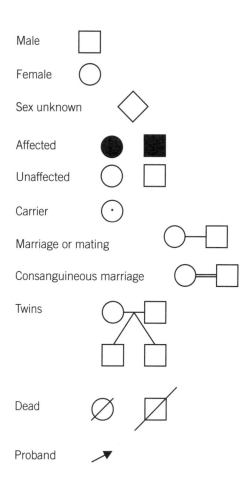

Greenwood Genetic Center, 1995

2. Normally, individuals have 46 chromosomes; 22 pairs of autosomes and 2 sex chromosomes.

   a. Each female normally has two X chromosomes.

   b. Each male normally has one X and one Y chromosome.

3. Problems or defects can be caused by abnormalities in the number or structure of chromosomes.

4. Abnormalities in chromosome number (aneuploidy)

   a. Cause a characteristic pattern of malformations.

   b. Associated with mental or physical disability or both.

   c. May involve autosomes or sex chromosomes.

d. Usually there is not a family history of the disorder.

e. Most common is trisomy (Cassidy & Allanson, 2001; Jorde, Carey, Bamshad, & White, 2003; Lewis, 2003; Seashore & Wappner, 1996)

    i. Trisomy 21—Down syndrome

        a. Complete extra chromosome 21

        b. Incidence: 1 in 770 births

        c. Risk of conceiving a child with trisomy 21 increases with maternal age

            1. Under age 30 the risk is 1 in 3,000.

            2. At age 35, the risk is 1 in 400.

            3. At age 40, the risk is 1 in 110.

            4. At age 45, the risk is 1 in 25.

        d. Phenotype—Major features include:

            1. Mental and physical retardation

            2. Short stature

            3. Straight line palmar crease

            4. Flat face with up slant eyes

            5. Protruding tongue, thick lips

            6. Sparse, straight hair

        e. Increased risk for health problems involving most body systems

            1. 40% have congenital heart disease.

            2. Thyroid problems

            3. Hearing problems

            5. Vision problems

    ii. Trisomy 13—Patau syndrome

        a. Complete extra chromosome 13

        b. Incidence: 1 in 10,000 births to 1 in 20,000 births (estimated)

        c. Rarely survives more than a few months

        d. Phenotype:

            1. Mental and physical retardation

            2. Skull and facial abnormalities

            3. Defects in all organ systems

            4. Cleft lip

            5. Large triangular nose

            6. Extra digits

      iii. Trisomy 18—Edwards syndrome

         a. Complete extra chromosome 18

         b. Incidence: 1 in 6,000 live births

         c. Rarely survives more than a few months; 95% die within first year

         d. Phenotype:

            1. Mental and physical retardation

            2. Skull and facial abnormalities

            3. Defects in all organ systems

            4. Extreme muscle tone

5. Abnormalities in chromosome structure (Jorde, Carey, Bamshad, & White, 2003; Lewis, 2003)

    a. Structural abnormalities involving only one chromosome

      i. Deletions—The loss of a portion of a chromosome. The structurally abnormal chromosome lacks whatever information was present in the lost fragment.

      ii. Duplications—The presence of part of a chromosome in duplicate.

         a. May involve whole genes, series of genes, or only a part of a gene.

         b. Duplications may be direct or inverted.

      iii. Paracentric inversions—An inverted chromosome segment in one arm of a chromosome that results from two breaks in a single chromosome, followed by reattachment of a deleted segment in inverted sequence.

      iv. Ring chromosomes—A type of deletion in which both ends of a chromosome have been lost and the two broken ends have reunited to form a ring.

      v. Isochromosomes—During cell division, the centromere of a chromosome sometimes mistakenly divides so that it separates the two arms rather than the two chromatids. The resulting chromosomes are isochromosomes.

    b. Structural abnormalities involving more than one chromosome (Jorde, Carey, Bamshad, & White, 2003; Lewis, 2003).

      i. Translocations—May be caused by exposure to viruses, drugs, or radiation but generally occur for no apparent reason.

         a. Balanced—The amount of genetic material is correct.

            1. The individual usually is phenotypically normal (has no clinical findings).

2. The individual with a balanced translocation is termed a "carrier."

b. Unbalanced—There is a loss or gain of genetic material that results in mental retardation and physical abnormalities

c. Reciprocal translocation—Part of one chromosome is transferred to another chromosome.

  1. There is an exchange of genetic material between chromosomes involved.

  2. The translocation is balanced when no genetic material is lost.

d. Robertsonian translocation—Usually involves the acrocentric chromosomes (chromosomes 13, 14, 15, 21, and 22)

  1. Breaks occur near the centromeres and whole chromosome arms are exchanged.

  2. The two acrocentric chromosomes fuse at the centromere.

  3. The short arms of both chromosomes are usually lost.

C. Single Gene Disorders (Mendelian Disorders)—Disorders caused by mutations at a single gene locus and inherited in characteristic patterns. The chromosome structure appears normal because the size of the area of faulty genetic information is so small that it is not visible even with powerful microscopes (Jorde, Carey, Bamshad, & White, 2003; Lashley, 1998; Lewis, 2003).

1. Common patterns of single gene inheritance

  a. Autosomal dominant inheritance (see Figure 5.2)

    i. Each child of an affected person has a 50% chance of being affected.

    ii. Male-to-male (father-to-son) transmission may occur.

    iii. Males and females have an equal chance of being affected.

    iv. Normal children of an affected parent will have normal children.

    v. Usually only one parent of an affected child is affected.

    vi. Individuals who have the disorder show varying degrees of severity (variable expression).

    vii. A person who inherits an autosomal dominant disorder may not demonstrate any of the physical or developmental characteristics of the condition (nonpenetrance). Nonpenetrant individuals have a 50% chance of passing the gene mutation on to their offspring.

    viii. Autosomal dominant disorders include:

      a. Neurofibromatosis—Signs and symptoms include brown skin spots and benign tumors under the skin.

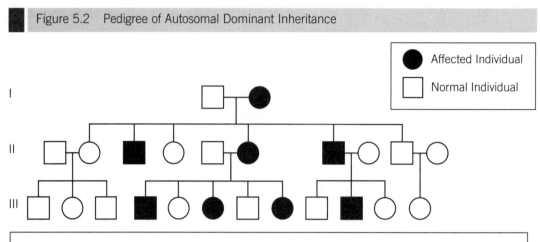

Figure 5.2   Pedigree of Autosomal Dominant Inheritance

CHARACTERISTICS OF AUTOSOMAL DOMINANT INHERITANCE

a. Multiple generations are affected.

b. Males and females are affected in equal proportion.

c. Male-to-male transmission does occur.

d. Each offspring of an affected parent has a 50% chance of being affected, 50% of being unaffected.

Greenwood Genetic Center, 1995

     b. Huntington disease—Signs and symptoms include uncontrollable movements and personality changes.

     c. Marfan syndrome—Long limbs, weakened blood vessels

     d. Achondroplasia—Dwarfism

b. Autosomal recessive inheritance (see Figure 5.3)

     i. Parents (heterozygous carriers) are clinically normal.

     ii. The rarer the gene, the greater likelihood that the parents are related.

     iii. Both parents must be carriers for an offspring to be affected.

     iv. Males and females have an equal chance of being affected.

     v. When both parents are carriers, each offspring has a 25% chance of being affected, a 50% chance of being a carrier, and a 25% chance of being a noncarrier, without the condition.

     vi. Autosomal recessive disorders include:

        a. Cystic fibrosis

        b. Tay-Sachs disease

        c. Sickle cell disease

        d. Phenylketonuria

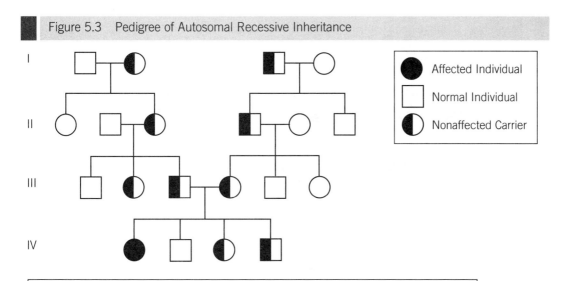

Figure 5.3   Pedigree of Autosomal Recessive Inheritance

- Affected Individual
- Normal Individual
- Nonaffected Carrier

CHARACTERISTICS OF AUTOSOMAL RECESSIVE INHERITANCE

a. Males and females are equally likely to be affected.

b. Both parents must be carriers of a single copy of the responsible gene in order for a child to be affected.

c. The recurrence risk is one in four (25%) for each offspring of carrier parents.

d. Certain autosomal recessive conditions are more common in specific ethinic groups.

e. Inquire about consanguinity, particularly if the condition is very rare.

Greenwood Genetic Center, 1995

    c. X-linked recessive inheritance (see Figure 5.4)

        i.   Much more common in males than females.

        ii. The probability of an affected male being born to a carrier mother is 50%.

        iii. The probability of a carrier female being born to a carrier mother is 50%.

        iv. All daughters of affected males will be carriers.

        v.   No male-to-male transmission.

        vi. X-linked recessive disorders include:

            a. Fragile X syndrome

            b. Hemophilia

            c. Duchenne muscular dystrophy

            d. Hunter syndrome

    d. X-linked dominant

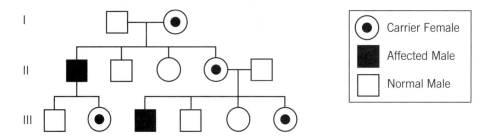

Figure 5.4   Pedigree of X-Linked Recessive Inheritance

CHARACTERISTICS OF X-LINKED RECESSIVE INHERITANCE

a. The incidence of the condition is much higher in males than females.

b. All daughters of affected males will be carriers.

c. Sons of carrier females have a 50% chance of being affected, 50% unaffected, in each pregnancy.

d. The condition is never transmitted directly from father to son.

Greenwood Genetic Center, 1995

    i.   An affected female has a 50% chance of passing on the gene mutation to a male or female child who would be affected.

    ii.   An affected female has a 50% chance of passing a normal gene to a male or female child who would be neither affected nor a carrier.

    iii.   X-linked dominant disorders tend to be much more severe in males than females.

    iv.   X-linked dominant disorders include:

        a.   Incontinentia pigmenti

        b.   Vitamin D–resistant rickets

D. Multifactorial Inheritance—Some conditions appear as the result of both genetic and environmental factors. While the specific contribution of each factor is not clearly defined, it is clear that each plays a role in the development of the disorder. The disorders tend to cluster in families but do not follow traditional laws of inheritance as seen with single gene disorders (Jorde, Carey, Bamshad, & White, 2003; Lewis, 2003).

    1. Multifactorial disorders include:

        a.   Neural tube defects

        b.   Cleft lip and palate

        c.. Pyloric stenosis

        d.   Congenital heart disease

        e.   Congenital hip dislocation

E. Mitochondrial Inheritance (see Figure 5.5)

    1. Gene mutations of mitochondrial DNA (mtDNA) cause a number of neuromuscular disorders that do not follow the typical patterns of inheritance.

        a. mtDNA is inherited only through the mother, because mitochondria are abundant in the ovum but not in sperm cells.

        b. Maternal inheritance—The female passes mtDNA to all offspring (male and female); however, only female offspring pass it on to their children.

        c. Inherited illnesses affect cells with abundant mitochondria, such as muscle cells.

        d. Mitochondrial inheritance disorders include:

            i. Leber's hereditary optic neuropathy (LHON)—Affects the optic nerve and results in sudden loss of central vision at about age 20.

           ii. Kearns-Sayre syndrome—Weakened heart muscle, degeneration of the retina, and skeletal muscle weakness in face, trunk, and extremities. (Jorde, Carey, Bamshad, & White, 2003; Lewis, 2003)

Figure 5.5   Pedigree of Mitochondrial Inheritance

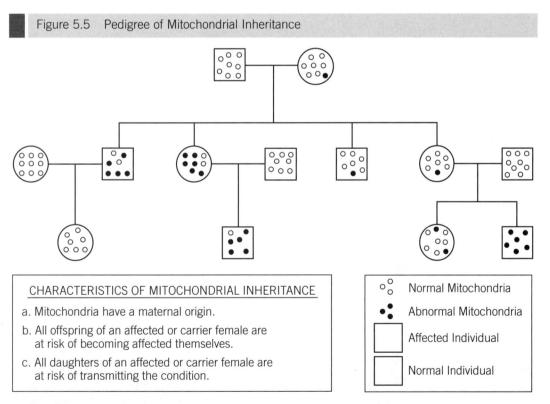

CHARACTERISTICS OF MITOCHONDRIAL INHERITANCE

a. Mitochondria have a maternal origin.

b. All offspring of an affected or carrier female are at risk of becoming affected themselves.

c. All daughters of an affected or carrier female are at risk of transmitting the condition.

°₀° Normal Mitochondria

•₀• Abnormal Mitochondria

☐ Affected Individual

☐ Normal Individual

Greenwood Genetic Center, 1995

    F. Chromosomal Mosaicism—Occurs when body cells contain two or more different chromosomal numbers or arrangements. Mosaicism is commonly caused by chromosomes failing to divide properly in early embryonic stages.

    G. Uniparental Disomy—When an offspring receives both chromosomes of a given pair from one parent and none of that pair from the other parent. Father-to-son transmission of hemophilia has been documented.

III. Genetic Screening, Evaluation, Diagnosis, and Counseling (Baker, Schuette, & Uhlmann, 1998; Curry et al., 1997; Lashley, 1998; Lea, Jenkins, & Francomano, 1998)

  A. Purpose

    1. To help families have healthy babies

    2. When children are not born healthy, to help them reach their fullest potential

    3. To help a family stay healthy as they adjust to their child's special needs

  B. Indications for Genetic Referral

    1. Child or individual has:

      a. Physical abnormalities

        i. Multiple congenital abnormalities (two or more physical abnormalities at birth)

        ii. Certain single physical abnormalities such as:

          a. Cleft lip and/or palate

          b. Neural tube defects such as

            1 Myelomeningocele

            2. Encephalocele

            3. Hydrocephalus

          c. Ambiguous external genitalia

        iii. Physical features associated with a specific genetic condition such as Down syndrome

      b. Growth problems

        i. Short stature

        ii. Failure to gain weight

      c. Developmental problems

        i. Delayed development

        ii. Mental retardation

        iii. Regression in mental function or in development

      d. Puberty problems

        i. Primary amenorrhea

        ii. Failure to develop secondary sexual characteristics (male or female)

        iii. Early or precocious puberty

  e. Specific known genetic disorder

        i. Child with chromosomal abnormality such as Down syndrome

        ii. Child with specific single gene disorders such as:

            a. Muscular dystrophy

            b. Cystic fibrosis

            c. Sickle cell disease

            d. Tay-Sachs disease

2. Couples who have pregnancy or reproductive problems

  a. Infertility

  b. Recurrent pregnancy losses (spontaneous abortions and/or stillbirths)

  c. Concerns about any of the following environmental exposures during pregnancy:

        i. radiation

        ii. infections

        iii. drugs

  d. Indications for considering chorionic villi or amniocentesis

        i. Increased risk for having infants with abnormal chromosomes

            a. Women 35 years or older

            b. Previous child with chromosomal disorder such as Down syndrome

            c. In certain cases, relatives of couples with a child with a chromosomal disorder

            d. Multiple spontaneous abortions (two or more)

        ii. Couples with a positive family history for neural tube defects

        iii. Couples at risk for having children with disorders for which molecular diagnosis is available, such as Duchenne muscular dystrophy, Fragile X syndrome, or cystic fibrosis

        iv. Couples at risk for having children with metabolic diseases, such as Tay-Sachs disease

        v. Previous child with multiple congenital abnormalities

        vi. Women who are at increased risk for having a child with a neural tube defect

3. Positive family history for:

  a. Certain chromosomal abnormalities

  b. Birth defects, such as neural tube defect

    c. Mental retardation

    d. Ethnicity with high risk for specific disorders such as:

        i. Tay-Sachs in the Jewish population

        ii. Sickle cell anemia in the black population

    e. Problems that "run in the family"

    f. Couples who are blood relatives (consanguinity)

C. Components of the Genetic Evaluation and Diagnostic Process—The following process is considered to be the mainstay of the genetic evaluation. These procedures are unlikely to be replaced by laboratory testing or screening methods. Longitudinal follow-up is very important, as it allows for individuals to be evaluated over time for physical and behavioral changes that may be significant in diagnosing many conditions.

    1. Clinical history including pre-, peri-, and post-natal history

    2. Family history and development of a three-history pedigree (see section D below)

    3. Physical and neurological examinations (see section E below) by experienced clinicians emphasizing assessment of

        a. Minor anomalies

        b. Growth

        c. Physical development

    4. Assessments of how the individual responds and interacts with others and the environment

D. Developing a Three-Generation Pedigree—(Special attention should be given to presence of individuals with learning problems, psychiatric disorders, autism, and mental retardation)

    1. Information is needed about the following:

        a. Patient (proband)

        b. All siblings

            i. living and dead

            ii. lost pregnancies

            iii. full siblings

            iv. note half siblings also

        c. Pregnancy losses

            i. miscarriages

            ii. stillborn children

            iii. neonatal deaths

        d. Parents

e. Father's siblings and their children

f. Father's parents

g. Mother's siblings and their children

h. Mother's parents

i. Any relative with a condition similar to proband's, including connecting relatives

j. Siblings and parents of affected relatives

k. When parents are blood relatives, draw in those who bridge that relationship.

2. What information needs to be recorded? (Symbols used in drawing a family history are shown in Overview section II A)

a. Proband's name

b. Proband's birth date

c. Proband's social security number

d. Date recorded

e. Ethnicity (explained below)

f. Consanguinity ("none" or specify relationship)

3. Proband

a. Mark with arrow

b. Note summary or clinical findings, history, and age of onset

4. Each individual in the family

a. Sex (square or circle)

b. Age

c. Health status (ask specifically about each person)

i. birth defects

ii. learning problems

iii. surgeries

iv. chronic health problems

d. If deceased, record age at time of death and cause of death

e. For those with symptoms (like or unlike proband's)

i. age at onset

ii. severity (e.g., for individuals with mental retardation: "Can she dress herself?")

iii. pertinent history (other unusual features, suspected causes)

5. Other family traits

6. Infertility problems

7. Gestational age for each miscarriage

8. Twins—Thought to be identical?

9. Consanguinity—Are parents of proband (or other affected individuals) blood relatives?

10. Ethnicity—be as specific as possible

   a. White, Black, Hispanic, etc.

   b. When known, include ancestry (e.g., English, Irish, German) or if unknown, the countries of family origin

E. Physical Assessment

1. Most patterns of physical abnormalities have been identified as genetic syndromes.

   a. A single, minor abnormal finding is not usually significant.

   b. Most people have one or more variations from normal.

   c. The total assessment of the individual is what is of importance.

2. Most genetic disorders disrupt growth and development.

   a. Monitoring growth and development is of prime importance.

   b. Growth parameters (height, weight, and especially head circumference) should be noted and compared to appropriate reference norms. When possible, earlier measurements should be obtained and compared to age-based normative data.

   c. Developmental assessment—Standardized tools include Denver Development Screening Test II, the Brazelton Neonatal Behavioral Assessment Scale, and the Bayley Scales of Infant Development.

   d. Significant variation from normal warrants referral for a more thorough evaluation.

3. Many observations of physical features can be made without touching a child.

   a. General body size for age

   b. Body shape

   c. Symmetry

   d. Movement

   e. Expression, etc.

4. Abnormal physical findings—A person should be referred for genetic evaluation if two or more unusual features are noted. Part of the genetic evaluation is to determine which features are variations from normal and which may reflect a more basic genetic disorder (see Table 5.1).

Table 5.1 Abnormal Physical Findings

BODY STRUCTURE	ABNORMAL FINDING
HEAD	Microcephaly
	Macrocephaly
	Frontal bossing
	Receding forehead
	Prominent or flat occiput
	Asymmetry
HAIR	Low hairline
	Excessive hair
	White forelock
	Bushy eyebrows
	Scalp defect
NOSE	Wide nasal bridge
	Short nose
	Depressed nasal bridge
	Bulbous nose
EYES	Downward slanting
	Upward slanting
	Ptosis
	Epicanthal folds
	Hypertelorism
	Nystagmus
	Strabismus
	Narrow palpebral fissures
	Microphthalmia
	Coloboma
MOUTH	Cleft lip and/or palate
	Micrognathia
	High arched palate
	Unusual contour of mouth (cupid bow, carp, thin upper lip)
	Large tongue
	Dental abnormalities
NECK	Short
	Webbed

(continues)

Table 5.1	Abnormal Physical Findings (*Continued*)
BODY STRUCTURE	**ABNORMAL FINDING**
HANDS and FEET	Syndactyly (fused fingers or toes)
	Polydactyly (extra digits)
	Clinodactyly (laterally bent fingers)
	Short first toe
	Club feet
	Deep flexion creases
	Four finger palmar crease
	Long or short fingers
	Wide space between toes
	Rockerbottom feet
	Abnormal thumbs
GENITALIA	Ambiguous
	Enlarged clitoris
	Small penis
	Bifid scrotum
	Undescended testicles
SKIN	Café au lait spots
	Port wine stain
	Dry, scaly skin
	Telangiectasia
	Too much or too little hair

F. Indications for Genetic Laboratory Studies

1. Chromosome analysis is considered a mainstay in the evaluation process. The following conditions do not always have a chromosomal etiology. However, if another cause is not evident, analysis to exclude a chromosome abnormality may be necessary.

a. Individuals with:

i. Suspected classic chromosomal syndrome (e.g., Down syndrome)

ii. Mental retardation

iii. Dysmorphic features (see II. E. Physical Assessment)

iv. Multiple congenital anomalies

v. Abnormalities of sexual development

a. Ambiguous genitalia

      b. Pubertal failure

   vi. Abnormalities of growth

  vii. Certain types of malignancies

  b. Couples with:

    i. Repeated spontaneous abortions

   ii. Infertility

  c. Family members:

    i. Both parents of a child who has a chromosomal duplication, deletion, translocation, or other rearrangement

   ii. All family members at risk of having a chromosomal rearrangement

  d. Products of pregnancy losses:

    i. Abortuses

   ii. Stillborn infants

      a. Malformed

      b. Undetermined etiology

2. Fragile-X analysis

  a. Confirmation of Fragile-X syndrome should be made by molecular analysis of the FRM1 gene. Cytogenetic studies are no longer appropriate to confirm Fragile-X syndrome.

  b. Diagnostic testing is relatively inexpensive.

  c. FRM1 testing is recommended for males and females with mental retardation of unknown etiology.

3. Neuroimaging

  a. Decisions regarding cranial imaging should be done after a thorough assessment, not before.

  b. MRI scan is generally superior to CT scan, although high quality CT imaging continues to be valuable.

  c. CT scan remains study of choice for individuals with suspected craniosynostatis or possible intracranial calcifications (e.g., congenital infections, tuberous sclerosis).

4. Evaluation for metabolic disorders

  a. Generally, infants and children with metabolic disturbances do not have birth defects or other dysmorphic features that are common in other genetic conditions, such as chromosomal abnormalities.

  b. Clues to the presence of such a defect may be largely limited to abnormalities of growth, development, or organ function. Signs and symptoms indicating the need for further testing are generally present in most infants and children with inborn errors of metabolism.

    c. It is not recommended that metabolic testing be performed routinely for patients with mental retardation, but used selectively for those individuals with a suspected category of disorder (Curry et al., 1997).

    d. The following is a selected list of abnormalities, which may indicate a need for metabolic testing:

       i. Failure to grow

       ii. Recurrent unexplained illness

       iii. Seizures

       iv. Ataxia

       v. Loss of psychomotor skills

       vi. Hypotonia

       vii. "Coarse" appearance

       viii. Eye abnormalities (cataracts, ophthalmoplegia, corneal clouding, abnormal retina)

       ix. Recurrent somnolence/coma

       x. Abnormal sexual differentiation

       xi. Arachnodactyly

       xii. Hepatosplenomegaly

       xiii. Metabolic/lactic acidosis

       xiv. Hyperammonemia

       xv. Low cholesterol

       xvi. Structural hair abnormalities

       xvii. Unexplained deafness

       xviii. Bone abnormalities

       xix. Skin abnormalities (angiokeratoma, "orange peel" skin, ichthyosis) (Curry et al., 1997, p. 474)

5. Molecular genetic testing

    a. Used for carrier testing, prenatal diagnosis, confirmation of a genetic diagnosis, and predisposition testing

    b. Direct molecular testing—A precise gene mutation has been identified in a family member, and other family members are tested for the presence of the gene mutation. Examples of genetic disorders where direct testing is used:

       i. Cystic fibrosis

       ii. Fragile X syndrome

       iii. Huntington's disease

c. Indirect genetic testing—A process accomplished by linkage analysis, which allows for indirect detection of a specific chromosome that contains a gene rather than identifying the gene mutation itself. The process requires complex interpretative analysis.

   i. Limitations:

      a. Generally, DNA must be available from at least one affected family member.

      b. Requires participation of family members across generations.

      c. Maternity and paternity must be known in order to interpret results correctly, and results may be inconclusive.

   ii. Used to detect conditions such as:

      a. Marfan syndrome

      b. Neurofibromatosis

      c. Other genetic conditions that may involve multiple mutations

d. Nurse's role in genetic testing

   i. Identify patients who may benefit from genetic testing. This may be based on nursing observation and family history or medical history.

   ii. Collaborate with other members of the health care team to provide information and support.

   iii. Discuss with patients and families the benefits and limitations of genetic testing.

   iv. Refer patients and families for evaluation and genetic counseling.

   v. Assure that patients understand the genetic testing process and that informed consent is obtained prior to testing.

   vi. Support the patient's right to choose or refuse to participate in genetic testing.

   vii. Support informed choice regarding reproductive and other health decisions.

   viii. Advocate for maintenance of confidentiality, privacy, and nondiscrimination regarding genetic information.

   ix. Provide case management services for individuals with genetic conditions.

   x. Assess the patient's and family's coping strategies. Provide support and further education about the testing process as needed.

e. Other health care professionals who are not experts in genetics should also have basic knowledge of genetic concepts and be able to refer an individual or family for genetic screening or testing when warranted. They can also serve as a support for families as they proceed through screening or testing and after the results are obtained and shared.

IV. Gene Therapy

A. Understanding the mechanism by which a gene or set of genes causes mental retardation and/or a specific condition that results in an intellectual and developmental disability (I/DD) supports the potential development of specific gene therapies to ameliorate or correct the condition.

B. Currently there is difficulty in identifying an appropriate vector or messenger for gene therapy that can successfully reach nervous tissue. The nervous system is affected in many conditions that result in mental retardation or I/DD and is therefore a future site for gene therapy. (Moser, 2000)

V. Ethical, Legal, and Social Issues (ELSI)

A. The results of the Human Genome Project will have a significant impact on individual and societal decision making in the future.

   1. A major goal of the project is to anticipate issues and develop guidelines or policies to address ethical, legal, and social concerns.

   2. About 5% of the Human Genome Project budget was dedicated to ELSI.

B. Ethical Considerations

   1. Genetic testing differs from other diagnostic tests.

      a. Permits diagnosis of the probability that a disorder may occur in an individual who has no symptoms.

      b. Identifies carriers who will not develop the disease but will transmit it to others.

      c. Genetic disorders, defects, and susceptibilities can be identified in unborn children.

      d. Provides personal information about blood relatives and raises the question of who has a right to know.

      e. Information received has the power to alter an individual's life as well as their family's lives.

   2. Privacy and confidentiality

   3. Discrimination—Has the potential to be misused in employment, insurance, or other societal situations (Hodge, 2004).

   4. Prenatal testing

      a. Currently, the ability to diagnose exceeds the ability to treat.

      b. When tests are positive for a genetic disorder, a decision must be made to terminate the pregnancy or to carry an affected child to term.

      c. Detailed information should be provided prior to prenatal testing about the type, quality, and meaning of the tests.

   d. Women may choose not to have tests done.

   e. Informed consent is necessary prior to testing.

C. Implications for Nursing and Health Care Professionals

   1. Increased demand for individuals trained in genetics

   2. Increased demand for interdisciplinary collaboration and communication among health disciplines

   3. Knowledge needed in informatics to collect, organize, interpret, and disseminate information

   4. Confidentiality issues regarding the "need and right to know" need to be resolved.

VI. Summary

It is essential that nurses and other health professionals who care for persons with I/DD have up-to-date knowledge on the basics of genetics, recent advances, and new technologies.

References

Baker, D. L., Schuette, J. L., & Uhlmann, W. R. (1998). *A guide to genetic counseling.* New York: John Wiley & Sons.

Cassidy, S. B., & Allanson, J. E. (2001). *Management of genetic syndromes.* New York: Wiley-Liss.

Curry, C. J., Aughton, D., Byrne, J., Carey, J. C., Cassiday, S., Cunniff, C., et al. (1997). Evaluation of mental retardation: Recommendations of a consensus conference, *American Journal of Medical Genetics, 72,* 468–477.

Greenwood Genetic Center. (1995). *Counseling aids for geneticists* (3rd ed.). Greenwood, SC: Jacobs.

Hodge, J. G. Jr. (2004). Ethical issues concerning genetic testing and screening in public health. *American Journal of Medical Genetics Part C (Seminars of Medical Genetics), 125C,* 66–70.

Human Genome Program. (2003). *Genomics and its impact in science and society: A 2003 primer.* U.S. Department of Energy. Retrieved May 20, 2004 from http://www.ornl.gov/sci/techresources/Human Genome/_publicat/_primer2001/2.shtml

Inlow, J. K., & Restifo, L. L. (2004). Molecular and comparative genetics of mental retardation. *Genetics, 166,* 835–881.

Jorde, L. B., Carey, J. C., Bamshad, M. J., & White, R. L. (2003). *Medical genetics.* St. Louis, MO: Mosby.

Lashley, F. R. (1998). *Clinical genetics in nursing practice.* New York: Springer.

Lea, D. H., Jenkins, J. J., & Francomano, C. A. (1998) *Genetics in clinical practice: New directions for nursing and health care.* Boston: Jones and Bartlett.

Lewis, R. (2003). *Human genetics: Concepts and applications* (5th ed.). Boston: McGraw-Hill.

Moser, H. W. (2000). Genetics and gene therapies. In M. L. Wehmeyer & J. R. Patton (Eds.). *Mental retardation in the 21st century* (pp. 235–250). Austin, TX: Pro-Ed.

National Human Genome Research Institute (2003). *About the Human Genome Project.* Retrieved May 20, 2004, from http://www.genome.gov

Seashore, M. R., & Wappner, R. S. (1996). *Genetics in primary care and clinical medicine.* Stamford, CT: Appleton & Lange.

Acknowledgment

The author wishes to thank Roger E. Stevenson, MD, founder and director of the Greenwood Genetic Center, Greenwood, South Carolina, for review, revisions, and recommendations for this chapter. You may learn more about the Greenwood Genetic Center by visiting their website at http://www.ggc.org.

Nursing and Health Care Professionals' Roles in the Field of Intellectual and Developmental Disabilities

IV

Roles and Responsibilities of Nurses and Other Health Care Professionals

6

J. Carolyn Graff, PhD, RN; Toni Whitaker, MD;
Laura Murphy, EdD; Susan McFadden, MEd, OTR/L

Objectives

At the completion of this chapter, the learner will be able to:

1. Identify the various settings in which persons with intellectual and developmental disabilities (I/DD) receive health-related services.

2. Describe overall responsibilities for nurses and health care professionals specializing in I/DD in these settings.

3. Describe the responsibilities of nurses and health care professionals specializing in I/DD in their roles as administrators, consultants, educators, and researchers.

4. Identify formal education needed by nurses and health care professionals specializing in I/DD in their various roles.

5. Discuss the changing roles and responsibilities of nurses and health care professionals working with persons with I/DD across the lifespan.

Key Points

- The settings in which persons with I/DD live and are supported determine to some extent the responsibilities assumed by nurses and health care professionals specializing in I/DD.

- The changing strengths and needs of persons with I/DD and their families lead to changing roles, responsibilities, and challenges for nurses and health care professionals.

- Health care professionals require ongoing education to ensure that their skills and knowledge are appropriate to provide the needed services for persons with I/DD.

- Advanced educational preparation and extensive experience may be required for nurses and health care professionals providing direct and indirect services to persons with I/DD.

I.   Introduction

A. Nurses and health care professionals specializing in I/DD work in settings where children and adults with I/DD live, go to school, work, play, and receive health care.

B. Of the over 4 million persons with I/DD in the U.S., 88% live with their families or in their own households (Administration on Developmental Disabilities, 2000).

C. Children with I/DD should live with their families, attend neighborhood schools, and participate in community recreation with children without disabilities. Adults with I/DD should live in the home of their choosing, and participate in meaningful work, inclusive recreation, and other leisure activities (American Association on Mental Retardation (AAMR) and The Arc of the United States, 2002).

D. As persons with I/DD grow, develop, and mature, their strengths and needs change. Likewise, the supports and types of professionals providing these supports may change.

E. A family-centered, continuous, comprehensive, coordinated, compassionate, and culturally competent care system for persons with I/DD represents the gold standard toward which professionals should strive (American Academy of Pediatrics, American Academy of Family Physicians, and American College of Physicians-American Society of Internal Medicine, 2002).

II.   Continuum from Birth to Adulthood and Home to School to Community Settings

A. Early Intervention Programs (Birth to 3 Years)

1. These programs offer services to meet the developmental needs of an infant or toddler with a disability in physical, cognitive, communication, social, emotional, and/or adaptive development (National Early Childhood Technical Assistance Center, n.d.).

2. Professionals work with children with I/DD and their families in family homes, community agencies, or community clinics to maximize the child's development.

3. Children under age three years should receive services in "natural environments" or "settings that are natural or normal for the child's age peers who have no disabilities" (*IDEA '97 Final Regulations*, 1999).

B. Preschool Programs (3 to 5 Years)

1. Preschool programs offer services to meet the developmental needs of preschool children with hearing impairment, visual impairment, preschool moderate to severe delay, or preschool speech/language delay.

2. Health care professionals work with children in preschools, family homes, community agencies, or community clinics to meet the developmental and health needs of children and to strengthen family members' support of each other.

C. Public and Private Schools (5 to 21 Years)

1. Schools offer services to meet the educational needs of students and to ensure success for each student in an inclusive setting with same-age peers.

2. Health care professionals should assure that needed school and community supports are available to prepare all students to participate fully in society.

D. Hospitals and Specialty Clinics (Infancy through Adulthood)

1. Hospitals and clinics offer health care services that include extensive inpatient and/or outpatient services for children and adults.

2. Health care professionals should provide high quality care to persons with I/DD and their families and ensure that services are based on individual need, preference, and choice (AAMR and The Arc of the United States, 2002).

E. Mental Health Centers (Infancy through Adulthood)

1. Mental health centers offer comprehensive, specialized mental health services to persons with I/DD.

2. Professionals working in mental health centers should provide high quality care to ensure that their services provide

   a. Access to supports that are based on individual need

   b. Opportunities for social integration

   c. Alternatives to challenging behaviors (AAMR and The Arc of the United States, 2002)

F. University Centers for Excellence in Developmental Disabilities, Education, Research, and Service (UCEDD)

1. UCEDDs offer interdisciplinary, family-centered, culturally competent, and state-of-the-art evaluations and treatment to children and adults with I/DD and their families (Association of University Centers on Disabilities, 2001).

2. The network of centers provides interdisciplinary training of students and fellows and conducts research related to I/DD (Administration on Developmental Disabilities, 2000).

G. Community-Based Living Options (Birth through Adulthood)

1. Community-based living options include

   a. Family homes

   b. Supported living arrangements

  c. Residential programs

 2. Professionals should provide high quality health care to ensure that persons with I/DD participate fully in social, educational, work, and community activities.

 3. Professionals should ensure that the needs of persons living in a residential facility can be met through services provided by that facility.

 4. Supported living arrangements may include a person's

  a. Own home

  b. Apartment

  c. Group home

III. Roles and Responsibilities of Nurses and Health Care Professionals: Administrator

A. In all settings, nurse administrators and administrators in other health professions may be involved in a continuum of services that are direct and indirect.

B. Direct administrative services may have a crisis emphasis, while indirect services may have an emphasis on prevention.

C. Indirect services include:

 1. Recruiting and hiring to ensure adequate staff

 2. Budgeting and managing supplies and materials

 3. Supervising staff who provide the day-to-day services that meet the goals of the organization

 4. Contributing to the professional development of those being supervised

 5. Collaborating with other managers and administrators

D. Additional responsibilities may include developing and implementing:

 1. Policies and procedures to ensure consistency in practice and outcomes

 2. Performance indicators used to evaluate competencies of persons providing nursing and health-related care

 3. Quality assurance activities to determine if staff activities are being performed effectively

E. In all settings, administrators may be responsible for a variety of reports, such as

 1. Monthly activity reports

 2. Rationale for productivity statistics

 3. Annual reports highlighting activities for the fiscal year

 4. Proposal or request for a program, personnel, equipment, and space

F. In a community setting, nurses may supervise case coordinators (also referred to as case managers), with clinical and personnel oversight as well as information management and programmatic operations responsibilities

G. Generally, health care professionals in administrative roles have masters or doctoral degrees.

IV. Roles and Responsibilities of Nurses and Health Care Professionals: Consultant

A. Consultants share the expertise of their disciplines to aid in evaluation, treatment, and planning for and with persons with I/DD.

B. Consultations typically result in professional advice or opinion, and may vary in scope and type of service.

   1. Consultations may be provided along a continuum of direct and indirect services.

      a. Direct consultations are usually crisis-oriented and focus on the person with I/DD.

      b. Indirect consultations are usually preventive and focus on the person's environment and caregivers (Erchul & Martens, 2002).

   2. Along this continuum, professionals' roles may be blurred as they are broadened and/or focused to address particular health issues that change over time.

   3. Consultation services may be provided in a single encounter or multiple encounters, when ongoing monitoring or treatment is required.

   4. Professionals providing consultations to persons with I/DD may include

      a. Audiologists

      b. Educators

      c. Nurses

      d. Nutritionists

      e. Occupational therapists

      f. Physical therapists

      g. Primary care physicians

      h. Psychologists

      i. Social workers

      j. Speech language pathologists

      k. Specialty physicians

         i. Behavioral pediatricians

         ii. Developmental pediatricians

         iii. Geneticists

         iv. Neurologists

         v. Ophthalmologists

         vi. Orthopedic surgeons

       vii. Otolaryngologists

       viii. Psychiatrists

C. In addition to the settings described previously, nurses and health care professionals provide consultations to community support and government facilities and agencies.

D. The consultant's role may include care coordination with other service providers or consultants (American Academy of Pediatrics, Committee on Children with Disabilities, 1999).

   1. In the health care system, care coordination may involve

      a. Planning treatment

      b. Monitoring health care financing

      c. Coordinating specialty health care

      d. Sharing pertinent health information

      e. Planning hospitalizations and emergency services

      f. Facilitating access to services

   2. In the educational system, care coordination may include

      a. Identifying needs for testing and educational services

      b. Clarifying plans as outlined in individual family service plans (IFSPs), individual educational plans (IEPs), or individual health plans (IHPs)

      c. Gaining access to transportation and assistive technologies

   3. Care coordination in the home setting may include elements of both the health and educational systems, as needed.

E. Comprehensive health-related services for persons with I/DD include input from many disciplines. Professionals may be enlisted as consultants to

   1. Screen for I/DD to identify children with or at risk for I/DD

   2. Diagnose the type, scope, and etiology of I/DD

   3. Treat primary and associated medical conditions to minimize additional health burdens

   4. Provide therapy on a short-term basis or monitor and assess therapy efficacy over time.

F. Appropriate educational placement and special education services

   1. Educators may rely on consultants to provide information on current or changing educational needs in a person whose I/DD affects educational achievement (American Academy of Pediatrics, 2001).

   2. Consultants may conduct initial evaluations regarding specific I/DD as well as measure progress over time.

      a. Updated standardized testing for academic and/or functional abilities will help educators assess progress.

   b. Medical conditions that interfere with learning should be monitored for potential deterioration.

G. Family-centered consultations occur in the natural environment of a person with I/DD.

   1. Children may be evaluated for early-intervention services in their home setting.

      a. Assessments done in a familiar rather than unfamiliar and potentially frightening setting may result in better compliance and performance on testing measures.

      b. Caregivers may benefit from support provided in the home setting by professionals who assess specific concerns in the natural environment and tailor recommendations to address these concerns.

   2. Older children and adults may receive assessments and/or services in their home setting based on level and type of I/DD.

      a. Individuals with significant medical or behavioral problems that limit their ability to seek care outside of the home will benefit from home services.

      b. Direct-care providers may benefit from a consultant's observation in the natural setting where specific triggers precipitate problem behaviors.

H. Nurses and health care professionals providing consultation services to persons with I/DD should have at least a baccalaureate degree in an area related to their professional expertise. Most consultants have graduate degrees (e.g., master of arts or MA, master of science or MS, doctor of philosophy or PhD) or professional degrees (e.g., doctor of medicine or MD).

   1. Generalist nurse consultants specializing in I/DD should have a baccalaureate degree in nursing (BSN).

   2. Advanced practice nurse consultants specializing in I/DD are masters or doctorally prepared (Nehring et al., 1998).

V. Roles and Responsibilities of Nurses and Health Care Professionals: Educator

A. More than other health care professionals, school nurses spend significant amounts of time educating students, teachers, parents, and others about the health needs of students and their implications for a student's success in the school setting.

   1. School nurses take the lead in

      a. Assessing a student's health to include immunization status

      b. Day-to-day health care monitoring of students

      c. Identifying health problems that may prevent educational progress

      d. Collaborating with family, physicians, public health, and social service agencies

    e.   Identifying health problems that may prevent educational progress

    f.   Participating in the planning and implementation of the individualized family service plan (IFSP), individualized education plan (IEP), and/or individualized health plan (IHP; may also be an individualized habilitative plan) (American Academy of Pediatrics, 2001).

2. The nurse develops IHPs for children with I/DD such as

    a. Hearing impairment

    b. Low vision

    c. Multiple disabilities

    d. Orthopedic impairment

    e. Traumatic brain injury

    f. Visual impairment

    g. Other physical impairments

3. The IHP and IEP are collaborative efforts among the nurse, special education teacher, general education teacher, administrator, parent, and others (e.g., family members, friends, or other professionals). Each situation will be unique and prescriptive to the needs of the individual child.

    a. The nurse and parent often take the lead in developing the IHP.

    b. The special education teacher and parent often take the lead in the development of the IEP.

    c. The school nurse's participation in the IEP or IFSP increases the potential that the IHP goals will be met.

4. Nurses in the educational setting help develop and implement health plans for children with I/DD who also have concurrent health needs such as

    a. Attention deficit hyperactivity disorder

    b. Diabetes

    c. Feeding problems

    d. Metabolic problems

    e. Seizure disorders

    f. Tic disorders

5. School nurses may serve as direct service providers or consultants to other educators for such procedures as nasogastric feedings, tracheostomy suctioning, and ventilator care.

    a. Nurses collaborate with special educators and general educators to facilitate the delivery of these services to children with I/DD.

    b. In situations where nurses do not provide direct services, they train others to provide these services and delegate certain responsibilities, while maintaining responsibility and accountability for this care as allowed by the nurse practice act in each state.

6. As team members, school nurses educate parents, teachers, support staff, and children with I/DD about activities that prevent serious side effects or complications. For example, exercise is important to reduce the likelihood of obesity that is often associated with diabetes and certain genetic disorders (e.g., Prader-Willi syndrome).

B. Nurses and health care professionals educate others about I/DD and the health care needs of persons with I/DD in community settings other than schools.

1. Nurses monitor immunization status in community clinics.

2. Nurses consult with parents, caregivers, and persons with I/DD about the importance of preventive medical care, such as visits for health surveillance.

3. Nurses and health care professionals are involved in educating both direct and indirect service providers about the disability and the health-related accommodations needed to ensure inclusion and optimal health of persons with I/DD.

VI. Roles and Responsibilities of Nurses and Health Care Professionals: Researcher

A. Nurses and health care professionals conduct research in all settings where persons with I/DD live, work, and receive health services. This most often includes

1. Health care settings where nurses and health care professionals provide direct and indirect services to persons with I/DD

2. Universities or other academic institutions

B. Professionals working in hospitals, clinics, and other health-related settings recruit persons with I/DD and their family members to participate in research activities after a thorough explanation of the study and obtaining informed consent.

C. Nurses and health care professionals may be involved with data collection, data analysis, and manuscript preparation. Research assistants often assist with data collection and data analysis.

D. Professionals may conduct research at one site (location) or multiple sites (locations). Researchers may represent one discipline such as nursing or several disciplines.

E. Research is often collaborative and includes researchers representing several disciplines at several locations within or outside the United States.

F. A professional's focus of research is related to that professional's area of expertise. For example, an audiologist may conduct research related to hearing and hearing loss, yet collaborate with speech language pathologists, developmental pediatricians, neurologists, nurses, and special educators.

G. Some examples of research that may be conducted by professionals working with persons with I/DD include:

1. Developmental medicine and behavioral pediatrics—Medication management and behavioral strategies that will be useful for managing behavior problems

2. Educators—Strategies that encourage persons with I/DD to participate fully in the community, benefit from the educational system, and reach their maximum potential

3. Geneticists—Identification and treatment of a genetic disorder, genetic cause of an I/DD, patterns of inheritance of a genetic disorder, and risk for family members

4. Nurses—Strategies that improve and enhance the health of persons with I/DD, quality of care for persons with I/DD, and methods of educating nurses working with persons with I/DD

5. Nutritionists—Nutritional needs and the health and quality of life of persons with I/DD

6. Neurologists—The neurological system, to include the brain, the nervous system, nerve function, and neurologic disorders

7. Psychiatrists—Mental health of persons with I/DD that includes assessment and intervention (e.g., medication, consultation)

8. Psychologists—Learning, behavior, and development of persons with I/DD and their families

9. Social workers—Social functioning of persons with I/DD in the context of their families and community

10. Speech language pathologists—Communication skills of persons with I/DD

H. Professionals should have up-to-date knowledge of the research being conducted in their areas of expertise so they can refer persons with I/DD and their families to the most appropriate research study. Information about current clinical research studies can be found at the National Institutes of Health website, http://clinicalstudies.info.nih.gov.

I. All professionals have responsibilities to ensure that the rights of research participants are protected and that the integrity of the research is sound. The Office for Human Research Protections, U.S. Department of Health and Human Services (n.d.) establishes policy and provides guidance on protecting the welfare of persons participating in research studies. Specific information about protecting the rights of persons with I/DD who participate in research can be found at http://ohrp.osophs.dhhs.gov/irb/irb_chapter6.htm.

J. Nurses and professionals conducting research have graduate degrees in their respective disciplines. Nurse researchers typically have doctoral degrees in nursing and may collaborate with experienced researchers during the early part of their research careers. Nurses should participate in research at a level appropriate to their education (Aggen et al., 1995).

VII. Summary

Nurses and health care professionals work in settings that encompass the lifespan of an individual with I/DD. Roles include administrator, consultant, educator, and researcher. Such professionals interact on a daily basis to provide essential services to individuals with I/DD and their families.

References

Administration on Developmental Disabilities. (2000). *Public law 106-402*. Retrieved December 13, 2003, from http://www.acf.gov/programs/add/DDA.htm

Aggen, R. L., Debennaro, M. D., Fox, L., Hahn, J. E., Logan, B. A., Von Fumetti, L., et al. (1995). *Standards of developmental disabilities nursing practice*. Eugene, OR: Developmental Disabilities Nurses Association.

American Academy of Pediatrics. (2001). *The role of the school nurse in providing school health services*. Retrieved September 16, 2003, from http://www.aap.org/policy/re0050.html.

American Academy of Pediatrics, American Academy of Family Physicians, and American College of Physicians-American Society of Internal Medicine. (2002). A consensus statement on health care transitions for young adults with special health care needs. *Pediatrics, 110*, 1304–1306.

American Academy of Pediatrics, Committee on Children with Disabilities. (1999). Care coordination: Integrating health and related systems of care for children with special health care needs. *Pediatrics, 104*, 978–981.

American Association on Mental Retardation and The Arc of the United States. (2002). *The Arc and AAMR Position Statements*. Retrieved December 14, 2003, from http://www.thearc.org/position-statements.htm

Association of University Centers on Disabilities. (2001). *Association of University Centers on Disabilities: Mission and vision*. Retrieved September 16, 2003, from http://www.aucd.org/about/mission/htm

Erchul, W. P., & Martens, B. K. (2002). *School consultation: Conceptual and empirical bases of practice*. New York: Plenum.

IDEA '97 Final Regulations. (1999). 34 CFR Part 300, Assistance to States for the Education of Children with Disabilities (Part B of the Individuals with Disabilities Education Act). Retrieved December 13, 2003, from http://www.ed.gov/offices/OSERS/Policy/IDEA/regs.html

National Early Childhood Technical Assistance Center. (n.d.). *Full text of P.L. 105-17 Individuals with Disabilities Act amendments of 1997, Part C, Section 619*. Retrieved December 13, 2003, from http://www.nectac.org/idea/105-17PartC.asp

Nehring, W. M., Roth, S. P., Natvig, D., Morse, J., Savage, T., & Krajicek, M. (1998). *Statement on the scope and standards for the nurse who specializes in developmental disabilities and/or mental retardation*. Washington, DC: American Nurses Publishing and American Association on Mental Retardation.

Office for Human Research Protections, U.S. Department of Health and Human Services. (n.d.). *Institutional review board guidebook: Chapter VI, Special classes of subjects*. Retrieved December 13, 2003, from http://ohrp.osophs.dhhs.gov/irb/irb_chapter6.htm

Health Promotion

Wendy M. Nehring, RN, PhD, FAAN, FAAMR and Melissa Faulkner, RN, PhD

7

Objectives

At the end of this chapter, the learner will be able to:

1. Identify key national health promotion goals for persons with intellectual and developmental disabilities (I/DD) in *Healthy People 2010*.
2. Discuss health promotion strategies for persons with I/DD as identified by the national blueprint from the former Surgeon General, Dr. David Satcher.
3. Discuss the current research literature on health promotion topics that involved research participants with I/DD.
4. Analyze current genetic knowledge on health promotion for persons with I/DD.
5. Describe levels of intervention by primary care providers.

Key Points

- Health promotion for persons of all ages with I/DD is an emerging public health area of concern (U.S. Department of Health and Human Services, 2000).
- Increased numbers of health professionals, in all disciplines, must be educated to care for persons of all ages with I/DD and their families in the present and future.
- Strategic community-based health promotion plans that are culturally relevant are necessary to reduce health disparities in persons with I/DD.
- Future scientific inquiry should be guided by conceptual models to explore the interrelated influences of level and type of disability, sociodemographic factors, access to services and technology, health promotion, the development of secondary conditions, and overall health status.

I.   Introduction

Health promotion is the science and art of helping people change their lifestyle to move toward a state of optimal health (*American Journal of Health Promotion,* 1989, p. 5).

A. Health is achieved through a balance of intellectual, physical, social, spiritual, and emotional health.

B. Internal and external factors influence healthy practices. Internal factors include, for example, desire, cognitive abilities, and the willpower to maintain healthy practices. External factors include, for example, support systems and programs or facilities that provide supportive environments.

II.   *Healthy People 2010*

Healthy People 2010 (U.S. Department of Health and Human Services, 2000) is a federal document that provides a vision for a healthy America. In this document, Chapter 6: Disability and Secondary Conditions was devoted to persons with disabilities. This was the first major attempt by the federal government to address the health of persons with disabilities. The specific objectives that were addressed in this chapter are:

A. Objective 1: All *Healthy People 2010*–related surveys should include a number of questions that can identify individuals with disabilities.

1. There is not a standardized definition of disability (see Chapter 2).

2. People with disabilities have not been included as a separate group in national surveys.

3. Recommendations include hiring people with I/DD to work in public health agencies and to consult on health promotion issues, presenting information on I/DD and health care concerns in public health curricula across all disciplines, and increasing and improving health promotion and health education materials for persons of all ages with I/DD (Seltser, 2001).

B. Objective 2: Decrease the proportion of sad, depressed, or unhappy children and adolescents with disabilities. In 1997, 31% reported unhappiness according to the National Health Interview Survey. The target is a reduction in reported unhappiness to 7% of respondents.

1. Recommendations would include providing more emphasis on developmental and situational mental and emotional health in children in didactic content and clinical experiences in undergraduate and graduate education across disciplines (Seltser, 2001). This also applies to adults (see the next objective).

C. Objective 3: Decrease the percentage of adults with disabilities who are sad, depressed, or unhappy, and as a result, do not keep active. In 1997, according to the National Health Interview Survey, 28% reported negative feelings that prevented activity. The target is a reduction in reported negative feelings to 7% of respondents.

D. Objective 4: Raise the percentage of adults with disabilities who are socially active. In 1997, according to the National Health Interview Survey, 95.4% participated in social activities. The target is an increase to 100% of adults with disabilities who participate in social activities.

E. Objective 5: Raise the percentage of adults with disabilities who have adequate formal and informal social support. In 1998, the Behavioral Risk Factor Surveillance System results showed that 71% had sufficient emotional support. The target is to increase this percentage to 79%.

F. Objective 6: Raise the percentage of adults with disabilities who are satisfied with life. In 1998, the Behavioral Risk Factor Surveillance System results showed that 87% were satisfied with their lives. The target is to increase this percentage to 96%.

G. Objective 7: Decrease the number of individuals with disabilities who reside in congregate care facilities who do not need to live in these settings.

    1. The target is to achieve a 50% reduction in the number of adults living in congregate care facilities.

    2. The target is also to achieve total reduction in the number of children living in congregate care facilities.

    3. Develop increased family support programs and facilities that support life in the community for all family members. Some options include personal care, personal assistance, respite care, supported employment, specialized foster care, alternative family arrangements (e.g., shared parenting), specialized day care, mental health support, and health promotion programs (Seltser, 2001).

H. Objective 8: Eradicate the disparity between the numbers of adults without disabilities who work and the numbers of adults with disabilities who work. The target is 82% of adults with disabilities are employed. In 1994–1995, the results of the Survey of Income and Program Participation showed that 52% of adults with disabilities were employed.

I. Objective 9: Raise the percentage of children and adolescents who participate in regular education (inclusion) to 80% or higher. The current target is 60%. In 1995–1996, the results of the Data Analysis System of the U.S. Department of Education found that 45% of school-age children were in regular education 80% or more of the time.

J. Objective 10: Raise the percentage of wellness and health and treatment facilities and programs that deliver full access for individuals with I/DD. This is a developmental objective in that there is no current research to provide statistics for the prevalence of full-access wellness and health and treatment facilities and programs in existence.

1. Keep in mind that the person with I/DD has a right to choose what activities they wish to participate in. Issues of healthy living and choices must be explored in persons with I/DD (Sutherland, Couch, & Iacono, 2002).

K. Objective 11: Decrease the percentage of individuals with I/DD who do not report adequate technology and assistive devices to meet current support needs. This objective is also developmental.

L. Objective 12: Decrease the percentage of individuals with I/DD who report environmental barriers that prevent participation in any type of activity outside the home. This objective is also developmental. Full participation must be a goal for everyone.

M. Objective 13: Raise the prevalence of states, tribes, and the District of Columbia that have health promotion and public health surveillance programs for individuals, of all ages, with I/DD and their caregivers. This objective is developmental for tribes, but in 1999, there were 14 such programs in the states and Washington, D.C.

1. The health and quality of life of family caregivers is a major public health concern.

III. A Plan to Reduce Health Disparities in Persons with I/DD

Former Surgeon General David Satcher (U.S. Public Health Service, 2002) outlined a national blueprint to reduce health disparities in persons with mental retardation. Six goals were proposed. Information specific to health promotion for each goal follows:

A. Goal 1: Health promotion should be integrated in community settings where persons with I/DD reside, work, and socialize.

1. Action steps involve developing health and wellness programs for persons with I/DD based on successful models for persons without I/DD, evaluating existing health promotion education materials and media, developing strategies for reducing turnover rates in nonfamily caregivers, developing strategies to reduce the caregiving burden and stress inherent in the role, developing strategies to eliminate health hazards and increase safety in workplace environments, and assessing the effect of wellness and health promotion activities on morbidity, mortality, and quality of life.

B. Goal 2: Advance understanding and knowledge of I/DD and health, ensuring that the knowledge is made understandable, accessible, culturally relevant, and accurate.

1. Research must be conducted to advance our knowledge of the interaction between health and I/DD. This involves the assessment of morbidity and mortality studies, secondary health conditions, mental health, and service needs of persons of all ages with I/DD.

2. As information is available, persons with I/DD, their family members, care providers, and health care professionals must be informed in a way that is understandable, practical, useable, culturally sensitive, and accurate. This information must cover the areas of diagnosis, treatment, health promotion, and disease prevention.

3. Persons with I/DD and/or their family members should be involved as a member of the research team or an advisory committee to the researchers to provide input.

4. Health care professionals who specialize in I/DD and are experts in their respective disciplines should continue to convene on a regular basis to identify a research agenda concerning health and persons with I/DD. The Arc of the United States sponsored a national meeting in January 2003 from which the proceedings are available (see http://www.thearc.org).

5. Researchers should also examine health services utilization and costs for health care for persons with I/DD, either noncategorically or by specific diagnosis, age, funding source, or geographical location.

6. Health care professionals should help persons with I/DD and their family members to examine the research literature on best practices to assist them in decision making.

7. Encourage increased numbers of graduates in all disciplines that provide health services to persons of all ages with I/DD.

8. Encourage health care professionals to conduct research and publish research results or clinical experiences. There is an urgent need to address the health care disparities for persons of all ages with I/DD.

C. Goal 3: Enhance health care quality for persons with I/DD.

1. Standards of health care, including health promotion, based on scientific evidence must be developed and made available. Until the evidence is available, consensus standards should be developed.

2. The best practices of care for specific conditions, age groups, and different settings must be defined.

3. Examine health across the lifespan, not just pediatric or adult, condition-specific, or by specialization.

4. Develop curricula across disciplines on health care needs and issues of disparity for persons of all ages with I/DD.

D. Goal 4: Provide new and additional didactic instruction and clinical experiences for health care professionals in the care of persons of all ages with I/DD.

1. Instruction should involve interdisciplinary experiences.

2. Develop scope and standards of practice for each discipline. Nursing is the only discipline to have done so (Nehring, Roth, Natvig, et al., 1998; Nehring et al., in press).

3. Instruction should also have a continuing education component.

4. University Centers of Excellence in Developmental Disabilities (UCEDD) are an excellent resource for such interdisciplinary didactic and clinical experiences (see http://www.aucd.org).

E. Goal 5: Appropriate health outcomes are affected by appropriate health care financing opportunities.

1. Health promotion activities should be included in service packages.

F. Goal 6: Health care services should be available and accessible.

1. Primary and specialty health care services are often fragmented and unavailable geographically, especially mental health professionals and dentists who are knowledgeable in the care of persons with I/DD.

2. It is important to increase the numbers of health professionals in all disciplines across the country to provide health care to persons with I/DD of all ages. This includes professionals who represent different ethnicities, speak different languages, and live across urban and rural settings.

3. Health care services must be accessible and less complicated for persons with I/DD to obtain. Care coordination is a recommended service.

4. Health care services, including health promotion activities, should be integrated in existing community programs and settings.

5. Develop health passports (see Chapter 12).

IV. Research Evidence on Health Promotion Topics Involving People with I/DD

The American Association on Mental Retardation, Health Promotion and Prevention Committee sponsored a national preconference on "Health Promotion for Persons with Intellectual/Developmental Disabilities: The State of Scientific Evidence" in June 2004. Research involving persons with I/DD on specific health promotion topics was reviewed by national experts in their fields. Findings are reported by topic.

A. Hypertension (Draheim, 2004)

1. Hypertension rates are similar to the general population, but there are some exceptions:

    a. Hypertension rates are lower in Down syndrome.

    b. Hypertension rates are higher in Williams syndrome.

    c. Hypertension rates may be lower in Prader-Willi syndrome, but the research is inconclusive.

2. Lifestyle modifications recommended by the Seventh Report of the Joint National Committee on Prevention, Detection, Evaluation, and Treatment of High Blood Pressure should be followed (National Heart, Lung, and Blood

Institute, 2003). These include weight management, physical activity, and dietary practices.

3. Research is primarily cross-sectional without a consistent definition of hypertension. Additional research using other research methodologies, including random controlled trials, is warranted.

4. Medication interactions need to be considered.

B. Obesity (Bandini, 2004)

1. Obesity is a problem for both children and adults with I/DD.

2. Prevalence of obesity and risk factors for obesity in persons with I/DD need to be explored.

3. Identify appropriate means to assess for being overweight and obesity in persons with different conditions with I/DD.

4. Identify factors that lead to the development of obesity.

5. Examine whether intervention programs to reduce being overweight and obesity should be integrated in other community programs, such as Weight Watchers, or should be designed and offered specifically for persons with I/DD.

6. Persons with I/DD living in the community are more likely to be overweight and to want to lose weight than those living in residential centers (Lewis, Lewis, Leake, King, & Lindemann, 2002).

C. Respiratory Health, Nutrition, and Associated Swallowing Behaviors (Lefton-Greif, 2004; Sheppard, 2004) (see Chapter 17)

1. Scientific research is limited in the areas of:

   a. Medication ingestion

   b. Prevention

   c. Professional and career training

   d. Daily management

   e. Interactions and adverse effects of nutritional problems and respiratory and/or gastrointestinal conditions

   f. Swallowing and feeding problems by age and development

   g. Terminology is not consistent between research studies.

2. Need to identify best practices, examining populations and costs.

3. Need to explore the effects of having feeding and swallowing problems as a child on later development of "adult onset" respiratory disorders.

4. Need to explore the additive effects of having physiological consequences as a result of childhood feeding and swallowing problems to later development of "adult onset" respiratory disorders.

D. Mental Health (Benson, 2004) (see Chapters 18 and 19)

1. There are many diagnostic issues in identifying mental health problems in persons with I/DD.

2. Need to develop specific tools, both pediatric and adult, to identify and assess mental health problems in persons with I/DD.

E. Physical Activity (Rimmer, 2004)

1. Random controlled trials need to be completed on specific conditions and/or secondary conditions.

2. Cross-sectional and prospective observational research needs to be completed on comparisons of different levels and length of exercise activity. Variables of interest include gender, secondary conditions, etiology, activity limitations, and physiological and psychosocial measures.

3. Identify gold standards for physical activity for persons with I/DD.

4. Examine personal and environmental factors that influence participation in exercise.

5. Describe and use new and emerging technology in measuring physical activity.

F. Reproductive Health Care (White-Scott, 2004) (see Chapter 13)

1. Limited scientific evidence for guideline development. Some evidence to support that women with I/DD have lower incidence of cervical cancer.

2. Areas where little research exists for persons with I/DD include: osteoporosis; rates of sexually transmitted diseases and treatment outcomes; rates of contraceptive use; screening for testicular, prostate, and breast cancer; and menopause.

3. Sex education programs need to be developed specifically for women with I/DD. It has been proven that adolescents and adults with I/DD know less about sexual and reproductive health issues than adolescents and adults without I/DD.

4. Current research is based on small sample sizes and limited use of control groups.

5. Health care providers often have a lack of accessible equipment and provide inadequate assistance during the health care visit. They also may lack knowledge about I/DD and have inappropriate or negative attitudes about persons with I/DD.

6. Health care providers may not provide adequate information to persons with I/DD on reproductive health or intimacy.

G. Violence (Sobsey, 2004)

1. Violence is the cause of I/DD in as much as 10% of all cases (e.g., abuse towards a child, abuse toward pregnant mother resulting in child with I/DD).

2. Violence is a health problem for persons with I/DD, including mental health issues.

H. Substance Abuse/Tobacco Use (Minihan, 2004)

   1. Adults with I/DD often experience the same or greater negative outcomes as misusers without I/DD.

   2. Adults with I/DD who are misusers have fewer opportunities to access treatment programs for substance abuse problems.

   3. Adolescents with I/DD may be abusing illegal substances at the same rate as adolescents without I/DD.

   4. Services for persons with I/DD are not recognizing this problem. Methods to identify at-risk individuals with I/DD and service availability, if a problem, must be developed and made available.

   5. Prevalence studies should be completed to examine for misuse and patterns of use of illegal substances and tobacco.

   6. Qualitative studies should be completed to understand why some persons with I/DD use and others do not. The consequences of using and the meaning use has for the person with I/DD should be determined.

   7. Need to determine whether treatment programs should segregate or integrate persons with I/DD from misusers without I/DD. This would include smoking cessation programs.

   8. Need to identify what interventions for smoking cessation and substance abuse are most effective and why. Also include barriers to treatment.

   9. Need to identify how substance abuse interacts with medications taken for symptoms of the condition causing I/DD or secondary conditions.

I. Theoretical Applications for Health Promotion (Cerrito, 2004)

   1. Health promotion research should involve conceptual frameworks that are based on health promotion behaviors.

   2. For example, Wilber et. al. (2002) developed the Massachusetts Survey of Secondary Conditions conceptual framework in 1995. Figure 7.1 illustrates an adaptation of this conceptual framework for persons of all ages with I/DD.

      a. This conceptual framework was developed to examine secondary conditions and their epidemiology; in particular, environmental influences that can be intervened through public health activities. The literature on health promotion for persons with and without I/DD was reviewed in the development of the original model.

      b. The model proposes that good health can be determined by the interactions among the diagnosis and needed supports, sociodemographic factors, and mediating factors. Mediating factors include adequate supports (personal and technological), adequate access to all facets of life, health promotion and healthy living, and other factors such as employment and social support.

Figure 7.1   Adaptation of the Massachusetts Survey of Secondary Conditions Conceptual Framework*

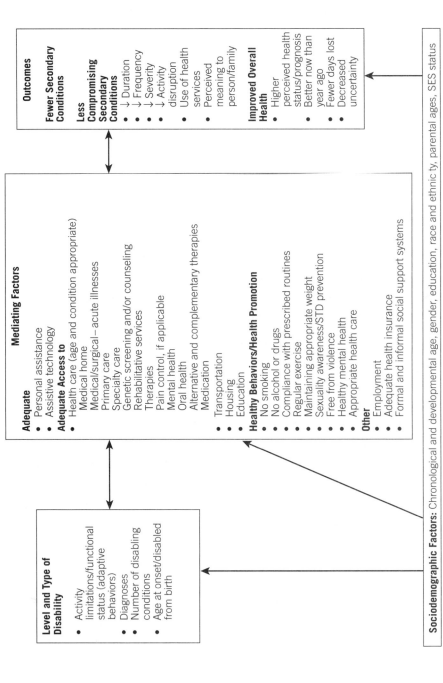

Level and Type of Disability

- Activity limitations/functional status (adaptive behaviors)
- Diagnoses
- Number of disabling conditions
- Age at onset/disabled from birth

Mediating Factors

Adequate
- Personal assistance
- Assistive technology

Adequate Access to
- Health care (age and condition appropriate)
  Medical home
  Medical/surgical – acute illnesses
  Primary care
  Specialty care
  Genetic screening and/or counseling
  Rehabilitative services
  Therapies
  Pain control, if applicable
  Mental health
  Oral health
  Alternative and complementary therapies
  Medication
- Transportation
- Housing
- Education

Healthy Behaviors/Health Promotion
- No smoking
- No alcohol or drugs
- Compliance with prescribed routines
- Regular exercise
- Maintaining appropriate weight
- Sexuality awareness/STD prevention
- Free from violence
- Healthy mental health
- Appropriate health care

Other
- Employment
- Adequate health insurance
- Formal and informal social support systems

Outcomes

Fewer Secondary Conditions

Less Compromising Secondary Conditions
- ↓ Duration
- ↓ Frequency
- ↓ Severity
- ↓ Activity disruption
- Use of health services
- Perceived meaning to person/family

Improved Overall Health
- Higher perceived health status/prognosis
- Better now than year ago
- Fewer days lost
- Decreased uncertainty

Sociodemographic Factors: Chronological and developmental age, gender, education, race and ethnic ty, parental ages, SES status

*Adapted from Wilber et al (2002). Disability as a public health issue: Findings and reflections from the Massachusetts survey of secondary conditions. The Milbank Quarterly, 80, 393–421.

    c. It is also proposed that developing and maintaining health promotion behaviors (e.g., access to health care and transportation) will decrease the occurrence of or exacerbation of secondary conditions and increase quality of life.

V. Genetic Advances

Advances in genetic knowledge and screening technologies will impact how we plan and implement interventions for health promotion (Wilkinson & Targonski, 2003).

A. We will learn more about how the environment and our genotype influence disease onset or exacerbation of diseases.

B. We will need to specifically examine how this interaction affects persons with I/DD.

C. Additional ethical questions will arise, such as whether persons with I/DD will be discriminated from receiving new screening tests as they become available.

D. Health care professionals must alter curriculums to include the new genetic knowledge and technology.

E. New standards of health care will be required.

VI. Levels of Intervention in Primary Care

Primary care providers for both children and adults often have challenging experiences with persons with I/DD. Multiple health diagnoses, medications, treatments, multisystem coordination, and needed services characterize health care management. Allen (2004) proposed a hierarchic intervention framework for primary care providers caring for children with chronic conditions. This framework has been adapted for the lifespan and includes health promotion.

A. Level 1—Ongoing health care management for persons without I/DD.

    1. The knowledge base includes regular health care maintenance and illness management, including screening, as prescribed by national and federal sources (see Green & Palfrey, 2002; U.S. Preventive Services Task Force, 1996, 2004a, 2004b).

B. Level 2—Task-oriented provision of care for individuals with I/DD. Primary and specialty care is provided by other professionals. An example of this type of care is drawing blood for tests or screening.

C. Level 3—Management of well and acute illnesses. Specific care related to the I/DD or secondary conditions is collaborated on with a specialist in that area or referred out.

1. Knowledge of the pathophysiology of the condition and specific health care guidelines (see Chapters 10, 12, and 14) are necessary. The primary care provider should also be aware of the individual with I/DD's and family members' reactions to the diagnosis and the meaning of the condition. An assessment of how the condition affects the person's quality of life and development is also important, taking into consideration the person's religious views and ethnicity. Last, the primary care provider should have a list of specialists, clinics, and community agencies to which the individual with I/DD and family can be referred.

D. Level 4—Comprehensive health care management of the person with I/DD. This involves providing the person with I/DD with a medical home (see American Academy of Pediatrics webpage: http://www.aap.org).

1. More in-depth knowledge is needed on current research on I/DD (e.g., understanding of the condition, including etiology; genetic knowledge, if applicable; prognosis; care management; secondary conditions; trajectory across the lifespan; developmental issues; family issues; Medicare and Medicaid laws and additional federal legislation affecting persons with I/DD; available interdisciplinary consultants and local and state resources for health, education, financial, residential, and social/recreational purposes.

E. Level 5—Care coordination for the individual with I/DD.

1. All of the above knowledge is required, plus information related to systems coordination, team coordination, processing requirements for federal and state funding, and outcome measures. This care should be person-centered when possible and, certainly, family-centered and culturally sensitive.

2. The primary care provider must be able to be an advocate for the person with I/DD.

F. Level 6—Serving as an advocate for the individual with I/DD.

1. The primary care provider must be knowledgeable of the legislative and due processes at all levels and be able to work for the rights of his or her patients with I/DD. This could involve city, state, or national governments; school systems; and area agencies. The primary care provider at this level may be a state or national leader in the field of I/DD and should be knowledgeable of all evidence-based practice for specific conditions leading to I/DD.

VII. Summary

Successful health promotion is a lifelong, multi-layered process that involves conscious effort and the support of others.

A. Living a healthy life involves cognitive, physical, spiritual, social, and emotional factors.

B. Recently, federal and national organizations that serve persons with I/DD and their families have emphasized the need for increased efforts in planning for and implementing information and programs for health promotion for persons with I/DD.

C. Federal documents have also provided recommendations for improvements.

D. Currently, research in health promotion topics involving persons with I/DD is not sufficient to develop standards of care, but efforts should be made to develop consensus guidelines for specific topics.

E. Finally, health care providers, whether primary or specialized, should include health promotion information and screening, as appropriate, in their daily practices for persons with I/DD.

References

Allen, P. J. (2004). The primary care provider and children with chronic conditions. In P. J. Allen & J. A. Vessey (Eds.). *Primary care of the child with a chronic condition* (4th ed., pp. 3–22). St. Louis, MO: Mosby.

American Journal of Health Promotion. (1989). Definition of health promotion. Retrieved June 25, 2004, from http://www.healthpromotionjournal.com

Bandini, L. (2004, June). *Obesity*. Paper presented at the American Association on Mental Retardation Preconference "Health Promotion for Persons with Intellectual/ Developmental Disabilities: The State of Scientific Evidence," Philadelphia, PA.

Benson, B. (2004, June). *Mental health*. Paper presented at the American Association on Mental Retardation Preconference "Health Promotion for Persons with Intellectual/ Developmental Disabilities: The State of Scientific Evidence," Philadelphia, PA.

Cerrito, M. (2004, June). *Conceptual health promotion models*. Paper presented at the American Association on Mental Retardation Preconference "Health Promotion for Persons with Intellectual/Developmental Disabilities: The State of Scientific Evidence," Philadelphia, PA.

Draheim, C. (2004, June). *Hypertension*. Paper presented at the American Association on Mental Retardation Preconference "Health Promotion for Persons with Intellectual/Developmental Disabilities: The State of Scientific Evidence," Philadelphia, PA.

Green, M., & Palfrey, J. S. (Eds.). (2002). *Bright futures: Guidelines for health supervision of infants, children, and adolescents* (2nd ed., rev.). Arlington, VA: National Center for Education in Maternal and Child Health.

Lefton-Greif, M. (2004, June). *Feeding/swallowing disorders in children*. Paper presented at the American Association on Mental Retardation Preconference "Health Promotion for Persons with Intellectual/ Developmental Disabilities: The State of Scientific Evidence," Philadelphia, PA.

Lewis, M. A., Lewis, C. E., Leake, B., King, B. H., & Lindemann, R. (2002). The quality of health care for adults with developmental disabilities. *Public Health Reports, 117*, 174–184.

Minihan, P. (2004, June). *Substance abuse/tobacco use*. Paper presented at the American Association on Mental Retardation Preconference "Health Promotion for Persons with Intellectual/Developmental Disabilities: The State of Scientific Evidence," Philadelphia, PA.

National Heart, Lung, and Blood Institute. (2003). *The seventh report of the Joint National Committee on prevention, detection, evaluation, and treatment of high blood pressure (JNC 7)*. Retrieved June 30, 2004, from http://www.nhlbi.nih.gov/guidelines/hypertension

Nehring, W. M., Roth, S. P., Natvig, D., Betz, C. L., Savage, T., & Krajicek, M. (in press). *Scope and standards for the nurse who specializes in intellectual and developmental disabilities.* Washington, DC: American Nurses Publishing and American Association on Mental Retardation.

Nehring, W. M., Roth, S. P., Natvig, D., Morse, J. S., Savage, T., & Krajicek, M. (1998). *Statement on the scope and standards for the nurse who specializes in developmental disabilities and/or mental retardation.* Washington, DC: American Nurses Publishing and American Association on Mental Retardation.

Rimmer, J. (2004, June). *Physical activity.* Paper presented at the American Association on Mental Retardation Preconference "Health Promotion for Persons with Intellectual/Developmental Disabilities: The State of Scientific Evidence," Philadelphia, PA.

Seltser, R. (2001). Where do we go from here? In National Center on Birth Defects and Developmental Disabilities. (Ed.). *Healthy people 2010.* (pp. 145–165). Atlanta, GA: Centers for Disease Control and Prevention.

Sheppard, J. (2004, June). *Swallowing behaviors in adults.* Paper presented at the American Association on Mental Retardation Preconference "Health Promotion for Persons with Intellectual/Developmental Disabilities: The State of Scientific Evidence," Philadelphia, PA.

Sobsey, R. (2004, June). *Violence.* Paper presented at the American Association on Mental Retardation Preconference "Health Promotion for Persons with Intellectual/Developmental Disabilities: The State of Scientific Evidence," Philadelphia, PA.

Sutherland, G., Couch, M. A., & Iacono, T. (2002). Health issues for adults with developmental disabilities. *Research in Developmental Disabilities, 23,* 422–445.

U.S. Department of Health and Human Services. (2000). *Healthy people 2010* (2nd ed.). Washington, DC: U.S. Government Printing Office.

U.S. Preventive Services Task Force. (2004a). *Clinical preventive services for children and adolescents (birth to 18 years).* Retrieved June 20, 2004, from http://www.ahrq.gov/clinic/ppipix.htm

U.S. Preventive Services Task Force. (2004b). *Clinical preventive services for normal-risk adults recommended by the U.S. Preventive Services Task Force.* Retrieved June 20, 2004, from http://www.ahrq.gov/clinic/ppipix.htm

U.S. Preventive Services Task Force. (1996). *Guide to clinical preventive services* (2nd ed.). Retrieved June 20, 2004, from http://www.ahrq.gov/clinic/cpsix.htm

U.S. Public Health Service. (2002). *Closing the gap: A national blueprint for improving the health of individuals with mental retardation. Report of the Surgeon General's conference on health disparities and mental retardation.* Washington, DC: Author.

White-Scott, S. (2004, June). *Reproductive health.* Paper presented at the American Association on Mental Retardation Preconference "Health Promotion for Persons with Intellectual/Developmental Disabilities: The State of Scientific Evidence," Philadelphia, PA.

Wilber, N., Mitra, M., Walker, D. K., Allen, D., Meyers, A. R., & Tupper, P. (2002). Disability as a public health issue: Findings and reflections from the Massachusetts survey of secondary conditions. *The Milbank Quarterly, 80,* 393–421.

Wilkinson, J. M., & Targonski, P. V. (2003). Health promotion in a changing world: Preparing for the genomics revolution. *American Journal of Health Promotion, 18,* 157–161.

Early Intervention Services for Infants and Their Families

Mary Beth Bruder, PhD

8

Objectives

At the completion of this chapter, the learner will be able to:

1. Discuss the history and background of early intervention.
2. List the services and professionals addressed in Part C of the Individuals with Disabilities Education Act (IDEA).
3. Describe the philosophical foundations of early intervention.
4. Define family-centered practices.
5. Describe team process.
6. Define natural environments and how they help a child to learn.
7. Describe service delivery components under Part C of IDEA.
8. Discuss early identification strategies and the entry process into early intervention.
9. Describe the role of the service coordinator under Part C of IDEA.
10. List the components of the individualized family service plan (IFSP).
11. Describe the importance of transition.
12. Define the role of the health care provider under Part C of IDEA.
13. Describe the role of the nurse and the health care provider in the medical home.

Key Points

- Early intervention has a rich history and legislative requirements that govern its implementation.
- Early intervention is based on a philosophical foundation that revolves around family-centered practices, team process, and the delivery of services in natural environments.

Key Points *(continued)*

- Part C of IDEA requires a number of service delivery components including early identification and entry into the system, service coordination, an IFSP, and transitions.
- Nurses and other health care professionals play an integral role in early intervention, in particular providing procedures to enable a child to benefit from early intervention and serving as a liaison and coordinator of the child's medical home.

I.   Background and Definitions

A. History

1. Fifty years of research supports the effectiveness of early intervention (Gallagher, 2000; Guralnick, in press; Kirk, 1958).

2. Early intervention efficacy studies have been criticized because of methodological limitations (e.g., heterogeneity of the population, lack of control groups, narrowly defined outcome measures, inappropriateness of standardized measures of intelligence for the population) (Guralnick, 1998; Roberts, Innocenti, & Goetze, 1999).

B. Benefits

1. The earlier a child is identified as having an intellectual and developmental disability (I/DD), the greater the likelihood the child will benefit from intervention strategies designed to compensate for the child's needs.

2. Families benefit from the support given to them through the intervention process.

3. Schools and communities benefit from a decrease in costs because more children arrive ready for school.

C. Definitions

1. The provision of educational or therapeutic services to children under the age of 8 years (Sigel, 1972).

    a. *Early intervention* describes the years birth to 3 years.

    b. *Early childhood special education* or *preschool special education* describes the period of the preschool years (ages 3–5 years).

    c. Individuals with Disabilities Education Act (IDEA) (1997), Part C, covers services for children age birth to 3 years and their families.

D. Part C of IDEA

  1. Each state provides services under a lead agency authorized by the governor.

  2. States decide eligibility criteria.

     a. Significant variations in eligibility definitions create a marked variability in the percent of children served.

  3. Each state must offer services as listed on Table 8.1.

  4. Each state must use professionals to provide these services as listed on Table 8.2.

II. Philosophical Foundation

A. There are service delivery differences between infants and toddlers and older pediatric populations.

  1. Infants and toddlers develop and learn in the context of their families (Bruder, 2000).

  2. Early development necessitates a focus that integrates learning across domains requiring a team of professionals (Bruder, 1996).

  3. Infants and toddlers have a low tolerance for time-intensive interventions, necessitating that intervention be integrated into their everyday routines and activities (Bruder, 2001).

Table 8.1   IDEA Part C Program Services
• family training, counseling, and home visits
• special instruction
• speech pathology and audiology
• occupational therapy
• physical therapy
• psychological services
• case management services
• medical services only for diagnostic or evaluation purposes
• early intervention, screening, and assessment services
• health services necessary to enable the infant or toddler to benefit from the other early intervention services
• social work services
• vision services
• assistive technology devices and assistive technology services
• transportation and related costs that are necessary to enable an infant or toddler and the infant's or toddler's family to receive early intervention services

Individuals with Disabilities Education Act, 1997

Table 8.2   Professional Disciplines in Early Intervention

Audiologist

Family therapist

Nurse

Nutritionist

Occupational therapist

Orientation and mobility specialist

Pediatrician and other physicians

Psychologist

Physical therapist

Social worker

Special educator

Speech and language pathologist

B. Family-centered orientation

   1. The caregiving family is the constant in the child's life and the primary unit for service delivery (Shelton, Jeppson, & Johnson, 1987).

   2. Families are heterogeneous, varying by background, economics, structure, cultures, and ethnicity (Lynch & Hanson, 2004).

   3. Families have a powerful effect on their children. The following factors have influenced children's development:

       a. Parents' education, socioeconomic status, and home environment (Garbarino, 1990; Werner, 1990)

       b. Parental attitudes and beliefs, including parents' beliefs about children's social competence (Guralnick, 1997, 1999; Mills & Rubin, 1992; Mize, Pettit, & Brown, 1995), the child's need for early intervention (Affleck et al., 1989), and cultural beliefs (Chen, Brekken, & Chan, 1997; Dunst, Trivette, Hamby, Raab, & Bruder, 2000; Turnbull, Blue-Banning, Turbiville, & Park, 1999)

       c. Family-orchestrated learning that occurs in the home and community (Dunst, Bruder, Trivette, Raab, & McLean, 1998; Guralnick, 1998)

       d. Parent–child interaction patterns (Barnard, 1997; McCollum & Hemmeter, 1997)

       e. Parents' ability to follow intervention recommendations for facilitating child development (Kaiser, Hancock, & Hester, 1998; Mahoney, Boyce, Fewell, Spiker, & Wheeden, 1998; Mahoney et al., 1999)

f.   The availability of social support for families, such as informal support networks (Dunst, Trivette, & Jodry, 1997)

4.   Early intervention should provide families with a sense of confidence and competence about their children's current and future learning and development (Bailey et al., 1998; Turnbull & Turnbull, 1997).

5.   The use of family-centered practices have proven to facilitate family–child competence (Bruder, 2001; Dunst, 1999; Dunst, Brookfield, & Epstein, 1998; Dunst, Trivette, Boyd, & Hamby, 1996; Mahoney et al., 1998; McWilliam, Tocci, & Harbin, 1998; Santelli, Turnbull, Marquis, & Lerner, 2000; Thompson et al., 1997; Trivette & Dunst, 1998). These practices include:

a.   Treating families with dignity and respect.

b.   Being culturally and socioeconomically sensitive to family diversity.

c.   Providing choices to families in relation to their priorities and concerns.

d.   Fully disclosing information to families so they can make decisions.

e.   Focusing on a range of informal, community resources as sources of parenting and family support.

f.   Employing help-giving practices that are empowering and enhance competency, including the provision of parent-to-parent models.

C. Team process

1.   Various personnel having medical, therapeutic, educational/developmental, and social-service expertise are involved in providing early intervention.

2.   Service providers may have different philosophies, training requirements, licensing or certification requirements, treatment modalities, and specific professional organizations (Bruder, 1994).

3.   Researchers suggest that most university training programs for professionals providing early intervention have little coursework and practica specific to infants, toddlers, and their families (Kilgo & Bruder, 1997; Stayton & Bruder, 1999).

4.   Early intervention requires a team approach to meet the needs of children (Hanson & Bruder, 2001).

5.   There are three types of teams used in early intervention:

a.   Multidisciplinary

b.   Interdisciplinary

c.   Transdisciplinary

6.   The transdisciplinary team model has been recommended for early intervention (Hanson & Bruder, 2001).

a.   The transdisciplinary approach consolidates interventions across developmental areas.

      b. The purpose of the transdisciplinary approach is to integrate the expertise of multiple team members with different professional backgrounds to meet the comprehensive needs of infants and toddlers (Bruder, 1996).

      c. The transdisciplinary approach requires continuous communication, teaching, and consultation among the members of the team (McWilliam, 1996).

D. Natural environments

  1. Natural environments are required by Part C of IDEA.

  2. Natural environments have been defined by IDEA as those places where the child would be had he or she not had an I/DD, for example, the home or other environments with their same-age peers. (34 CFR §303.18)

  3. Researchers support the use of natural environments for learning (Bruder & Staff, 1998; Odom, 2000).

  4. The use of natural environments has been cited as a quality indicator of early intervention (Division for Early Childhood, 1993).

  5. The challenge of using natural environments is to take advantage of learning opportunities (both short- and long-term planning) that happen with a child in all the environments in which they spend time (Bruder, 2001; Dunst, 2001).

III. Service Delivery Components

A. Early identification and entry into intervention

  1. Research has found 300 categories of eligibility criteria used for children enrolled in Part C (Hebbeler, Simeonsson, & Scarborough, 2000).

  2. Children in Part C are usually identified and referred by someone close to them (parent, pediatrician, etc.).

      a. Developmental questionnaires completed by parent or health care provider have been used extensively as an identification tool (Bricker, Squires, & Kaminski, 1988; Glascoe, 1991; Squires, 1996).

      b. Anticipatory guidance has been suggested as a strategy for health care providers to identify developmental concerns (Dworkin, 1989).

  3. An initial evaluation is completed on any child who is referred into Part C to see if the child qualifies for services.

      a. The evaluation usually uses standardized assessment instruments that address domains of behavior, cognition, fine and gross motor skills, receptive and expressive language, social-emotional development and self-help, and/or adaptive skills (McLean, Wolery, & Bailey, 2003).

      b. The evaluation must be done by a multidisciplinary team (at least two disciplines represented) as required by Part C regulations.

4. If a child is determined to be eligible for Part C services, assessment continues in order to assist the IFSP team to develop a valid and meaningful IFSP.

B. Service coordination

1. Part C requires the designation of a service coordinator for each eligible family.

2. Part C establishes requirements for service coordinators (see Table 8.3).

3. The complexity of service coordination varies as a result of needs of families, needs of children, state and local service systems, funding streams (Akers & Roberts, 1999; McCollum, 2000; Striffler, Perry, & Kates, 1997), and expanding systems reform in welfare (Janko-Summers & Joseph, 1998; Ohlson, 1998; Rosman & Knitzer, 2001), child care (Kagan, 1996; Spencer, Blumenthal, & Richards, 1995), health care (Braddock & Hemp, 1996; Lobach, 1995) and mental health (Knitzer, 2000; Knitzer & Page, 1998).

Table 8.3 Service Coordination under IDEA Part C

QUALIFICATIONS ➝	RESPONSIBILITIES ➝	TASKS ➝	OUTCOME
Knowledge and understanding about: • Infants and toddlers who are eligible under Part C; • Part C of the act and its regulations; and • The nature and scope of services available under the state's early intervention program, the system of payments for services in the state, and other pertinent information	Assisting parents of eligible children in gaining access to the early intervention services and other services identified in the IFSP Coordinating the provision of early intervention services and other services (such as medical services for other than diagnostic and evaluation purposes) so that the child's needs are being provided for Facilitating the timely delivery of available services Continuously seeking the appropriate services and situations necessary to benefit the development of each child being served for the duration of the child's eligibility	Coordinating the performance of evaluations and assessments Facilitating and participating in the development, review, and evaluation of IFSPs Assisting families in identifying available service providers Coordinating and monitoring the delivery of available services Informing families of the availability of advocacy services Coordinating with medical and health providers Facilitating the development of a transition plan to preschool services, if appropriate	Children and families receive appropriate supports and services that meet their individual needs

4. Factors have been identified that facilitate service coordination (Harbin, 1996; Harbin, McWilliam, & Gallagher, 2000; Harbin & West, 1998):

   a. State and community context

   b. State policy

   c. Service delivery model

   d. Leadership

   e. Service provider skills and characteristics

   f. Family characteristics

   g. Service provider/family relationships

5. Effective service coordination is associated with the amount and type of partnerships that are demonstrated between agencies, services, families, and service providers (Bruder, in press; Summers et al., 2001).

C. The individualized family service plan (IFSP)

1. The IFSP is a planning document to shape and guide the day-to-day provision of early intervention services.

2. An IFSP is required for each eligible child and family.

3. The IFSP consists of requirements from the federal legislation (see Table 8.4).

4. The IFSP should contain individualized outcomes, objectives, and strategies that are functional and embedded within daily activity settings delivered according to the family's wishes (Bruder, 1995; Kramer, McGonigel, & Kaufmann, 1991).

   a. The assessment process should focus on identifying family activity settings and learning opportunities for the child (Bruder, 2001).

Table 8.4   Requirements of the IFSP

- A statement of the child's present level of functioning in cognitive development, communication development, social or emotional development, physical development, and adaptive development
- A statement of the family's resources, priorities, and concerns
- A statement of expected intervention outcomes, including criteria, procedures, and timelines
- A description of the services that the child and family need including method, frequency, and intensity
- A statement of the natural environments in which early intervention services shall be provided
- Projected dates for initiation of services and expected duration
- The name of the service coordinator who will be responsible for implementation of the plan and coordination with other agencies and persons
- The procedures to ensure successful transition from infant services to preschool programs

      b. Specific intervention strategies should be embedded within the family's activity settings (Dunst, 2001; Halvorsen & Sailor, 1990).

   5. The IFSP is developed as part of a team process across disciplines including the family (Bruder, 2000).

D. Transition

   1. Transition is a series of well-planned steps to facilitate the movement of the child and family into another setting (Guralnick, 2001).

   2. Successful transitions are one of the primary goals of early intervention (Bruder, in press; Guralnick, in press).

   3. Transition is dynamic, occurring anytime a family moves in or out of service delivery (Bruder & Chandler, 1996).

   4. Transition is the responsibility of all those involved with a family.

   5. A transition team should be developed at least six months before a child is scheduled for a planned transition, according to Part C.

   6. A good transition is guided by a plan to ensure continuity of services and to minimize disruption to the family (Bruder & Chandler, 1996; Wolery, 1989).

IV. The Role of the Nurse and Other Health Care Professionals in Early Intervention (see Table 8.5 from Bruder, M. B. (2004))

A. Part C requires health services to enable the infant or toddler to benefit from other early intervention services.

Table 8.5 Service Delivery Components and Potential Roles for Nurses

SERVICE DELIVERY COMPONENT	ROLE OF NURSES
Early identification and entry into early intervention	• Conduct developmental screening and/or medical evaluation • Education of parents during evaluation process • Referral of children into the early intervention system
Service coordination	• Serve as service coordinator • Liaison with other care coordinators including Title V
Individualized family service plan	• Informant of child's medical needs and assessments • Participant in development of collaborative goals and objectives • Consultant to early intervention team or others providing intervention
Transitions	• Identification of potential placements for child and family • Informant of child's future medical and developmental needs

1. This will include procedures and care conducted in accordance with nursing and medical guidelines such as administration of medications, wound care, and medical procedures such as catheterization or suction (Browne, Langlois, Ross, & Smith-Sharp, 2001).

2. Certain health care assessments must be conducted by medical personnel in order to determine a child's needs for the IFSP.

B. Liaison with medical home

1. Health care providers including nurses can provide continuity with a child's medical home (American Academy of Pediatrics, 2002; Nickel, Cooley, McAllister, & Samson-Fang, 2003).

2. Each child should have a medical home that is comprehensive, coordinated, family centered, and community based (Koop, 1987).

V. Summary

Early intervention programs have positively influenced the development of children with I/DD and their families. Such programs provide comprehensive, culturally sensitive, and coordinated services preferably by a transdisciplinary team.

References

Affleck, G., Tennen, H., Rowe, J., Roscher, B., Walker, L., & Higgins, P. (1989). Effects of formal support on mothers' adaptation to the hospital-to-home transition of high risk infants: The benefits and costs of helping. *Child Development, 60,* 488–501.

Akers, A. L., & Roberts, R. N. (1999). The use of blended and flexible funding in Part C programs at the community level. *Infants and Young Children, 11*(4), 46–52.

American Academy of Pediatrics. (2002). Policy statement: The medical home. *Pediatrics, 110*(1), 184–186.

Bailey, D. B., Jr., McWilliam, R. A., Darkes, L. A., Hebbeler, K., Simeonsson, R. J., Spiker, D., et al. (1998). Family outcomes in early intervention: A framework for program evaluation and efficacy research. *Exceptional Children, 64,* 313–328.

Barnard, K. E. (1997). Influencing parent–child interactions for children at risk. In M. J. Guralnick (Ed.) *The effectiveness of early intervention* (pp. 249–270). Baltimore: Paul H. Brookes.

Braddock, D., & Hemp, R. (1996). Medicaid spending reductions and developmental disabilities. *Journal of Disability Policy Studies, 7,* 2–31.

Bricker, D., Squires, J., & Kaminski, R. (1988). The validity, reliability, and cost of a parent-completed questionnaire system to evaluate at-risk infants. *Journal of Pediatric Psychology, 13*(1), 55–68.

Browne, J., Langlois, A., Ross, E., & Smith-Sharp, S. (2001). BEGINNINGS: An interim Individualized Family Service Plan for use in the intensive care nursery. *Infants and Young Children, 14*(2), 19–32.

Bruder, M. B. (1995). Early intervention. In J. W. Wood & A. M. Lazzari (Eds.) *Exceeding the boundaries: Understanding exceptional lives* (pp. 534–569). Fort Worth, TX: Harcourt Brace.

Bruder, M. B. (2000). Family-centered early intervention: Clarifying our values for the new millennium. *Topics in Early Childhood Special Education, 20*, 105–115.

Bruder, M. B. (2001). Infants and toddlers: Outcomes and ecology. In M. J. Guralnick (Ed.) *Early childhood inclusion: Focus on change* (pp. 203–228). Baltimore: Paul H. Brookes.

Bruder, M. B. (1996). Interdisciplinary collaboration in service delivery. In R. A. McWilliam (Ed.) *Rethinking pull-out services in early intervention: A professional resource* (pp. 27–48). Fort Worth, TX: Harcourt Brace.

Bruder, M. B. (in press). Service coordination and integration in a developmental systems approach to early intervention. In M. J. Guralnick (Ed.) *A developmental systems approach to early intervention: National and international perspectives.* Baltimore: Paul H. Brookes.

Bruder, M. B. (2004). The role of the physician in early intervention for children with developmental disabilities. *Connecticut Medicine, 68*, 507–518.

Bruder, M. B. (1994). Working with members of other disciplines: Collaboration for success. In M. Wolery & J. S. Wilbers (Eds.) *Including children with special needs in early childhood programs* (pp. 45–70). Washington, DC: National Association for the Education of Young Children.

Bruder, M. B., & Chandler, L. (1996). Transition. In S. Odom & M. McLean (Eds.) *Early intervention/early childhood special education: Recommended practices* (pp. 287–307). Austin, TX: ProEd.

Bruder, M. B., & Staff, I. (1998). A comparison of the effects of type of classroom and service characteristics on toddlers with disabilities. *Topics in Early Childhood Special Education, 18*(1), 26–37.

Chen, D., Brekken, L. J., & Chan, S. (1997). Project CRAFT: Culturally responsive and family-focused training. *Infants and Young Children, 10*(1), 61–73.

Division for Early Childhood (Ed.). (1993). *DEC recommended practices: Indicators of quality in programs for infants and young children with special needs and their families.* Reston, VA: Council for Exceptional Children.

Dunst, C. J. (2001). Participation of young children with disabilities in community learning activities. In M. J. Guralnick (Ed.) *Early childhood inclusion: Focus on change* (pp. 307–333). Baltimore: Paul H. Brookes.

Dunst, C. J. (1999). Placing parent education in conceptual and empirical context. *Topics in Early Childhood Special Education, 19*, 141–146.

Dunst, C. J., Brookfield, J., & Epstein, J. (1998). *Family-centered early intervention and child, parent and family benefits.* (Final report).

Dunst, C. J., Bruder, M. B., Trivette, C. M., Raab, M., & McLean, M. (1998). *Increasing children's learning opportunities through families and communities: Early childhood research institute.* Year 2 Progress Report submitted to the U.S. Department of Education.

Dunst, C. J., Trivette, C. M., Boyd, K., & Hamby, D. (1996). Family-oriented program models, helpgiving practices, and parental control appraisals. *Exceptional Children, 62*, 237–248.

Dunst, C. J., Trivette, C. M., Hamby, D., Raab, M., & Bruder, M. B. (2000). Family ethnicity, acculturation and enculturation, and parent beliefs about child behavior, learning methods and parenting roles. *Journal of Early Intervention, 23*, 151–164.

Dunst, C. J., Trivette, C. M., & Jodry, W. (1997). Influences of social support on children with disabilities and their families. In M. J. Guralnick (Ed.) *The effectiveness of early intervention* (pp. 499–522). Baltimore: Paul H. Brookes.

Dworkin, P. H. (1989). British and American recommendations for developmental monitoring: The role of surveillance. *Pediatrics, 84,* 1000.

Gallagher, J. J. (2000). The beginnings of federal help for young children with disabilities. *Topics in Early Childhood Special Education, 20*(1), 3–6.

Garbarino, J. (1990). The human ecology of early risk. In S. J. Meisels & J. P. Shonkoff (Eds.) *Handbook of early childhood intervention* (pp. 78–96). New York: Cambridge University Press.

Glascoe, F. (1991). Developmental screening: Rationale, methods, and application. *Infants and Young Children, 4*(1), 1–10.

Guralnick, M. J. (Ed.). (in press). *A developmental systems approach to early intervention: National and international perspectives.* Baltimore: Paul H. Brookes.

Guralnick, M. J. (2001). A developmental systems model for early intervention. *Infants and Young Children, 14*(2), 1–18.

Guralnick, M. J. (1998). Effectiveness of early intervention for vulnerable children: A developmental perspective. *American Journal on Mental Retardation, 102,* 319–345.

Guralnick, M. J. (1999). Family and child influences on the peer-related social competence of young children with developmental delays. *Mental Retardation and Developmental Disabilities Research Reviews, 5,* 21–29.

Guralnick, M. J. (1997). Second generation research in the field of early intervention. In M. J. Guralnick (Ed.) *The effectiveness of early intervention* (pp. 3–20). Baltimore: Paul H. Brookes.

Halvorsen, A., & Sailor, W. (1990). Integration of students with profound disabilities: A review of the research. In R. Gaylord-Ross (Ed.) *Issues and research in special education* (Vol. 1, pp. 110–172). New York: Teacher's College Press.

Hanson, M. J., & Bruder, M. B. (2001). Early intervention: Promises to keep. *Infants and Young Children, 13*(3), 47–58.

Harbin, G. L. (1996). The challenge of coordination. *Infants and Young Children, 8*(3), 68–76.

Harbin, G. L., McWilliam, R. A., & Gallagher, J. J. (2000). Services for young children with disabilities and their families. In J. P. Shonkoff & S. J. Meisels (Eds.) *Handbook of early childhood intervention* (pp. 387–415). New York: Cambridge University Press.

Harbin, G. L., & West, T. (1998). *Early intervention service delivery models and their impact on children and families.* Chapel Hill, NC: Early Childhood Research Institute on Service Utilization, Frank Porter Graham Child Development Center, University of North Carolina at Chapel Hill.

Hebbeler, K., Simeonsson, R. J., & Scarborough, A. (2000). *Describing disability in young children: A national study of early intervention eligibility.* Paper presented at Conference on Research in Early Intervention 2000, San Diego, CA.

Individuals with Disabilities Education Act (IDEA), Pub. L. No. 105–17, 111 Stat. 37 (1997).

Janko-Summers, S., & Joseph, G. (1998). Making sense of early intervention in the context of welfare to work. *Journal of Early Intervention, 21,* 207–210.

Kagan, S. L. (1996). Looking backward–looking forward: The state of early childhood policy. *Dimensions of Early Childhood, 24,* 3–4.

Kaiser, A. P., Hancock, T. B., & Hester, P. P. (1998). Parents as co-interventionists: Research on applications of naturalistic language teaching procedures. *Infants and Young Children, 10*(4), 36–45.

Kilgo, J., & Bruder, M. B. (1997). Creating new visions in institutions of higher education: Interdisciplinary approaches to personnel preparation in early intervention. In P. J. Winton, J. McCollum, & C. Catlett (Eds.) *Reforming personnel preparation in early intervention: Issues, models, and practical strategies* (pp. 81–102). Baltimore: Paul H. Brookes.

Kirk, S. A. (1958). *Early education of the mentally retarded: An experimental study.* Urbana, IL: University of Illinois Press.

Knitzer, J. (2000). Early childhood mental health services: A policy and systems development perspective. In J. P. Shonkoff & S. J. Meisels (Eds.) *Handbook of early childhood intervention* (2nd ed., pp. 416–438). New York: Cambridge University Press.

Knitzer, J., & Page, S. (1998). *Map and track: State initiatives for young children and families.* New York: National Center for Children in Poverty, Columbia School of Public Health.

Koop, C. E. (1987). *Surgeon General's report: Children with special health care needs—campaign '87—commitment to family-centered, coordinated care for children with special health care needs.* Washington, DC: U.S. Department of Health and Human Services.

Kramer, S., McGonigel, M. J., & Kaufmann, R. K. (1991). Developing the IFSP: Outcomes, strategies, activities, and services. In M. J. McGonigel, R. K. Kaufmann, & B. H. Johnson (Eds.) *Guidelines and recommended practices for the individualized family service plan* (2nd ed., pp. 57–66). Bethesda, MD: Association for the Care of Children's Health.

Lobach, K. S. (1995). Health policy in the Family Support Act of 1988. In P. L. Chase-Lansdale & J. Brooks-Gunn (Eds.) *Escape from poverty: What makes a difference for children?* (pp. 159–169). New York: Cambridge University Press.

Lynch, E. W., & Hanson, M. J. (Eds.). (2004). *Developing cross-cultural competence: A guide for working with children and their families.* Baltimore: Paul H. Brookes.

Mahoney, G., Boyce, G., Fewell, R. R., Spiker, D., & Wheeden, C. A. (1998). The relationship of parent–child interaction to the effectiveness of early intervention services for at-risk children and children with disabilities. *Topics in Early Childhood Special Education, 18*(1), 5–17.

Mahoney, G., Kaiser, A., Girolametto, L., MacDonald, J., Robinson, C., Safford, P., et al. (1999). Parent education in early intervention: A call for renewed focus. *Topics in Early Childhood Special Education, 19,* 131–140.

McCollum, J. A. (2000). Taking the past along: Reflecting on our identity as a discipline. *Topics in Early Childhood Special Education, 20,* 79–86.

McCollum, M., & Hemmeter, M. L. (1997). Parent–child interaction intervention when children have disabilities. In M. Guralnick (Ed.) *The effectiveness of early intervention* (pp. 549–576). Baltimore: Paul H. Brookes.

McLean, M., Wolery, M., & Bailey, D. (2003). *Assessing infants and preschoolers with special needs* (3rd ed.). Columbus, OH: Merrill/Prentice Hall.

McWilliam, P. J. (1996). Collaborative consultation across seven disciplines: Challenges and solutions. In R. A. McWilliam (Ed.). *Rethinking pull-out services in early intervention: A professional resource* (pp. 315–340). Baltimore: Paul H. Brookes.

McWilliam, R. A., Tocci, L., & Harbin, G. L. (1998). Family-centered services: Service providers' discourse and behavior. *Topics in Early Childhood Special Education, 18,* 206–221.

Mills, R. S. L., & Rubin, K. H. (1992). A longitudinal study of maternal beliefs about children's social behaviors. *Merrill-Palmer Quarterly, 38,* 494–512.

Mize, J., Pettit, G. S., & Brown, E. G. (1995). Mothers' supervision of their children's peer play: Relations with beliefs, perceptions, and knowledge. *Developmental Psychology, 31,* 311–321.

Nickel, R. E., Cooley, W. C., McAllister, J. W., & Samson-Fang, L. (2003). Building medical homes for children with special health care needs. *Infants and Young Children, 16,* 331–341.

Odom, S. L. (2000). Preschool inclusion: What we know and where we go from here. *Topics in Early Childhood Special Education, 20*(1), 20–27.

Ohlson, C. (1998). Welfare reform: Implications for young children with disabilities, their families, and service providers. *Journal of Early Intervention, 21,* 191–206.

Roberts, R. N., Innocenti, M. S., & Goetze, L. D. (1999). Emerging issues from state level evaluations of early intervention programs. *Journal of Early Intervention, 22,* 152–163.

Rosman, E. A., & Knitzer, J. (2001). Welfare reform: The special case of young children with disabilities and their families. *Infants and Young Children, 13*(3), 25–35.

Santelli, B., Turnbull, A., Marquis, J., & Lerner, E. (2000). Statewide parent-to-parent programs: Partners in early intervention. *Infants and Young Children, 13*(1), 74–86.

Shelton, T., Jeppson, E., & Johnson, B. (1987). *Family-centered care for children with special health care needs* (2nd ed.). Washington, DC: The Association for the Care of Children's Health.

Sigel, I. (1972). Developmental theory: Its place, the relevance in early intervention programs. *Young Children, 27*, 364–372.

Spencer, M. B., Blumenthal, J. B., & Richards, E. (1995). Child care and children of color. In P. L. Chase-Lansdale & J. Brooks-Gunn (Eds.) *Escape from poverty: What makes a difference for children?* (pp. 138–158). New York: Cambridge University Press.

Squires, J. (1996). Parent-completed developmental questionnaires: A low-cost strategy for child-find and screening. *Infants and Young Children, 9*(1), 16–28.

Stayton, V., & Bruder, M. B. (1999). Early intervention personnel preparation for the new millennium: Early childhood special education. *Infants and Young Children, 12*(1), 59–69.

Striffler, N., Perry, D. F., & Kates, D. A. (1997). Planning and implementing a finance system for early intervention systems. *Infants and Young Children, 10*(2), 57–65.

Summers, J. A., Steeples, T., Peterson, C., Naig, L., McBride, S., Wall, S., et al. (2001). Policy and management supports for effective service integration in Early Head Start and Part C programs. *Topics in Early Childhood Special Education, 21*(1), 16–30.

Thompson, L., Lobb, C., Elling, R., Herman, S., Jurkiewicz, T., & Hulleza, C. (1997). Pathways to family empowerment: Effects of family-centered delivery of early intervention services. *Exceptional Children, 64*(1), 81–98.

Trivette, C. M., & Dunst, C. J. (1998). *Family-centered helpgiving practices.* Presentation made at the 14th Annual Division for Early Childhood International Conference on Children with Special Needs, Chicago, IL.

Turnbull, A., & Turnbull, H. (1997). *Families, professionals and exceptionality: A special partnership.* (3rd ed.). Upper Saddle River, NJ: Prentice Hall.

Turnbull, A. P., Blue-Banning, M., Turbiville, V., & Park, J. (1999). From parent education to partnership education: A call for a transformed focus. *Topics in Early Childhood Special Education, 19*, 164–172.

Werner, E. E. (1990). Protective factors and individual resilience. In S. J. Meisels & J. P. Shonkoff (Eds.) *Handbook of early childhood intervention* (pp. 97–116). New York, NY: Cambridge University Press.

Wolery, M. (1989). Transition in early childhood special education: Issues and procedures. *Focus on Exceptional Children, 22*, 1–16.

Preschool and Early Childhood

Dalice L. Hertzberg, FNP-C, MSN and
Marilyn J. Krajicek, RN, EdD, FAAN

9

Objectives

At the completion of this chapter, the learner will be able to:

1. Identify the most common developmental issues experienced by children with intellectual and developmental disabilities (I/DD) in this age group.

2. List the family concerns that commonly arise during this developmental period.

3. Identify the federal laws that impact services for the 3- to 5-year-old child with I/DD.

4. Differentiate the standards for the individualized education plan (IEP) from the standards for the individual family service plan (IFSP).

5. Discuss common challenges that families encounter when obtaining and maintaining services for their preschool-aged child.

6. Discuss nursing and other health professional roles in providing services and supports for preschool-aged children with I/DD.

Key Points

*   Best practices for the preschool-aged child with I/DD and their family recommend that services are interdisciplinary in nature.

*   The child and family are the most important members of the interdisciplinary team.

*   Services are family-centered, coordinated, community-based, comprehensive, culturally sensitive, inclusive, and continuous across all levels and sites of care.

*   Services take into account the unique nature of each individual child's and family's strengths and challenges.

*   Services are designed to maximize the child's potential and promote options for the child and family.

I.   Definitions

A. The preschool years are from 3 through 5 years of age.

B. The National Association for the Education of Young Children (NAEYC) and the Division of Early Childhood define early childhood (for the purpose of defining early childhood programs) as birth through 8 years of age (NAEYC, 1996).

C. The issues and care of children 3 through 5 years of age will be addressed in this chapter.

II.   Developmental Issues

A. I/DD may be recognized and diagnosed during this age period (Batshaw, 2002). Examples include:

1. Hearing deficit and speech/language disorders

2. Some types of muscular dystrophies

3. Intellectual disability

4. Autism spectrum disorders

5. Chronic illness such as asthma or juvenile diabetes mellitus

6. Mental health disorders including attention deficit disorder

7. Late identification of developmental delay, which began earlier

B. Developmental screening is particularly important during this period to pick up any delays or conditions that were missed earlier or that develop at a later age. This is a common period for identifying speech/language and hearing problems (Krajicek, Hertzberg, Sandall, & Anastasiow, 2003).

1. Screening tools such as the Denver Developmental Screening Test II, the Miller Preschool Screening Test, and the First Step screening test may be used to assess gross and fine motor skills, mental status, expressive and receptive language, and abnormal movements or behavior.

2. Developmental surveillance is a method used by pediatric health care providers to "spot check" for delays at regular well-child care visits (American Academy of Pediatrics (AAP), 2001).

C. Secondary conditions may be recognized and treated during this period. Prevention of secondary conditions that may complicate the original disability is very important (Sulkes, 1995).

1. Motor problems such as spasticity and delayed gross and fine motor skills

2. Growth failure, obesity, or feeding disorders

3. Seizures

4. Gastrointestinal problems such as constipation, malabsorption, or gastro-esophogeal reflux

5. Sensory impairments such as vision and hearing

6. Speech disorders

7. Attention problems

8. Condition-specific problems such as mild congenital heart disease not recognized earlier, growth disorders such as obesity, acquired thyroid disease, and chronic otitis media in children with Down syndrome (Van Riper & Cohen, 2001).

D. Behavioral difficulties are often identified at this time (Merrell & Lea, 1997).

1. What earlier appeared to be minor behavioral variations can become significant challenges for the child and service provider (Keenan, Shaw, Delliquadri, Giovannelli, & Walsh, 1998).

2. Behavioral challenges may become less amenable to routine interventions and require professional consultation and therapy.

3. Screening tools such as the Child Behavior Checklist may be used (AAP, 2001).

4. Referrals to developmental psychologists or an interdisciplinary diagnostic team can lead to a specific diagnosis for the child and a treatment program.

E. For a review of typical development see Table 9.1.

III. Health Considerations

AAP has issued policy statements on a number of I/DD that provide health guidelines across the pediatric years (e.g., Down syndrome, Fragile X) (see http://aappolicy.aappublications.org/policy_statement/index.dtl).

IV. Risk Factors

A. Intrinsic vulnerabilities may result in acquired disability (Hertzberg, 1999). These include:

1. Less mature immune system, which can result in severe infection resulting in central nervous system infection such as meningitis or transverse myelitis.

2. Exposure to other children in group situations at preschool and child care, which may result in frequent and more severe infections, including ear infections potentially resulting in hearing loss and speech and language delay (National Institute of Child Health and Human Development Early Child Care Research Network, 2001).

3. Increased independence and activity level of the preschool child, which can lead to accidents such as poisoning; falls; automobile-pedestrian accidents; automobile accidents (unrestrained in car); aspiration of foreign objects; entrapment in automobile trunks, discarded refrigerators, or other unsafe objects; and drowning and near drowning (Crawley-Coha, 2001).

Table 9.1	Summary of Development from 3 through 5 Years of Age
Developmental task	Development of a sense of initiative. Piaget's pre-operational period of intellectual development.
Physiological	More slender and proportioned than infant. Visual acuity matures. Has all deciduous teeth.
Motor	Both fine and gross motor skills improve. The 3-year-old can jump, run backwards, climb steps, and pedal a tricycle, and can undress independently, but needs help dressing. The older preschooler has enough coordination to dance and roller skate. The 5-year-old is independent in dressing and undressing.
Cognitive	The preschooler is more aware of self and others, and shows increasingly complex mental representations. More independence develops. Language skills increase from using about 900 words at age 3 to more than 2100 words at age 5, in complex, meaningful sentences. The 5-year-old is usually able to count to 10, has an awareness of cultural differences, and has a well-established sense of gender. At 3 years, the child is egocentric and does not understand anticipatory explanations (e.g., in preparing for a procedure). Rituals are important, and maintaining consistent mealtimes, toys, and caregivers enables the child to cope with change. A strong sense of body image and body boundaries enables the preschooler to separate self from the environment.
Play	The 3-year-old cooperates and takes turns, and participates in simple games with others. Imaginative play is frequent, with attention span increasing from 4 to 5 years of age. Preschoolers like being read to, listening and singing along with music, and rhythmic play. The 5-year-old enjoys gross motor play.
Safety	All sources of water present a risk of drowning. The home should be child proofed, relative to the child's age and size (e.g., ability to climb, open containers). Preschoolers must be closely monitored and taught to avoid unsafe areas such as drainage pipes and old buildings. Car seats and seat belts should be used, according to the child's age and weight. Four-year-olds and up can understand basic safety teaching about poisons and other dangers. Five-year-olds can understand how to safely cross streets, not to speak to strangers, and can learn how to swim.
Challenges for preschool-age children with I/DD	May have less energy, motivation, and ability to learn about the environment. May be less able to develop a positive self-concept and sense of mastery; more vulnerable to negative messages. Stuttering may be noticed during this age period. Challenging behavior may emerge. Preschool-age children who have conditions requiring personal physical care (e.g., urethral catheterization) may be less aware of privacy and more at risk for sexual abuse. Developmentally, the preschooler with physical disabilities may fear they are to blame for their condition(s). Need safety instruction designed for their developmental level.

Adapted from Betz, Hunsberger, & Wright, 1994; Hertzberg, 1999; Vessey & Rumsey, 2003.

4. During the early years from birth through 5 years of age, children are most vulnerable to abuse and neglect that may result in developmental delay and disability.

5. Children who are in the foster care system, and who do not receive adequate permanency planning, may experience negative emotional and psychological effects.

V. Family Concerns

A. Families of children with I/DD are faced with a new service system when their child turns 3 years of age, leaving the individualized family service plan and starting the individualized educational plan (Krajicek et al., 2003).

   1. Lack of good transition services at this time can leave services in chaos, and cause major disruption to families.

   2. The child enters the school system and may leave more secure or familiar environments such as child care, family child care, or an early intervention center.

   3. Families must adjust to less frequent services in the school setting, such as physical, occupational, and speech therapy, and are often faced with obtaining private pay services to meet their child's therapy needs. Different funding sources may pay for different services, leaving the family to sort out who will pay for which therapy.

B. Families of children with multiple medical needs may find their insurance has reached, or will soon reach, lifetime limits of service, and need to pursue other funding opportunities.

C. Managed health care systems such as Medicaid managed care or private systems may change benefits and providers yearly, disrupting continuity of care. Children with autism, children with complex health conditions, children whose siblings have disabilities or chronic health conditions, and parents who have health problems experience increased barriers to access to specialty medical care (Krauss, Gulley, Sciega, & Wells, 2003).

D. Primary care providers, private therapists, school therapists, and consultants may not communicate changes in the child's treatment or recommendations to one another.

E. Families may find the task of service coordination for their child becomes more complex if there are additional systems involved with the care of their child as he or she enters the school system, and may require additional support from professionals and/or parent advocacy groups.

F. Families adopting children with I/DD from within and outside the United States may receive varying amounts of assistance, ranging from limited Medicaid funding to no assistance or support.

G. Families who adopted younger children who did not have I/DD may find the child is now identified as having an I/DD, and must adjust emotionally and financially. Periodic reassessments for the child are necessary.

H. Families who adopted children from orphanages or specialized programs in other countries may find the child is now identified as having an I/DD, and must adjust emotionally and financially to the changed image of the child and to the ongoing assessments and treatments that are necessary.

I. Some parents will experience crises at times of key transition for their child—such as entering the school system at age 5 or 6 years—and relive feelings of loss. Other parents deny experiencing these feelings (National Information Center for Children and Youth with Disabilities, 1997; Youngblood, 1999).

J. As children fail to achieve expected milestones, exhibit challenging behaviors, or are diagnosed as having an I/DD, families may experience cultural stigma at the child's changed status, which can further stress the family. Some cultures exhibit a collectivist view, which indicates that an I/DD in the family reflects upon the entire family, not just the individual with an I/DD (Jezewski & Sotnik, 2001).

K. Connecting families with parent-to-parent support groups can be helpful to provide unique support for parents of preschool children with I/DD (Lin, 2000; Olsen, Marshall, Mandleco, Allred, Dyches, & Sansom, 1999).

VI. Interdisciplinary Care

A. Best practices dictate the interdisciplinary nature of services for children with I/DD.

B. The interdisciplinary team (see Chapter 6) collaborates and shares expertise to achieve optimal outcomes. Team members and responsibilities in providing services for the preschool child include:

1. Family—The family is ultimately responsible for the child's care, and their concerns and priorities should be reflected in team goals. Family members actively participate in team meetings and are the primary service coordinator for their child.

2. Physician—Responsibilities for the preschool-age child include provision of primary health care, including immunizations. Behavioral pediatricians and pediatric physiatrists are actively involved with rehabilitation services and follow-up regarding developmental problems.

3. Nurse—Nurses function as advocates for the child and family, providing leadership, policy development, and systems change on behalf of the child and family. They provide teaching to the child and family and may function as service coordinators, particularly during the transition phase from early intervention programs to the school system. Direct hospital care is provided by nurses during in-patient stays. Continuity of care in the community occurs in the school system and public health in the maternal and child

health system. Nurse practitioners provide primary health care, administer developmental screening, and refer for specialty treatment. Nurses may also function as consultants in child care and preschool (Youngblood, 1999).

4. Physical therapists—Physical therapists (PTs) assist the child and family with gross motor testing and functional restoration. Treatment focuses on achieving and maintaining strength, range of motion, and developmental milestones in the motor areas. In the preschool age group, PTs may visit the child at home, in the preschool setting, or in a free-standing clinic. PTs participate in evaluation and diagnosis of motor problems in the preschool aged child.

5. Occupational therapists—Occupational therapists (OTs) are concerned with activities of daily living and self-care activities typical at the preschool developmental age. They also focus on fine motor issues, perceptual motor problems, and sensory integration issues. Particularly in children with autism, who generally lack gross motor problems, the OT is extensively involved in daily care and environmental issues for the child. The OT is an important team member in the evaluation and diagnosis of preschool-aged children for fine motor, perceptual, and sensory problems, which may be very subtle in this age group.

6. Speech therapists—The speech therapist participates in the evaluation and diagnosis of the preschool-aged child, and engages in speech and language therapy with the child. Speech therapists specialize in speech production and articulation as well as receptive and expressive language. They also participate extensively in intellectual testing, which may be limited by the child's speech and language skills.

7. Psychologist—In the preschool age group, child psychologists may be involved with developmental and intellectual testing of the child, as well as in evaluation and treatment of any behavioral problems that might arise. They also may diagnose any mental health problems that may arise in this developmental period.

8. Social worker—Assistance with financial support, family support, and eligibility for state programs is a role of the social worker. Social workers also participate in family assessment during evaluation.

9. Other professionals may be called in for specific cases as needed for their expertise (e.g., nutritionists, physiatrists).

VII. Specific Legislation for this Age Group

A. The Individuals with Disabilities Education Act (IDEA)—IDEA mandates that all children with I/DD receive a free and appropriate public education. Children must be identified and evaluated to determine if they are eligible for services through the local public school (Krajicek et al., 2003).

1. Children younger than 3 years of age who are identified with an I/DD, or who are at risk of developing an I/DD, are served under Part C of IDEA, the early intervention section of the law. They may receive an individualized family service plan (IFSP), which focuses on the crucial role of the family in the education of the very young child, and provides family support as well as educational and early intervention services to the child and family.

2. Part B of IDEA describes entitlements and safeguards for children ages 3 through 21 years, so preschool-aged children fit within this section of the law. Children in Part B of IDEA receive an individualized educational plan (IEP), which focuses on the education, and related service needs of the child in the school setting (Krajicek et al., 2003).

B. The Developmental Disabilities Assistance and Bill of Rights Act defines developmental disabilities for funding purposes and provides funding for developmental disabilities programs at the state level, such as developmental disabilities planning councils, protection and advocacy programs (legal protection), university centers of excellence in developmental disabilities, and special grant projects (Developmental Disabilities Assistance and Bill of Rights Act (P.L. 106-402), 2000).

C. The Technology-Related Assistance for Individuals with Disabilities Act (Tech Act) Amendments facilitate access to assistive technology for children and adults with I/DD and their families by funding programs in the states. The law authorizes a competitive grant program enabling states to designate lead agencies to facilitate access to, and provision of, assistive technology devices and services (Lange, 2000).

1. The Tech Act supports the IDEA provision of assistive technology services and supports for preschoolers with I/DD in the school setting.

2. An assistive technology device is one that is used to increase, maintain, or improve the functional capacity of a child with an I/DD (Lange, 2000).

3. Assistive technology services directly assist a child with an I/DD in the selection, acquisition, or use of an assistive technology device.

4. The need for assistive technology services and devices is established in the child's IEP.

D. The Americans with Disabilities Act (ADA) prohibits discrimination against people with I/DD. Enacted in 1991, the ADA affects preschoolers and their families by requiring that public accommodations (such as child care centers, preschools, doctors' offices, pharmacies, and retail stores) do not discriminate (Krajicek et al., 2003).

1. Other components of the ADA that may affect children ages 3 through 5 years include:

   a. transportation (such as public buses, trains, or airplanes)

   b. telecommunications (appropriate equipment must be provided by telephone companies to individuals who are deaf or hard of hearing)

    c.   auxiliary aids and services (designed to accommodate individuals with a lost of hearing or vision, or other disabilities)

E.   The federal Center for Medicare and Medicaid Services mandates early periodic screening, diagnosis, and treatment (EPSDT) for all children covered by state Medicaid programs. EPSDT provides screening for and treatment of developmental and mental health problems, which may be detected in the preschool age group.

F.   State and local regulations vary from state to state. Examples of regulations that may affect preschoolers with I/DD and their families include:

   1.   State child care and preschool regulations, such as child care licensing laws, may require a child entering preschool to be potty trained, and training for child care providers administering medications.

   2.   Social services and child welfare systems that administer child protection programs and foster care programs may or may not provide for special training or health care funding for foster parents who take preschoolers with I/DD.

   3.   Child welfare systems that administer crisis nurseries may service preschoolers with I/DD.

   4.   State nurse practice acts may state whether or not a registered nurse may delegate specific nursing tasks (such as invasive health procedures and administration of medications, which are required by some preschoolers with I/DD) to child care or preschool staff.

VIII. Service Systems

Preschoolers with I/DD and their families interact with a variety of service systems. Agencies and systems providing services to this population may not adhere to the values of family-centered, community-based, accessible, culturally sensitive, collaborative, continuous (providing continuity), and inclusive care and services. Frequently, children receive services through different agencies that do not communicate with one another, resulting in fragmentation and duplication of services (Edwards, 1999a).

A.   Heath care systems

   1.   Private primary health care offices staffed with pediatricians, family practice physicians, and/or nurse practitioners may not have experience or knowledge about I/DD, and may take only a small number of clients who are insured by Medicaid or other public funding sources.

   2.   Pediatricians, much less developmental pediatricians, may not be available in rural areas.

3. Community hospitals may not have pediatric units, nor experience with young children with I/DD. Specialty children's hospitals are often in large urban areas, and although they have the necessary expertise to care for young children with I/DD, services are costly and access may be limited.

4. Families may lack knowledge of accessible health and education systems and may not understand their rights.

5. Specialized developmental clinics are often available only in urban areas.

6. Home care staff often lack experience with children with I/DD, unless they specialize in pediatric home care.

B. Education (Krajicek et al., 2003).

1. Public preschool services are available in most states, and in most areas of states. Schools are instructed by IDEA to provide inclusive services wherever possible; however, resources vary. Special education services are provided, as are related services including nursing, through IDEA.

2. Public preschool programs generally only last part of the day, and may only be available to the family for 2–3 days a week, leaving them to find alternative care for the child the remainder of the time.

3. Preschool services are available at variable cost through private programs. The ADA instructs that no child be turned away on the basis of disability, unless undue burden can be demonstrated. Programs that receive federal funding are instructed to include preschoolers with specific classifications of I/DD.

4. Each state department of education has child find services, which identify children who qualify for special education services.

C. Head Start programs serve socially and economically disadvantaged children ages 3 through 5 years. Head Start is mandated to provide services for children with I/DD.

1. Programs provide comprehensive health, nutrition, education, and social services for children to give them an educational and social advantage upon starting public school.

2. Health services are available in the form of nurse consultants who may provide medication and special care, as well as some limited service coordination.

3. Head Start has an active program, which solicits families to enroll their children, as well as family support programs.

D. Child welfare and child protection systems operate social services departments, which monitor and act upon incidents of abuse and neglect for all children, including monitoring and operating foster care programs and permanency planning.

1. Preschoolers with I/DD and their families may become involved in the system due to abuse, neglect, or suspicion of abuse. Preschoolers with I/DD may experience delayed permanency planning.

E. State and federal funding agencies (Edwards, 1999b).

1. The Child Health Insurance Program (CHIP) is federally mandated and state run, and provides low-cost health insurance for uninsured children and families. Limited disability-related services such as physical, occupational, or speech therapy and specialty medical care may or may not be provided.

2. Medicaid provides health insurance for low income groups, families with dependent children (birth through 6 years), the elderly poor, and people with I/DD. Prenatal care is also funded. Disability-related services are funded, but at lower reimbursement rates for health care providers. Medicaid is a federal and state funded program, administered by the states.

3. State Title IV services provide funding and other special programs for children with I/DD and their families, such as therapy, durable medical equipment, and specialty medical services for families who qualify on the basis of income.

4. Title V programs also provide service coordination, and advocate and act upon policy on behalf of children with I/DD and their families.

5. Private insurance provides a variety of plans at various costs to children and families. Disability-related services may or may not be included.

F. Natural supports are resources and strategies that enable families to access resources, information, and relationships that promote integration, and which result in enhanced independence, productivity, community integration, and satisfaction (Ohtake & Chadsey, 2001).

1. Natural supports differ from formal supports (e.g., counselors, health and human service system staff, other service providers) in that they do not result from paid relationships, but from natural relationships within the community, such as those formed with neighbors, friends, relatives, fellow worshipers, and other community members.

2. For preschoolers, this might include neighborhood playgroups, babysitters, private preschools, or family home child care.

3. Service coordination is an important concern as preschoolers enter more complex systems of service.

    a. Many agencies offer service coordination, and a child and family may have more than one service coordinator.

    b. Current best practice focuses on supporting the family to be their own service coordinator and advocate as much as they are able, and providing resources to the family toward that goal.

G. Transition services are recommended by IDEA.

1. Transition services are a coordinated set of activities for a student, designed with an outcome-oriented process, which promotes movement between service systems such as Part C and/or private child care to Part B services (Barnes, 2001).

2. Activities are based on the individual child's needs, the IFSP, and components of the IEP.

3. Transition services ease the many changes a child and family experience when changing service systems, and are designed to ensure continuity of services and supports.

IX. Summary

The preschool and early childhood years are important years for screening in all developmental domains and prevention of secondary conditions if prevailing I/DD are present. During this period, the child and his or her family become involved in more complex systems. It is important that parents become educated in the child's condition(s), health, and developmental needs, and be able to advocate for present and future needs. Knowledge of legislation, child rights, and ways to acquire needed professional expertise and services is essential.

References

American Academy of Pediatrics (AAP). (2001). Developmental surveillance and screening of infants and young children. *Pediatrics, 108*(1), 192–196.

Barnes, E. (2001). Paving the way to kindergarten: Timelines and guidelines for preschool staff working with young children with special needs and their families. Retrieved January 28, 2003 from http://soeweb.syr.edu/thechp/PavingTheWay.pdf

Batshaw, M. L. (Ed.). (2002). *Children with disabilities* (5th ed.). Baltimore: Paul H. Brookes.

Betz, C. L., Hunsberger, M., & Wright, S. (1994). Growth and development of the preschooler. In C. L. Betz, M. Hunsberger, & S. Wright (Eds.). *Family-centered nursing care of children* (2nd ed., p. 236). Philadelphia: W. B. Saunders.

Crawley-Coha, T. (2001). Childhood injury: A status report. *Journal of Pediatric Nursing, 16,* 371–374.

Developmental Disabilities Assistance and Bill of Rights Act (2000). Pub. L. No. 106-402, 114 Stat. 1677 (2000).

Edwards, P. (1999a). Community based health care delivery systems. In P. Edwards, D. Hertzberg, S. Hays, & N. Youngblood. (Eds.) *Pediatric rehabilitation nursing* (pp. 31–39). Philadelphia: W. B. Saunders.

Edwards, P. (1999b). Financing health care. In P. Edwards, D. Hertzberg, S. Hays, & N. Youngblood (Eds.). *Pediatric rehabilitation nursing* (pp. 52–61). Philadelphia: W B. Saunders.

Hertzberg, D. (1999). Child growth, development, and maturation. In P. Edwards, D. Hertzberg, S. Hays, & N. Youngblood (Eds.). *Pediatric rehabilitation nursing* (pp. 144–199). Philadelphia: W B. Saunders.

Jezewski, M., & Sotnik, P. (2001). *Culture brokering: Providing culturally competent rehabilitation services to foreign-born persons.* CIRRIE Monograph Series, John Stone (Ed.). Buffalo, NY: Center for International Rehabilitation Research Information and Exchange, University at Buffalo, State University of New York.

Keenan, K., Shaw, D., Delliquadri, E., Giovannelli, J., & Walsh, B. (1998). Evidence for the continuity of early problem behaviors: Application of a developmental model. *Journal of Abnormal Child Psychology, 26,* 441–455.

Krajicek, M., Hertzberg, D., Sandall, S., & Anastasiow, N. (2003). *First start: Care of infants, toddlers, and young children with disabilities and chronic conditions.* San Antonio: Pro-Ed.

Krauss, M., Gulley, D., Sciega, M., & Wells, N. (2003). Access to specialty medical care for children with mental retardation, autism, and other special health care needs. *Mental Retardation, 41,* 329–339.

Lange M. L. (2000). Focus on . . . EADLs and young children . . . electronic aids to daily living. *OT Practice, 5*(24), 19–21.

Lin, S. (2000). Coping and adaptation in families of children with cerebral palsy. *Exceptional Children, 66,* 201–218.

Merrell, K. H., & Lea, M. L. (1997). Social-emotional behavior of preschool-age children with and without developmental delays. *Research in Developmental Disabilities, 18,* 393–405.

National Association for the Education of Young Children. (1996). Developmentally appropriate practice in early childhood programs serving children from birth through age 8. Retrieved January 28, 2003 from http://www.naeyc.org/resources/position_statements/dap1.htm

National Institute of Child Health and Human Development Early Child Care Research Network. (2001). Child care and common communicable illnesses: results from the National Institute of Child Health and Human Development Study of Early Child Care. *Archives of Pediatrics & Adolescent Medicine. 155,* 481–488.

National Information Center for Children and Youth with Disabilities. (1997). Parenting a child with special needs: A guide to reading and resources. *NICHCY Digest,* (2nd Ed.) News Digest 20. Retrieved January 28, 2003 from http://www.nichcy.org/pubs/newsdig/nd20txt.htm

Ohtake, Y. & Chadsey, J. G. (2001). Continuing to describe the natural support process. *Journal of the Association for People with Severe Handicaps, 26*(2), 87–95.

Olsen, S. F., Marshall, E. S., Mandleco, B. L., Allred, K. W., Dyches, T. T., & Sansom, N. (1999). Support, communication, and hardiness in families with children with disabilities. *Journal of Family Nursing, 5,* 275–291.

Sulkes, S. B. (1995). MD's DD basics: Identifying common problems and preventing secondary disabilities. *Pediatric Annals, 24,* 245–252, 254.

Van Riper, M., & Cohen, W. (2001). Caring for children with Down syndrome and their families. *Journal of Pediatric HealthCare, 15,* 123–131.

Vessey, J., & Rumsey, M. (2003). Chronic conditions and child development. In P. Allen & J. Vessey (Eds.). *Primary care of the child with a chronic condition* (4th ed., pp. 44–59). St. Louis, MO: Mosby.

Youngblood, N. (1999). Models for practice and service. In P. Edwards, D. Hertzberg, S. Hays, & N. Youngblood (Eds.). *Pediatric rehabilitation nursing* (pp. 113–126). Philadelphia: W. B. Saunders.

School-Age and Adolescence

10

Wendy M. Nehring, RN, PhD, FAAN, FAAMR and Sandra A. Faux, RN, PhD

Objectives

At the completion of this chapter, the learner will be able to:

1. Discuss the prevalence of intellectual and developmental disabilities (I/DD) in children aged 6 to 21 years of age.

2. List normal developmental issues for children during their middle childhood (6 to 12 years) and adolescent (13 to 21+ years) periods.

3. Synthesize physical, health, cognitive, and psychosocial influences on normal middle childhood and adolescent development due to having an identified I/DD.

4. Describe federal legislation that impacts school-age children with I/DD.

5. Discuss developmental screening and testing during the school-age years for children with I/DD.

6. Analyze the individualized education plan (IEP) and related school issues for children with I/DD.

Key Points

- Health care professionals must work as interdisciplinary teams collaboratively with children with I/DD and their families to identify educational issues and problems and to achieve successful educational experiences.

- School-age children with I/DD must have an IEP that is comprehensive, coordinated, culturally sensitive, family- and person-centered, and community-based, and that is re-evaluated on an annual or more frequent basis in order to provide the optimal experience.

- Developmental assessments must be chronologically and developmentally appropriate.

- Health care professionals should assist adolescents with I/DD (and their parents, if applicable) to become an advocate for their health and developmental needs.

I.   Introduction

The school-age years are significant because this is the first experience for parents in launching their children to the outside world. Although children with I/DD may have been in child care, day care, preschool, and/or early intervention experiences, sending a child to school is an initial experience in saying, "This is my child, and he or she belongs here, and is more similar to than different from your child." For the child with I/DD, this is a time to fit in and belong. It is important that the school years are as successful as possible because experiences in school, whether academic or social, stay with a person throughout their life.

A. The school-age and adolescent years, for the purposes of this chapter, are from ages 6 through 21 years.

B. Specific transition issues, occurring from approximately ages 14 through 21 years are covered in Chapter 11.

II.   Statistics

A. Based on the results of the 1992 to 1994 National Health Interview Survey, 6.5% of all children under the age of 18 years were diagnosed with a disability (4.4 million children) (Newacheck & Halfon, 1998).

1. Diagnosis of speech, special sense, or intelligence impairments was identified in 1,696 per 100,000 children.

B. In an analysis of children ages 5 to 20 years from the 2000 U.S. census, 5.2 million children (1 in 12 children) had either a mental or physical disability (Cohn, 2002).

C. Health care and technological advances have improved the life expectancy of children with disabling chronic conditions, such as children born extremely premature (Allen, 2004).

D. Emerging chronic childhood conditions are present, such as long-term adverse effects of treatments for cancer in childhood, exposure to environmental toxins, and survival from pediatric HIV/AIDS (Allen, 2004; Woodruff, Axelrad, Kyle, Nweke, & Miller, 2003).

E. The number of U.S. children (ages 6 to 21 years) in special education during the 2001–2002 academic year was approximately 5.9 million (U.S. Department of Education, Office of Special Education Programs, 2002).

III.   Normal Developmental Issues During Middle Childhood (6–12 years)
(Feldman, 2003)

A. Physical Development

1. Growth—May vary as a result of race, socioeconomic level, nutrition, and/or presence of a chronic condition that affects growth (e.g., spina bifida).

    a. Continue to use standardized growth charts. In addition, when available, use specific growth charts for certain chronic conditions, such as Down syndrome and cerebral palsy.

2. Weight—Growing epidemic of obesity in children. May be exacerbated by presence of an I/DD, such as Prader-Willi syndrome that affects weight.

3. Exercise—Important for healthy body and developing healthy habits. May begin involvement in Special Olympics.

4. Safety—Need for health education regarding alcohol, drugs, and tobacco, but also for reducing risky behavior. Accidents are the leading cause of death, specifically being hit by a car.

5. Early puberty

    a. Average puberty for girls is approximately 10 years. African American girls can begin puberty 1–2 years earlier than girls from other ethnic groups. Girls begin puberty before boys.

    b. Boys begin puberty on average at 12 years.

6. Body image and self-esteem—As early as the primary grades, children begin to compare themselves with others, often stating that they are "stupid," "fat," or "ugly," either because they perceive themselves to be that or someone has called them that name. Assisting to build self-esteem and a good body image must begin during these years, if not before.

B. Motor Development

1. Fine and gross motor skills are similar for boys and girls.

2. Motor development continues at a steady and slow pace during these years.

3. Children enjoy board or card games and sports activities that have rules.

C. Cognitive Development

1. Piaget—Concrete operational period (5–7 to 11 years).

    a. Characteristics of this period include development of logic, mathematical understanding, conservation, seriation, spatial relations, and class inclusion.

2. Vygotsky—Development of inner speech.

3. Flavell—Development of domain-specific knowledge and information-processing abilities.

4. Language development includes increased ability to initiate and maintain conversations.

5. Kohlberg's moral development—Moving from obeying rules and external control (preconventional morality: 4–10 years) to obeying rules to maintain order and to please others; having a social conscience (conventional morality: 10–13 years).

6. Use of standardized intelligence tests in school.

7. Memory development for success in academic work.

8. School issues, such as labeling, report cards, teachers, and favorites, and type of schooling (e.g., home, charter, parochial, specialized school).

D. Psychosocial Development

1. Development of independence and mastery over their environment.

2. Gaining social skills.

3. Maintaining a healthy self-esteem and coping with disappointment and stress.

4. Friendships and best friends.

5. Participation in organizations (e.g., Girl or Boy Scouts, religious groups, sports groups) (Feldman, 2003).

IV. Normal Developmental Issues During Adolescence (13–21+ years) (Feldman, 2003)

Adolescence has historically ended at age 18 or 21 years. In the past, many people of that age were leaving school, getting jobs, getting married, and living independently of their parents. Today, young people are not becoming independent until often their mid- to late twenties. Federal laws, which will be discussed later, extend childhood or pediatric services until age 21 or 22 years, depending on the law and definition for persons with I/DD.

A. Physical Development

1. Second greatest period of physical growth next to infancy.

2. First signs of puberty are increased hormone production (e.g., smelly feet, body odor, aggression in boys, and moodiness in girls).

3. Puberty involves the growth spurt, the start of menstruation in girls, production of sperm in males, maturation of reproductive organs, development of pubic hair, a deeper voice, and muscular growth.

4. Exercise

5. Nutrition—Eating a healthy diet, staying away from junk food, and eating disorders.

6. Sleep—Need for adequate hours of sleep.

7. Safety—Continuing to avoid alcohol, drugs, and tobacco. Being aware of STDs and HIV/AIDS. Education about gun control. Avoiding risky behavior and behaving in a safe and responsible manner.

B. Cognitive Development

1. Piaget—Formal operational period (11–15+ years) characterized by abstract thought, perception of the future, scientific method, taking the perspective of others, imaginary audience, egocentrism, personal fable, and overthinking.

2. Academic issues focus on school performance, grade progression, and career and vocational development.

C. Psychosocial Development

1. Freud—Genital phase, which examines the balance between love and work and sexual intimacy.

2. Erikson—Identity versus role confusion that focuses on place in society and value system, occupational and/or educational choices, and developing a sexual identity.

3. Cultural identity development; for example, what it means to a person to be a Chinese American.

4. Kohlberg's moral development—Many only reach the conventional morality stage, but the last stage is postconventional morality (characterized by democratically accepted law and universal principles).

   a. Women and men differ in their moral development as women are more caring and want to avoid harm, whereas men are more justice oriented.

5. Friendships and peer groups—Building lifelong relationships.

6. Dating and intimacy (see Chapters 13 and 24).

7. Sibling and parental relationships—During adolescence, there is much testing of boundaries; by late adolescence, relationships will be developed that may last through adulthood (see Chapter 24).

8. Personality development.

9. Future plans for career, vocation, marriage, and family (Feldman, 2003).

V. Influences on Normal Development Due to Having an I/DD

A. Physical Development and Health

1. Health care guidelines for specific conditions need to be followed when available (e.g., Down syndrome, Prader-Willi syndrome, Fragile X), as well as age-appropriate screening (see Allen & Vessey, 2004a; Batshaw, 2002; Green & Palfrey, 2002; and the American Academy of Pediatrics webpage: http://aappolicy.aappublications.org/policy_statement/index.dtl).

2. Prevention or identification of secondary conditions should occur. When present, provide appropriate management and education.

3. Severity of the condition, whether health or mobility related, will affect development.

4. Provide anticipatory guidance concerning specific I/DD. Assist the child, especially the adolescent, and family members to understand the diagnosis, any required medical treatments/procedures, and lifespan projections.

5. Health care professionals need to keep abreast of best practices for the specific I/DD. Knowledge must also include unproven therapies so that counseling and information can be shared with families. Complementary and

alternative medicine approaches should also be considered and weighed for efficacy when families inquire about their usefulness (American Academy of Pediatrics, Committee on Children with Disabilities, 2001).

6. Beginning around age 7 years, teach the child to complete own self-care concerning health care management of condition. For example, the child with spina bifida may learn and do their own self-catheterization.

7. Identify appropriate health care professionals to meet health needs. Insurance coverage will dictate extent of available services. Even when covered, it is often difficult to identify appropriate health care professionals, such as dentists and mental health professionals (see Chapters 18 and 23).

   a. Continuity and coordination of care also becomes important as health care needs may become more complex with additional health care concerns and need for additional specialists, such as a gynecologist who has equipment for examination of a woman with cerebral palsy who has contractions and mobility concerns.

   b. Families may also experience health care professionals lacking appropriate knowledge of certain conditions necessary to provide optimal care (U.S. Public Health Service, 2002).

   c. The American Academy of Pediatrics, Maternal and Child Health Bureau, and Family Voices collaborated on a 10-year plan to achieve a comprehensive, community-based service system for children with special health care needs (Maternal and Child Health Bureau, Health Resources and Services Administration, 2001). The goals of this plan are:

      i. Families will be active partners in the interdisciplinary team and experience satisfaction in their child's care. This should include the child whenever possible.

      ii. Families will have access to a "medical home" in which comprehensive, continuous, family-centered, and coordinated quality health care is delivered. A better name for such care would have been a "health care home," considering the interdisciplinary and full spectrum care that is provided (Allen, 2004).

      iii. Each child should have adequate and appropriate public and/or private health care insurance.

      iv. Ongoing health care includes appropriate screening and/or treatment for comprehensive health and developmental concerns.

      v. Community-based services are accessible and available.

      vi. Health, social, educational, and vocational services for children with special health care needs also involve plans for transition to adulthood.

8. The child's future may be uncertain. The trajectory of many childhood chronic conditions resulting in I/DD throughout adulthood is unknown.

Additional research is warranted to describe health and developmental outcomes throughout adulthood and older adulthood (Nehring, Faux, Ito, & Braun, 2004).

B. Cognitive Development

1. Standardized intelligence testing (see Section VII of this chapter).

2. English as a second language may influence outcomes of standardized testing in the schools.

3. Acculturation in society—First determine whether a child is a first generation immigrant to the United States (see Chapter 25). Intelligence screening and testing must be culturally sensitive and the tester should not be culturally biased.

4. Type of test given—Standardized, norm-referenced test or regional test with less validity and reliability.

5. I/DD may be first diagnosed after school screening, but not obvious outside of school as adaptive functioning not affected.

6. Develop educational goals based on developmental, not chronological, age.

7. Assess child's emotional maturity.

8. Plan for future—Vocational and/or academic goals.

C. Psychosocial Development

1. Coping with labels based on diagnosis, appearance, and/or behavior. Help to eliminate stigmatization.

    a. Teasing—For example, children with spina bifida who are ambulatory, have balance problems, and are often teased and pushed to see them fall down.

    b. The junior high or middle school years are often the most difficult for children with I/DD. Experiences with teasing and bullying leave lifelong impressions (Nehring et al., 2004).

2. Identify strengths.

3. Assess for depression—By the junior high or middle school years, children with I/DD realize that they are different and may become depressed. It is important to look for signs of depression and intervene quickly. Many parents have also reported that their adolescent children have become depressed after they have been rejected for a date from a peer without an I/DD; children without an I/DD often believe it is alright to be a friend, but it is not alright to date a person with I/DD.

4. Assess for behavioral changes—Children with I/DD may show behavioral changes due to changes in their health condition, onset of a behavioral disability (e.g., Fragile X, ADHD), or school-related issues. It is important to obtain professional assistance if needed for appropriate diagnosis and/or treatment.

5. Be aware that children with I/DD whose disability is largely invisible (e.g., spina bifida occulta) may experience more psychological distress. Because their disability is not visible, they are expected to perform and behave normally.

6. Children with I/DD who are enrolled in inclusive schools experienced increased friendships with children both with and without I/DD, less abusive behavior, and greater advocacy from children without I/DD (Bunch & Valeo, 2004).

7. Help parents to balance their child's development of independence and being overprotective. In particular, parents have to understand their feelings about their child with I/DD being sexually active. The health care professional needs to ask: Does the parent need support in understanding those feelings, providing sex education to their child, and/or helping the child to plan for a future intimate relationship or not planning for such a relationship (see Chapter 13)?

8. Identification and use of support services:

    a. Vocational rehabilitation

    b. Therapies—physical, occupational, and/or speech

    c. Special transportation services

VI.   Federal Legislation

Since 1975, when the first educational law for children with I/DD was passed (Public Law 94-142: The Education for All Handicapped Children Act of 1975), children with I/DD have had the right to receive free and appropriate public education from the age of 3 through 21 years. Additional legislation over the years has also affected children with I/DD; each of these will be discussed in their present form. Health care professionals must be knowledgeable of federal legislation affecting children with I/DD and their families and be able to explain, advise, and counsel families as needed (American Academy of Pediatrics, Committee on Children with Disabilities, 2000).

A. Public Law 105-17: Individuals with Disabilities Education Act Amendments of 1997 (IDEA '97) (1997).

1. Part A discusses general provisions, the purpose of the act, the goals of the act, and definitions.

2. Part B is entitled "Assistance for Education of All Children with Disabilities," and describes the federal assistance that will be given to provide for the free and appropriate education of all children with I/DD, ages 3 to 21 years, including a section on the rights of children with I/DD and their families, including guardians where applicable. Additional provisions are given to describe how state agencies must monitor and supervise the statute.

3. Part C discusses the program that oversees children with I/DD from birth to 3 years.

4. Part D provides federal assistance for the preparation and credentialing of special educators.

5. Important provisions in this legislation are:

    a. Least restrictive environment—Providing education to the child in their optimal environment. Today, the majority of school-age students with I/DD participate in inclusion in which they are integrated with other students without I/DD in the classroom; this may involve all of their classes or a percentage of classes, including physical education. A small percentage of school-age students with I/DD that severely impact their intelligence and/or adaptive behaviors still receive their education in segregated, noninclusion classrooms.

    b. Parental rights as a full partner in determining educational decisions involving placement, curriculum, performance, and behavioral goals, and eligibility.

    c. Child find—A program to identify and evaluate all children for I/DD. Attention is given to ethnic diversity.

    d. Due process procedures to reduce or eliminate disagreements between parent(s) and the school system.

    e. Related services that include corrective, supportive, and developmental services; transportation; school health services; psychological support through school social workers; before and after school care; parent training and counseling; mobility services; accommodation supports; and transition services (see also Allen & Vessey, 2004b; Clair, Church, & Batshaw, 2002).

B. Public Law 106-402: Developmental Disabilities Assistance and Bill of Rights Act of 2000 (2000). This legislation was enacted in order to ensure access to appropriate community-based services, individualized supports, and other means of assistance to promote independence, self-determination, and inclusion in society. This legislation specifically provides for:

1. Rights of individuals with I/DD, including protection and advocacy support

2. Federal assistance to state councils on developmental disabilities

3. Federal assistance to develop and maintain a national network of university centers for excellence in developmental disabilities education, research, and service and projects of national significance

4. Federal assistance to provide adequate family support systems

5. Program for direct support workers, including scholarships and a curriculum for staff development

C. Section 504 of the Rehabilitation Act (PL 93-112, 1973). Discusses the importance of not discriminating against any child based on gender, ethnic origin, or race in acquiring education. The act also provides for classroom accommodation and educational supports. Other elements of the act concern parental notification of identification, developmental assessment, and consequent placement; periodic developmental evaluations; assistive technology; and other related services (Allen & Vessey, 2004b).

D. Americans with Disabilities (ADA) Act of 1990 (PL 101-336) prohibits discrimination against any individual with I/DD in all settings, telecommunications, transportation, and public accommodations.

VII. Developmental Screening and Testing

Developmental screening is a part of well-child care. It is essential when a developmental concern is identified by a health care or educational professional and/or parent that appropriate developmental screening and testing, if warranted, is completed. Waiting to see "if the child will grow out of it" may permanently impact optimal growth and development. A comprehensive list of instruments used for developmental screening and testing is found in Vessey and Rumsey (2004).

A. Developmental screening and testing during the school-age years focuses on associated learning, behavioral, language, and social limitations.

B. Physicians may be the primary health care professional to conduct such screening, but more likely such findings will be identified in the school setting.

C. School nurses should help parents to keep a record of all health and developmental findings so that such information can be shared between settings and not have to be repeated unnecessarily.

D. School nurses should assist in the child's transition back to school after absences due to illness and/or hospitalizations.

E. School nurses need to identify what responsibilities they will have in each particular school district (e.g., catheterizations, tube-feedings). In some cases, children with I/DD may have aides accompany them to school, and school nurses need to know what activities and responsibilities these aides have. School nurses also need to know the role that the parent will play and when the parent wants to be contacted.

F. Primary care providers, either physicians or nurse practitioners, must conduct full histories and physical examinations to rule out physiological reasons for symptoms. Psychosocial considerations for symptoms must also be considered and explored. It is important that "diagnostic overshadowing" does not occur (see Chapter 18). For example, an adolescent with Down syndrome who has a disagreement with her best friend is not depressed because of her diagnosis of Down syndrome.

G. Primary care providers and other health care professionals must be knowledgeable of providers and agencies for appropriate health and/or developmental referrals.

H. Health care professionals must be advocates for children with I/DD and, when appropriate, assist the adolescent to become an advocate for their own health and developmental needs as they age (American Academy of Pediatrics, Committee on Children with Disabilities, 1999).

VIII. Individualized Education Plan (IEP) and Related School Issues

The IEP is the hallmark of the education legislation for children with I/DD. Many of the school issues surround appropriate assessment, planning, implementation, and evaluation of the child with I/DD. The IEP must be person- and family-centered and involve the child, when appropriate, and the parent as full partners in the interdisciplinary team (Allen & Vessey, 2004b; American Academy of Pediatrics, Clair, Church, & Batshaw, 2002; Committee on Children with Disabilities, 1999).

A. The team that is involved in the development and implementation of the IEP includes at least one parent, the child (when appropriate), at least one of the child's regular teachers and a special education teacher, a school district representative, other professionals identified by the school who interpret the academic implications of the recent developmental evaluations, and other professionals identified by the parent. School nurses are often a member of a child's IEP team.

B. Measurable academic, behavioral, and/or social goals are developed on an annual basis. Yearly reports on the child's accomplishments and progress towards goals are required.

C. The IEP must contain the current level of academic performance, a list of measurable goals and objectives, criteria for successful accomplishment of the goals, a list of the accommodations and related services needed, placement, rationale for a lack of participation in segregated settings, and accommodations for standardized testing or rationale for why such testing is not possible.

D. When the child with I/DD reaches age 14 years, an individualized transition plan (ITP) must be developed (see Chapter 11).

E. Related services under IDEA '97 include medical (including nutrition), social work, psychological, audiology and speech-language, physical, and occupational therapy; counseling services; recreation programs; and mobility and orientation services (see Chapter 8).

F. Factors that may influence the child with I/DD's performance in the school setting include school absenteeism, mobility issues, fatigue, medications and treatments, and health management procedures. Additional psychosocial issues were discussed earlier in this chapter.

IX. Summary

School-agers with I/DD require coordinated, comprehensive, culturally sensitive, community-based, and family-centered health and developmental services. This requires interdisciplinary participation and collaboration. Federal legislation provides for free education from ages 3 through 21 years and details services and accommodations to provide for optimal educational and developmental experiences. Health care professionals must assist adolescents (and parents, if applicable) to be their own advocate for their health and developmental needs.

References

Allen, P. J. (2004). The primary care provider and children with chronic conditions. In P. J. Allen & J. A. Vessey (Eds.). *Primary care of the child with a chronic condition* (4th ed., pp. 3–22). St. Louis, MO: Mosby.

Allen, P. J., & Vessey, J. A. (Eds.). (2004a). *Primary care of the child with a chronic condition* (4th ed.). St. Louis, MO: Mosby.

Allen, P. J., & Vessey, J. A. (2004b). School and the child with a chronic condition. In P. J. Allen & J. A. Vessey (Eds.). *Primary care of the child with a chronic condition* (4th ed., pp. 71–87). St. Louis, MO: Mosby.

American Academy of Pediatrics, Committee on Children with Disabilities. (2001). Counseling families who choose complementary and alternative medicine for their child with chronic illness or disability. *Pediatrics, 107*, 598–601.

American Academy of Pediatrics, Committee on Children with Disabilities. (2000). Provision of educationally-related services for children and adolescents with chronic diseases and disabling conditions. *Pediatrics, 105*, 448–451.

American Academy of Pediatrics, Committee on Children with Disabilities. (1999). The pediatrician's role in development and implementation of an Individual Education Plan (IEP) and/or an Individual Family Service Plan (IFSP). *Pediatrics, 104*, 124–127.

Americans with Disabilities Act (ADA) of 1990, PL 101-336, 42 U.S.C. 12101 *et seq.* (1990).

Batshaw, M. L. (Ed.). (2002). *Children with disabilities* (5th ed.). Baltimore: Paul H. Brookes.

Bunch, G., & Valeo, A. (2004). Student attitudes towards peers with disabilities in inclusive and special education schools. *Disability & Society, 19*(1), 61–77.

Clair, E. B., Church, R. P., & Batshaw, M. L. (2002). Special education services. In M. L. Batshaw (Ed.). *Children with disabilities* (5th ed., pp. 589–606). Baltimore: Paul H. Brookes.

Cohn, D. (2002, July). U.S. counts one in 12 children as disabled. Census reflects increase of handicapped youth. *The Washington Post*, p. B1(2).

Developmental Disabilities Assistance and Bill of Rights Act of 2000, Pub. L. No. 106-402, 114 Stat. 1677 (2000).

Education for All Handicapped Children's Act of 1975, Pub. L. No. 94-142, 89 Stat. 773 (1975).

Feldman, R. (2003). *Child development* (3rd ed.). Upper Saddle River, NJ: Pearson Education.

Green, M., & Palfrey, J. S. (Eds.). (2002). *Bright futures: Guidelines for health supervision of infants, children, and adolescents* (2nd ed., rev.). Arlington, VA: National Center for Education in Maternal and Child Health.

Individuals with Disabilities Education Act Amendments of 1997, PL 105-17, 20 U.S.C. 1440 *et seq.* (1997).

Maternal and Child Health Bureau, Health Resources and Services Administration. (2001). *All aboard the 2010 express: A 10-year action plan to achieve community-based service systems for children and youth with special health care needs and their families.* Rockville, MD: Author.

Nehring, W. M., Faux, S. A., Ito, J., & Braun, P. A. (2004). *Transitional and health issues for adults with NTDs.* Unpublished manuscript.

Newacheck, P. W., & Halfon, N. (1998). Prevalence and impact of disabling chronic conditions in childhood. *American Journal of Public Health, 88,* 610–617.

Rehabilitation Act of 1973, PL 93-112, 29 U.S.C. 701 *et seq.* (1973).

U.S. Department of Education, Office of Special Education Programs. (2002). *Racial/ethnic composition (number) of students ages 6–21 served under IDEA, Part B by disability, during the 2001–2002 school year—All disabilities.* Retrieved August 31, 2003, from http://www.idea-data.org/tables25th/ar_aa15.htm

U.S. Public Health Service. (2002). *Closing the gap: A national blueprint for improving the health of individuals with mental retardation. Report of the Surgeon General's conference on health disparities and mental retardation.* Washington, DC: Author.

Vessey, J. A., & Rumsey, M. (2004). Chronic conditions and child development. In P. J. Allen & J. A. Vessey (Eds.). *Primary care of the child with a chronic condition* (4th ed., pp. 23–43). St. Louis, MO: Mosby.

Woodruff, T. J., Axelrad, D. A., Kyle, A. D., Nweke, O., & Miller, G. G. (2003). *America's children and the environment: Measures of contaminants, body burdens, and illness* (2nd ed.) (EPA 240-R-03-001). Washington, DC: U.S. Environmental Protection Agency.

Transition to Adulthood

Cecily Betz, RN, PhD, FAAN

11

Objectives

At the completion of this chapter, the learner will be able to:

1. Cite the factors that are important in preparing youth for transition to adulthood.
2. Discuss the relevance of adult outcomes to planning and implementing transition programs for youth.
3. Define transition as specified in federal legislation such as the Individuals with Disabilities Education Act (IDEA) and service systems.
4. Identify the relevance of federal legislation and its application to programs and services for youth in transition.
5. Discuss the factors that facilitate and hinder the transition to adulthood.
6. Describe the interagency services approach for facilitating successful transition from youth to the adult service systems.
7. Describe nurses' and other health care professionals' roles in facilitating the adolescent's transition to adulthood.
8. Describe methods of assessment to facilitate the adolescent's transition.
9. Describe models of intervention to facilitate the adolescent's transition.

Key Points

- Transition planning and implementation must be adolescent-centered and based upon the needs, interests, and preferences of the adolescent.
- Transition planning and implementation must be based upon the principles of self-determination and self-advocacy.
- Successful transition planning and implementation involves interagency collaboration.
- Transition planning and implementation will be more successful if based on the extent to which the adolescent can communicate wants and desires.

I.   Background Information

A.   Mortality and morbidity (Betz, 2003a; Hughes, 2001; Lewis, Lewis, Leake, King, & Lindemann, 2002)

1.   Medical and technological advances have improved the level of care provided to individuals with I/DD.

2.   Life expectancy of children with I/DD has improved dramatically, resulting in greater numbers living into their fifties and sixties.

3.   Extended life spans of individuals with I/DD have resulted in the development of secondary conditions and health problems related to the aging process.

B.   Service delivery (U.S. Public Health Service, 2001)

1.   Service need has developed for long-term, comprehensive services and support for individuals with I/DD due to their extended life expectancy.

2.   Services provided are based upon the best practices model that is adolescent-centered, coordinated, community-based, comprehensive, and culturally competent (Betz, 2003b; National Maternal and Child Health Bureau, 2004).

3.   Service system linkages are needed between service systems for children and adults (School to Work Interagency Transit Partnership Consumer/Parent/Family Coalition, 1996).

a.   Services for children can be clustered in one setting, such as school settings wherein the child can receive educational, health, habilitation, and work-based skills training.

b.   Pediatric health care service models for children and youth with I/DD are family-centered and interdisciplinary, in contrast to adult models that are specialty oriented and client-centered in approach.

c.   Interagency service system linkages are considered a model of "best practice."

i.   Interagency coordination is an ideal goal, yet difficult to achieve due to:

a.   Agency culture and requirements

b.   Lack of personnel and fiscal resources enabling interagency coordination

c.   Regulatory mandates preventing co-mixing of funds and shared authority for services

d.   Agency personnel resistance to interagency service coordination

e.   Lack of personnel skill in working collaboratively

f.   Lack of agency commitment and leadership to work collaboratively

4.   Interagency collaboration is needed to ensure the adolescent receives an array of transition services to achieve adult outcomes (Individuals with Disabilities Education Act Amendments of 1997, 1997).

    a. Adult service systems for youth with I/DD include:

        i.   Health care

        ii. I/DD

        iii. Rehabilitation

        iv. Job development

        v.   Education

        vi. Mental health

        vii. Community colleges/universities (disabled student services)

        viii. Social security

        ix. Community-based residential providers

        x.   Independent living centers

    b. Each agency has it own methods for determining eligibility, procedure for referral, and array of services, which can be overwhelming for the youth and family.

C. Scope of the problem: Statistics on employment, community living, social life, and leisure

   1. Social Security beneficiaries (U.S. General Accounting Office (GAO), 1998)

      a. 7.5 million persons with general disabilities receive income assistance.

      b. Supplemental Security Income (SSI)/Social Security Death Index (SSDI) program costs $73 billion annually.

      c. SSI/SSDI costs are projected to increase 6% per year.

      d. SSI/SSDI disability payments are the fourth largest federal entitlement expenditure.

      e. Less than one-half of 1% of beneficiaries leave Social Security rolls and become self-sufficient. Employment of 75,000, or just 1% of the 7.5 million people with disabilities, would amount to $3.5 billion in savings.

   2. Employment rates of individuals with disabilities (Disability Statistics Center, 1998; National Organization on Disability (NOD), 2002; NOD/Louis Harris & Assoc. Inc. (Harris), 2000; Stoddard, Jans, Ripple, & Kraus, 1998; U.S. GAO, 1996)

      a. 50% to 75% of people with all types of disabilities are unemployed.

      b. 32% of people with disabilities from 18 years to 64 years are employed full or part-time, compared to 81% of people without disabilities.

      c. Individuals with more severe disabilities are less likely to be employed than individuals with less severe disabilities.

      d. 35.1% of individuals with mental retardation are employed.

      e. Approximately 75% of people with developmental disabilities are unemployed.

f. Unemployment rates for individuals with developmental disabilities have not changed since 1911.

g. 10 million people with all disabilities report annual income of less than $10,000.

h. 25% of jobs held by people with disabilities are food preparation and service, sales, and machine operator jobs.

3. Community living outcomes (NOD/Harris, 2000)

a. 50% to 75% of the 300,000 students with disabilities who leave the public school system annually do not live independently.

b. 50% to 70% of individuals with severe disabilities live in various types of residential placements such as community care facilities (ranging from more than 50 beds to 15 beds), group homes (less than 6 beds), and supported and independent living arrangements (1–3 beds).

c. 30% to 40% of individuals with severe disabilities live with family members and relatives.

D. Socioeconomic status of working age individuals (NOD/Harris, 2000)

1. 29% of people with disabilities live on or below the poverty line, compared to 10% of people without disabilities.

2. 16% of people with disabilities live in households with incomes more than $50,000 annually, compared to 39% of people without disabilities.

II. Federal Legislation Relevant to Transition

A. Individuals with Disabilities Education Act (IDEA) (P.L. 105-17) (1997)

1. IDEA was enacted in 1990, expanding upon previous legislation (Public Law 94-142) designed in 1975 to provide educational opportunities for children with disabilities. It specifies that children with disabilities are entitled to free and appropriate education in the least restrictive setting.

2. This legislation specified transition services, meaning that individualized educational plans (IEP) were to include plans for the student's transition from school to work. If transition needs were not addressed in the IEP, then the school was considered to be out of compliance.

3. IDEA (P.L.105-17) was reauthorized June 4, 1997. Changes in the reauthorization became effective July 1, 1998 (IDEA '97 Final Regulations, 1998).

a. Section 602 (d) (Code of Federal Regulations 34CFR Part 300 Section 300.27). This section of the IDEA reauthorization provides a description of the intent of the law regarding IEP transition services. "Transition services refers to a coordinated set of activities for a student, designed within an outcome-oriented process, which promotes movement from school to post school activities." (IDEA, 1997, pp. 13–14)

    i. Coordinated set of activities refers to these areas:

      a. Instruction

      b. Related services

      c. Community experiences

      d. Employment and other post-school activities

    ii. Outcome oriented in terms of student achievement.

    iii. Post-school services and activities need to be included in the IEP.

    iv. Transition services must be based upon the student's preferences, interests, and needs.

  b. Section 300.347 (b)(1)(2). This section describes the changes in the IEP requirements for transition services. "Beginning at age 14, and updated annually, the IEP must include a statement of the transition service needs of the child under the applicable components of the child's IEP." Furthermore, "Beginning at age 16, (or younger if determined appropriate by the IEP), a statement of needed transition services for the child including, when appropriate, a statement of the interagency responsibilities or any needed linkages" (Authority: 20 U.S.C. 1414(d)(1)(A) and (d)(6)(A)(ii)) (IDEA, 1997).

  c. Section 300.344 (a). This section further clarifies the school's role in facilitating interagency linkages. "The public agency also shall invite a representative of any other agency that is likely to be responsible for providing or paying for transition services." Furthermore, "If an agency invited to send a representative to a meeting does not do so, the public agency shall take other steps to obtain participation of the other agency in the planning of any transition services" (Authority 20 U.S.C. 1401 (30), 1414 (d)(1)(A)(7), (b)) (IDEA, 1997).

B. Carl D. Perkins Vocational and Applied Technology Education Act of 1998 (P.L. 105-332) (Kilburn & Pittman, 1996)

  1. Provides legislative authority and funding for vocational and technical training and supported employment programs in each state that lead to high skill and high wage jobs.

  2. Students with I/DD are to be included in school district programs that receive Perkins funds.

  3. Funds can be used for the costs of vocational and technical education services identified in the student's IEP/504 Plan.

  4. Students with I/DD and their parents are to be informed of programs available prior to entering grade 9.

    a. Vocational educational opportunities available

    b. Eligibility requirements

    c. Courses available

      d. Available employment opportunities

      e. Job placements

C. School to Work Opportunities Act of 1994 (P.L. 103-239)

    1. Legislation provides funds for five years to states to create statewide partnerships among education, business, labor, and the community to prepare youth for jobs and careers of the future.

    2. Programs are based upon the principles of career awareness and planning, work- and school-based learning, and connecting activities between the school setting and business community (National Transition Alliance for Youth with Disabilities, 1996).

    3. School-to-work programs are to provide inclusive opportunities for students with disabilities—programs that are not segregated or separated from their peers without I/DD.

D. The Americans with Disabilities Act (ADA, 1990) (P.L. 101-336)

    1. This civil rights legislation extends protection against discrimination to individuals with disabilities. This legislation has important application for youth in transition and their families as it provides them rights and protections to ensure educational, community, and work settings are accessible and reasonable accommodations are provided if needed.

      a. Based upon principles of accessibility, reasonable accommodations, and nondiscrimination.

      b. Addresses four major areas of need: employment, public facilities, transportation, and communication.

      c. Educational institutions:

        i. Are required to make reasonable modifications in policies, practices, or procedures to prevent discrimination.

        ii. Must make physical modifications to ensure accessibility.

        iii. Must ensure participation in school activities (field trips, athletic events).

        iv. If student is involved in work-based learning, must make necessary accommodations to enable the student's full participation are needed.

        v. Private schools are expected to make reasonable accommodations and provide equal treatment for students with disabilities.

III. Obstacles to Transition (Betz, 2003a; Betz & Redcay, 2002; Geenen, Powers, & Sells, 2003; Harman, Bender, & Linden, 2000; McDonagh, Foster, Hall, & Chamberlain, 2000; Scal, 2002)

A. Intrapersonal factors

    1. No work-based experience prior to leaving school.

    2. Lack of skill training in self-care, community living.

B. Familial factors

1. Lack of family support.

2. Parental/caregiver overprotectiveness and having difficulty "letting go."

3. Lack of family resources for out of pocket expenses, replacement equipment and supplies, and newer technological aids such as computers

4. Cultural values and beliefs—may not believe independent living and employment are acceptable.

5. Single parent/caregiver.

6. Family coping and ability to access community services are inadequate.

C. Community factors

1. Lack of system coordination between agencies.

2. Lack of available community resources such as Section 8 housing, disability-related services and supports, and limited paratransit services.

3. Level of competency/knowledge of service provider is inadequate.

D. Resources

1. Adult service systems differ significantly from pediatric.

2. Service model differences (family-centered vs. individually-oriented).

3. Cumbersome eligibility determination process for adult services.

4. In contrast to pediatrics, state stipends go to agencies rather than families.

5. Agency cultures create barriers for families (unfamiliar terminology and regulations).

6. Adult service providers may be unfamiliar with pediatric condition and treatments.

IV. Factors That Impact Transition (Betz, 2003a; Blacher, 2001; Kagan-Krieger, 2001; Wehman, 1998)

A. Interpersonal factors

1. Level of motivation

2. Developmental readiness

3. Personality characteristics

4. Self-esteem

5. Coping ability

6. Level of functioning in terms of cognitive level

7. Limitations associated with disability such as gross and fine motor behaviors

8. Level of maturity

9. Previous life experiences

10. Level of self-sufficiency with activities of daily living

11. Level of independence in managing health care, self care, and long-term disability management

B. Familial factors

1. Family support

2. Family access to and use of community resources

3. Family's level of functioning

C. Community factors

1. Available community resources

2. Interagency service coordination.

V. Interagency Approach to Services (Betz, 2003b; DeStefamo & Hasazi, 2000)

Achievement of successful adult outcomes can be facilitated with an interagency approach. An interagency approach enables providers from different service systems to collaborate and formulate a comprehensive plan for determining future vocational training, employment, and community living.

A. Referrals to community services and supports will be dependent on the adolescent's needs, preferences, and interests as identified in the student's IEP.

1. IDEA specifies that the IEP includes information on interagency services by age 16 years. Interagency services can include:

a. Department of rehabilitation—Provides services in the areas of community life and employment in order to help the consumer to achieve economic self-sufficiency and independence.

i. After eligibility is determined and individualized plan for employment (IPE) is developed

ii. Services provided include:

a. Vocational training

b. Purchase of work-related equipment and supplies

c. Job search and placement

d. Job coaches

e. Work-site job training

b. Disabled student services (DSS)—Disability resource center on university and community college campuses that assists students with access and accommodations.

i. Student must provide documentation of disability. Type of documentation needed is dependent upon the type of disability. DSS campus office should be contacted to inquire about the type of documentation required as variations will exist at each campus.

    ii. Services provided include:

       a. Accessible parking

       b. Accessible campus housing

       c. Mobility assistance

       d. Interpreters

       e. Large print texts

       f. Alternative work assignments

       g. Accommodations for test taking

       h. Accommodations for work assignments

B. Workforce Investment Partnership Act (PL 105-220), enacted on August 7, 1998, created new provisions for serving adolescents ages 14 to 21 years. Programs funded by the Workforce Investment Act (WIA) are required to provide 10 core service elements to adolescents with I/DD that are designed to better prepare them for the workforce:

   1. Tutoring and study skills

   2. Alternate secondary school services

   3. Summer employment

   4. Paid and unpaid experiences

   5. Occupational skills training

   6. Support services

   7. Guidance and counseling

   8. Leadership development

   9. Adult mentoring

   10. 12-month post-program follow-up

C. Developmental disability service system—Provides case management services to individuals with I/DD using a person-centered approach to determine the array of services and supports needed to live in inclusive, community-based settings. The goal of services is to promote the independence, productivity, and inclusion of individuals with I/DD across the lifespan.

   1. Individualized, person-centered plan is developed based upon the individual's needs, preferences, and interests.

   2. Services provided include:

      a. Community skills training

      b. Vocational training

      c. Mobility training

      d. Social skills training

      e. Health care self-care skills training

      f. Residential services

      g. Transportation services

      h. Health care services

      i. Attendant services

D. Educational system—Transition services are provided that will help the student to access needed adult services and achieve optimal adult outcomes.

    1. Once the student reaches 14 years of age, an IEP is developed that addresses the need for transition planning.

    2. Transition planning can include the following services:

      a. Work-based experiences in community settings

      b. Learning of community living skills

      c. Mobility training

      d. Coordination with other community-based agencies (see Section 4, Betz, 1998b; Betz, 1998a; Betz, 2003a; Betz & Redcay, 2002)

E. Health care system—Facilitates the transition of individuals with I/DD from pediatric to adult health care settings (Betz, 1998b; Betz, 1998a; Betz, 2003a; Betz & Redcay, 2002).

    1. Preparation for transitioning to adult health care provider and health care services begins early in adolescence (Blum, 1995).

    2. Transition planning includes the following:

      a. Assessment of health care self-sufficiency conducted by the nurse or other health care professional (see Appendix 11.1)

        i. Identification of needs

        ii. Identification of acquired health care self-care skills

      b. Development of plan to acquire health care self-care skills

      c. Has access to primary and specialized adult health care services

VI. Key Indicators of Successful Transition as Evidenced by Successful Adult Outcomes

A. Employment—Participates in job training program or is employed in job of choice.

B. Residential options—Lives in an inclusive setting in community of choice.

C. Leisure—Participates in recreational and leisure activities of choice.

D. Health care—Demonstrates optimal health outcomes.

VII. Nurse's Role in Facilitating Transition (Betz, 1999)

A. Nurse's role will depend upon the service setting.

    1. School—The school nurse can serve as a member of the IEP team and provide input on the impact of health concerns upon the adolescent's needs, preferences, and goals for transition planning. The nurse can serve as a liaison between the youth's specialized medical team in the health care setting and the school setting.

    2. Secondary/Tertiary care settings—The pediatric nurse in acute care settings can reinforce and support the goals of the adolescent's ITP by identifying the health-related needs to consider for accommodation and for developing self-sufficiency competencies.

    3. Primary care setting—The nurse practitioner participates in the adolescent's transition in ways similar to nurses in tertiary care settings. Additionally, the nurse practitioner is in a pivotal position to refer the youth to community resources and agencies that will provide assistance in accessing adult programs and services.

B. Nursing process (Betz, 1998b, 1999)

    1. Assessment

        a. Assess adolescent readiness for transition (standardized tools can be used to assess components of transition readiness, see Appendix 11.1).

            i. Developmental readiness to assume increasing responsibility for self-care in managing health care needs

            ii. Previous experience in assuming responsibility

            iii. Ability to exercise mature judgement

            iv. Problem-solving ability

            v. Decision-making ability

            vi. Coping ability

            vii. Level of family support for assuming additional responsibility and becoming self-sufficient

        b. Assess current unmet health care needs and concerns.

        c. Assess need and extent to which transition planning has addressed adolescent's goals and dreams for the future.

    2. Planning and intervention—Based upon the needs identified during the assessment process, an intervention plan will be developed and implemented.

        a. Plan will be coordinated with other service agencies (see Section V) to achieve desired adult outcomes.

        b. Instruction in health care self-care skills will be implemented.

       c.　Referral to primary and specialized adult health care services will be made.

    3.　Evaluation—Achievement of IEP goals is identified as a component of transition planning and acquisition of desired adult outcomes.

       a.　Progress in achieving IEP goals will be assessed on an annual basis during IEP meetings.

       b.　The IEP will be revised/updated as needed.

VIII.　Other Health Care Professionals' Roles in Successful Transition

    A.　The health care professionals' role will reflect the service setting.

      1.　The role of the health care professional in a school setting will vary depending on his or her position within the school. The type and number of health care professionals involved in IEP transition planning will depend on the individualized needs of the student. Health care professionals who could be involved in IEP transition planning include the dietician, dentist, pediatrician, occupational therapist, physical therapist, social worker, audiologist, speech and language therapist, and psychologist. For example, if the occupational or physical therapist is employed by the school district, this professional would be more readily included as a member of the student's IEP team. However, if the occupational therapist or physical therapist was employed in a health care setting or program such as a pediatric hospital or state Title V program for children with special needs, then their role would be that of a consultant. As a consultant, this health care professional can serve as a liaison between the adolescent's specialized medical team in the health care setting and the school setting.

      2.　The health care professional can serve as a member of the IEP team or as a consultant and provide input on the impact of health concerns on the adolescent's needs, preferences, and goals for transition planning.

      3.　The health care professional in secondary/tertiary care settings can reinforce and support the goals of the adolescent's ITP by identifying the health-related needs to consider for accommodation and for developing self-sufficiency competencies. Examples of useful objectives for transition planning might include learning meal planning if being overweight or obese is a health concern, home physical therapy management program, learning transfer procedures with a new wheelchair, and learning to use a language augmentation devices.

      4.　The health care professional employed in primary care settings participates in the adolescent's transition in ways similar to health care professionals in tertiary care settings. Additionally, the health care professional is in an optimal position to refer the adolescent to community resources and agencies that will provide assistance in accessing adult programs and services such as parks and recreation programs, mental health services, food programs, and mobility training.

B. Transition service approaches (Betz, 1998a, 1999)

1. Assessment

   a. Assess adolescent readiness for transition (standardized tools can be used to assess components of transition readiness) (see Appendix 11.1).

      i. Developmental readiness to assume increasing responsibility for self-care in managing health care needs

      ii. Previous experience in assuming responsibility

      iii. Ability to exercise mature judgment

      iv. Problem-solving ability

      v. Decision-making ability

      vi. Coping ability

      vii. Level of family support for assuming additional responsibility and becoming self-sufficient

   b. Assess current unmet health care needs and concerns.

   c. Assess need and extent to which transition planning has addressed adolescent's goals and dreams for the future.

2. Planning and intervention—Based upon the needs identified during the assessment process, an intervention plan will be developed and implemented.

   a. Plan will be coordinated with other service agencies (see Section V) to achieve desired adult outcomes.

   b. Instruction in health care self-care skills will be implemented and coordinated with other members of the IEP/health care team.

   c. Referral to primary and specialized adult health care and therapy services will be made.

3. Evaluation—Achievement of IEP goals is identified as a component of transition planning and acquisition of desired adult outcomes.

   a. Progress in achieving IEP goals will be assessed on an annual basis during the IEP meeting. IEP will be revised/updated as needed.

IX. Summary

The transition from adolescence to adulthood is a critical period of development that requires individual, family, and professional cooperation and planning. It is important for adult health care professionals to be knowledgeable of conditions resulting in I/DD, the trajectory of these conditions throughout adulthood, and services needed and available in the community in which the individual with I/DD lives.

References

Americans with Disabilities Act of 1990 (ADA). Pub. L. No. 101-336. Title 42, USC 12101 *et seq: U.S. Statutes at Large, 104,* 327–378 (1990).

Betz, C. (1998b). Adolescent transitions: A nursing concern. *Pediatric Nursing, 24*(1), 23–28.

Betz, C. L. (1999). Adolescents with chronic conditions: Linkages to adult service systems. *Pediatric Nursing, 25,* 473–476.

Betz, C. L. (2000). California healthy and ready to work—Transition health care guide: Developmental guidelines for teaching health care. *Issues in Comprehensive Pediatric Nursing, 23,* 203–244.

Betz, C. L. (2003a). Creating healthy futures: An innovative nurse-managed transition clinic for adolescents and young adults with special health care needs. *Pediatric Nursing, 29*(1), 25–30.

Betz, C. L. (2004). CAHRTW: *Transition health care assessment.* Unpublished document.

Betz, C. L. (2003b). Nurse's role in promoting health transitions for adolescents and young adults with developmental disabilities. *Nursing Clinics of North America, 18,* 1–19.

Betz, C. L. (1998a). Facilitating the transition of adolescents with chronic conditions from pediatric to adult health care and community settings. *Issues in Comprehensive Pediatric Nursing, 21,* 97–115.

Betz, C. L., & Redclay, G. (2002). Lessons learned from providing transition services to adolescents with special health care needs. *Issues in Comprehensive Pediatric Nursing, 25,* 129–149.

Blacher, J. (2001). Transition to adulthood: Mental retardation, families, and culture. *American Journal of Mental Retardation, 106,* 173–188.

Blum, R. (1995). Transition to adult health care: Setting the stage. *Journal of Adolescent Health, 17*(1), 3–5.

Carl D. Perkins Vocational and Applied Technology Education Act of 1998. Pub. L. No. 105-332. 20 USC 2301 (1998).

DeStefamo, L., & Hasazi, S. (2000). *IDEA 1997: Implication of the transition requirements.* Minneapolis, MN: National Transition Network, University of Minnesota, The College of Education and Human Development.

Disability Statistics Center. (1998). Employment statistics. Retrieved September 24, 2003, from http://www.dsc.ucsf.edu/main.php

Geenen, S., Powers, L., & Sells, W. (2003). Understanding the role of health care providers during the transition of adolescents with disabilities and special health care needs. *Journal of Adolescent Health, 32,* 225–233.

Harmon, R., Bender, B., & Linden, M.(1998). Transition from adolescence to early adulthood: Adaptation and psychiatric status of women with 47, XXX. *Journal of the American Academy of Child and Adolescent Psychiatry, 37,* 286–291.

Hughes, C. (2001). Transition to adulthood: Supporting young adults to access social, employment, and civic pursuits. *Mental Retardation and Developmental Disabilities Research Reviews, 7*(2), 84–90.

IDEA '97 Final Regulations. (1998). 34 CFR Part 300, Assistance to states for the education of children with disabilities (Part B of the Individuals with Disabilities Education Act). Retrieved November 22, 2002 from http://www.ideapractices.org/law/regulations/index.php

Individuals with Disabilities Education Act Amendments of 1997 (IDEA). Title I-Amendments to the Individuals with Disabilities Education Act, Sec 101. 20 USC 1400 *et seq.* (1997).

Kagan-Krieger, S. (2001). Factors that affect coping with Turner Syndrome. *Journal of Nursing Scholarship, 33*(1), 43–45.

Kilburn, J., & Pittman, C. (1996). *Transition plans: Guide to the future*. Sacramento, CA: California Department of Education, Special Education Division.

Lewis, M. A., Lewis, C. E., Leake, B., King, B. H., & Lindemann, R. (2002). The quality of health care for adults with developmental disabilities. *Public Health Reports, 117,* 174–184.

Maternal Child Health Bureau. (2004). *Achieving and measuring success: A national agenda for children with special health care needs*. Retrieved October 25, 2004 from http://www.mchb.hrsa.gov/programs/specialneeds/measuresuccess.htm

McDonagh, J., Foster, H., Hall, M., & Chamberlain, M. (2000). Audit of rheumatology services for adolescents and young adults in the UK. British Paediatric Rheumatology Group. *Rheumatology, 39,* 596–602.

National Organization on Disability. (2002). *What is the employment gap?* Retrieved September 23, 2003 from http://www.nod.org/content.cfm?id=968

National Organization on Disability/Louis Harris and Associates, Inc. (NOD/Harris). (2000). *2000 NOD/Harris survey of Americans with disabilities*. Washington, DC: Author.

National Transition Alliance for Youth with Disabilities. (1996). School to Work Opportunities Act (STWOA). *Alliance: The Newsletter of the National Transition Alliance, 1*(2), 6.

Powers, L., Singer, G., & Sowers, J. (1996). *Promoting self-competence in children and youth with disabilities: On the road to autonomy*. Baltimore: Paul H. Brookes.

School to Work Interagency Transition Partnership Consumer/Parent/Family Coalition. (1996). *Best practices for transition services from school to adult life from the consumer/family viewpoint*. Sacramento, CA: Author.

School to Work Opportunities Act of 1994, Pub. L. No. 103–239, 108 Stat. 568 (1994).

Stoddard, S., Jans, L., Ripple, J., & Kraus, L. (1998). What occupations are held by people with a work disability who are employed? *Chartbook on Work and Disability in the United States, 1998*. Washington, DC: U.S. National Institute on Disability and Rehabilitation Research.

U.S. Department of Health and Human Services. (2002). *New Freedom initiative: Fulfilling America's promise to people with disabilities*. Retrieved December 1, 2002 from http://www.hhs.gov/newfreedom

U.S. General Accounting Office. (1996). Report to the Chairman, Subcommittee on Employer-Employee Relations, Committee on Economic and Educational Opportunities, House of Representatives. *People with disabilities: Federal programs could work together more efficiently to promote employment*. (Publication No. GAO/HEHS 96-126). Washington, DC: Author.

U.S. General Accounting Office. (1998). Report to the Chairman, Subcommittee on Social Security, Committee on Ways and Means, House of Representatives. *Social security disability insurance: Multiple factors affect beneficiaries' ability to return to work*. (Publication No. GAO/HEHS-98-39). Washington, DC: Author

Wehman, P. (1998). *Life beyond the classroom: Transition strategies for young people with disabilities* (2nd ed.). Baltimore: Paul H. Brookes.

Workforce Investment Partnership Act of 1998, Pub. L. No. 105-220, §401, 112 Stat. 1092 (1998).

California Healthy and Ready to Work
Transition Health Care Assessment

PLEASE CIRCLE ONE:

Yes   No   N/A   W/A*

Have knowledge of your health condition and how to take care of yourself:

1.   Do you understand what caused your medical condition?   Yes   No   N/A   W/A

2.   Do you understand the changes/symptoms caused by your medical condition?   Yes   No   N/A   W/A

3.   Do you manage your daily treatment needs?   Yes   No   N/A   W/A

4.   Do you have any problems with your daily treatment needs?   Yes   No   N/A   W/A

5.   Do you understand the action of the medications you take?   Yes   No   N/A   W/A

6.   Do understand the laboratory and diagnostic
       tests you have taken?   Yes   No   N/A   W/A

What you do to keep healthy:

1.   Do you have a primary care physician (PCP) that you see regularly?   Yes   No   N/A   W/A

2.   Are you up-to-date with immunizations and health care screenings?   Yes   No   N/A   W/A

3.   Do you use alcohol, cigarettes, drugs, or engage in unprotected sex?   Yes   No   N/A   W/A

4.   Do you use self-protection devices such as wearing orthotics/helmet?   Yes   No   N/A   W/A

5.   Do you wear a Medic-Alert bracelet/necklace?   Yes   No   N/A   W/A

6.   Do you exercise regularly?   Yes   No   N/A   W/A

7.   Do you see a dentist on a regular basis?   Yes   No   N/A   W/A

8.   Do you brush and floss your teeth?   Yes   No   N/A   W/A

9.   Do you know when you re getting sick, such as a cold or urinary tract infection?   Yes   No   N/A   W/A

What to do in an emergency:

1.   Do you have a phone to use in case of an emergency?   Yes   No   N/A   W/A

2.   Do you have the phone numbers of family and friends to call in
       emergencies?   Yes   No   N/A   W/A

3.   Do you have the phone numbers of health and nonhealth emergency
       services, and a poison control center?   Yes   No   N/A   W/A

4.   Do you know where the closest ER is?   Yes   No   N/A   W/A

5.   Have you notified the fire department of your special needs and
       developed an emergency evacuation plan?   Yes   No   N/A   W/A

6.   Have you notified the gas/electric companies of your additional service needs?   Yes   No   N/A   W/A

Have needed environmental modifications/accommodations:

1.   Do you have the electrical modifications or other durable equipment that you need?   Yes   No   N/A   W/A

*With Assistance

2. Do you have storage space for your supplies and equipment?   Yes   No   N/A   W/A

3. Does your home have wheelchair ramps and other modifications (doors, tubs)?   Yes   No   N/A   W/A

4. Are you able to properly and safely dispose of supplies (i.e., needles)?   Yes   No   N/A   W/A

Know how to monitor special health care needs:

1. Do you know when to see the doctor?   Yes   No   N/A   W/A

2. Can you recognize when you re getting ill?   Yes   No   N/A   W/A

3. Do you know what situations (increased elevations, large crowds, airport scanners) to avoid for health reasons?   Yes   No   N/A   W/A

Know how to manage your special health care needs:

1. Are you responsible for making appointments with specialty care provider(s)?   Yes   No   N/A   W/A

2. Are you responsible for refilling medications and supplies?   Yes   No   N/A   W/A

3. Do you know when to replace durable equipment?   Yes   No   N/A   W/A

4. Do you have extra/backup supplies or equipment?   Yes   No   N/A   W/A

5. Do you have an attendant(s), home health aide(s), school aide(s), interpreter(s)?   Yes   No   N/A   W/A

6. Are you responsible for their supervision?   Yes   No   N/A   W/A

7. Do you hire the personal attendants/assistants (PAs) that you need?   Yes   No   N/A   W/A

Know how to communicate effectively:

1. Do you know how to seek answers to health-related concerns?   Yes   No   N/A   W/A

2. Do you know how to ask questions of providers?   Yes   No   N/A   W/A

3. Do you know how to obtain appropriate communication devices/systems as needed?   Yes   No   N/A   W/A

4. Do you know how to make contact with teen/young adult support groups/camps?   Yes   No   N/A   W/A

Know how to use community resources:

1. Do you know how to get services in your area?   Yes   No   N/A   W/A

2. Have you used services in your community?   Yes   No   N/A   W/A

3. Are you able to use community transportation when you need it?   Yes   No   N/A   W/A

4. Do you have an individualized health plan developed by the school nurse that is used at your school?   Yes   No   N/A   W/A

Demonstrate responsible sexual activity:

1. Are you able to avoid dangerous situations (exploitation and victimization)?   Yes   No   N/A   W/A

2. Are you able to provide a reliable sexual history?   Yes   No   N/A   W/A

3. Do you know what an STD is and how it can affect you?   Yes   No   N/A   W/A

4. Do you have enough information about contraception and ways to prevent STDs?   Yes   No   N/A   W/A

Appendix 11.1   (*Continued*)

Obtain information and reproductive counseling when needed:
1.   Do you know when to seek reproductive counseling?   Yes   No   N/A   W/A

2.   Do you understand the problems associated with teenage/unplanned pregnancy?   Yes   No   N/A   W/A

3.   Do you think you understand the responsibilities of being a parent?   Yes   No   N/A   W/A

Keep track of health records:
1.   Do you have a copy of your health records?   Yes   No   N/A   W/A

2.   Does your doctor/therapist have a copy of your health records?   Yes   No   N/A   W/A

3.   Do you have an insurance card, or a copy of it?   Yes   No   N/A   W/A

4.   Do you have a method for keeping track of your health care appointments?   Yes   No   N/A   W/A

Have knowledge of health insurance concerns and issues:
1.   Do you know the eligibility requirements for your health insurance?   Yes   No   N/A   W/A

2.   Have you applied for income assistance (SSI) and other public services?   Yes   No   N/A   W/A

Demonstrate knowledge of rights and protections:
1.   Do you have the school/work setting accommodations that you need?   Yes   No   N/A   W/A

2.   Have you contacted the college/university Office of Disabled Students?   Yes   No   N/A   W/A

3.   Do you understand the rights you have under the Americans with Disabilities Act?   Yes   No   N/A   W/A

4.   Have you applied for other public services (social service, vocational rehabilitation)? Yes   No   N/A   W/A

Use transportation safely:
1.   Do you have a driver s license?   Yes   No   N/A   W/A

2.   Do you use buses, trains, or other types of public transportation?   Yes   No   N/A   W/A

3.   Do you use bus or other travel schedules for getting rides?   Yes   No   N/A   W/A

4.   Do you have the money you need to get bus passes/use your car?   Yes   No   N/A   W/A

5.   Do you have any problems in getting to your travel destinations?   Yes   No   N/A   W/A

6.   Do you know transportation etiquette: waiting one s turn,
         getting up for elderly?   Yes   No   N/A   W/A

7.   Do you use Dial-a-Ride, access van?   Yes   No   N/A   W/A

8.   Do you feel safe taking the bus, van, driving?   Yes   No   N/A   W/A

9.   Do you usually arrive and leave on time?   Yes   No   N/A   W/A

10. Do you avoid sitting next to passengers with colds, cough?   Yes   No   N/A   W/A

11. Do you know how you should interact with strangers when traveling/using public
         transportation?   Yes   No   N/A   W/A

12. Do you carry the phone number of friends/family when you travel/use transportation? Yes   No   N/A   W/A

13. Do you let others know when you take trips or leave the house?   Yes   No   N/A   W/A

' Cecily Betz, 2000, 2004

Adulthood

Wendy M. Nehring, RN, PhD, FAAN, FAAMR, and Laura Pickler, MD, MPH

12

Objectives

At the completion of this chapter, the learner will be able to:

1. Identify important elements of health promotion for the adult with intellectual and developmental disabilities (I/DD).
2. Discuss preventive aspects of the health examination for young and middle adults with I/DD.
3. Delineate special considerations for selected genetic conditions.
4. Synthesize factors needed for a successful and satisfactory adulthood.

Key Points

- Health promotion is an essential aspect of good health.
- Health care is comprehensive and involves more than a yearly physical examination from a primary care provider.
- Mental health, economics, informal and formal support systems, religion, and legal factors all impact upon good health throughout the adult years and must be explored in a comprehensive health examination for the person with I/DD.

I.   Health Care for Adults with Intellectual and Developmental Disabilities

All persons with I/DD have a right to receive health care in accordance with acceptable national guidelines according to age, although for certain conditions (e.g., Down syndrome) the guidelines may be altered. It is essential that nurses and other health care professionals follow national guidelines for the health care of all persons, and add criteria if such guidelines are available. Decisions regarding health care should be person-centered whenever possible.

A.   Health Promotion

1.   Health promotion is an important aspect of health care during the adult years (Marks & Heller, 2003).

a.   Education/Prevention—Information on health promotion activities and acute and chronic conditions must be written at a level that can be understood by persons with I/DD. Information written for people with low literacy skills can often be used or adapted when available. Such education can help a person with I/DD to be better informed to make appropriate decisions regarding their health and allow for greater and longer independence. When appropriate, education and health promotion efforts must be person-centered.

b.   Anticipatory guidance—Generally discussed for children, anticipatory guidance should be a part of adult health care. The following elements should be considered:

i.   Changes in physical endurance and mobility

ii.   Changes in weight patterns and bodily changes

iii. Informal and formal support systems

iv. Normal developmental changes in vision, hearing, and dentition

v.   Known condition-specific aging changes and/or normal developmental changes affected by the condition (e.g., premature aging in Down syndrome)

vi. Living arrangements

vii. Recreation

viii. Transportation issues

ix. Future plans, including living will

c.   Access to care issues

i.   Medical home—Every individual has a right to a primary care provider who will manage care across time. This primary care provider has the responsibility to advocate for the individual with I/DD and to coordinate care and billing with insurance programs, including Medicaid and Medicare. Appropriate referrals should be made as needed and include parent support groups and voluntary agencies, such as the United Cerebral Palsy Association and the Arc of the United States (American Academy of Pediatrics, Committee on Children with Disabilities, 1997).

ii.   Extra time is needed for health care appointments, procedures, tests, and education. Often a greater amount of time is needed to establish trust and to decrease fears related to the physical examination, tests, or procedures.

iii. Barriers can be physical, communication, attitudinal, insurance, administrative, and cultural. Often adult health care professionals do not have adequate education regarding the health of persons with I/DD and are unaware of what to ask in a history or what to look for in a physical examination.

iv. Health promotion activities are often omitted for persons with I/DD. For example, classes in smoking cessation are not offered for persons with I/DD; women with I/DD are not given Pap smears as directed by national guidelines.

v.   Diagnostic overshadowing occurs when a complaint is viewed as being related to the condition causing I/DD and not assessed for what is underlying the complaint. For example, a person with spina bifida who is depressed is assessed to be depressed because they have spina bifida, not because a grandparent recently died.

vi. Individuals with I/DD 36 years and older have been found to have choices in doctors, but less coverage for dental care. These individuals are also unlikely to report unmet health care needs, prescription medications, and/or mental health care (Anderson, Larson, Lakin, & Kwak, 2003).

d. Satisfaction with health care—Adults with I/DD need to be made aware of what they should expect from a primary care and/or specialist health care provider. Their satisfaction with care should be ascertained on a regular basis and, when applicable, persons with I/DD should be on advisory committees to clinics and hospitals.

i.   Individuals with I/DD have less positive experiences with health care than do people without I/DD, as reported by Anderson et al. (2003), using data from the 1994 and 1995 National Health Interview Survey.

e. Advocacy—Adults with I/DD have not been instructed on how to advocate for their health care needs, whether for health promotion or for the primary, secondary, or tertiary prevention of secondary conditions. It is important that nurses and health care professionals begin to address advocacy skills in adolescence so that these skills can be operationalized in adulthood. Contacts with individuals with I/DD or organizations that serve individuals with I/DD and/or specific conditions should be identified and contact information provided by health care professionals.

B. Periodic Comprehensive Health Examinations (Agency for Healthcare Research and Quality, 2003)—Many families have kept health records since birth. Some clinics have health records designed for persons with I/DD. If so, the record should continue to be maintained throughout the individual's life.

1. The young adult (20s and 30s)

    a. History—Include family history, birth history, health and school history, personal health habits (including hours and quality of sleep per night and exercise), stressors, age, gender, race/ethnicity, and mental health status or ability to respond to questions independently. Identify who, if anyone, accompanies the person with I/DD. Also identify likes and dislikes, hobbies, employment history, residential setting, and formal and informal support systems. Ask about safety practices (i.e., can call "911," knows CPR, emergency phone numbers, emergency contact info or home phone number, etc.).

    b. Physical examination

        i.   Time of peak strength, energy, and endurance.

        ii. Senses are functioning at sharpest level in life. Visual acuity is keenest during these years. Hearing loss, especially for high-pitched sounds, begins around age 25 years.

        iii. Males will show continued growth in their vertebrae until approximately 30 years.

        iv. Basal metabolic rate (BMR) begins to decline during the 20s, may show weight gain after 25 years.

        v.   Reaction time generally decreases between 20 and 30 years of age; may decrease earlier in certain conditions.

        vi. Hypertension may begin to appear.

    c. Laboratory work.

        i.   Cholesterol—Should be checked every 5 years beginning in males 35 years and older and in females 45 years and older. If risk factors for heart disease are present, such as a history of smoking, diabetes, high blood pressure, and/or a family history of heart disease, then regular cholesterol testing should begin after age 20 years and occur more frequently than every 5 years.

        ii. Fasting blood sugar—If risk factors for diabetes are present: overweight, diabetes during pregnancy, family history, and/or of African

American, Hispanic, American Indian, and/or Alaska Native descent, or taking atypical antipsychotics.

   iii. Prolactin—if on antipsychotics

   iv. TSH

   v. Electrolytes

   vi. HIV or HBV screening if necessary

   vii. Liver function tests—annually if Hepatitis B carrier

   viii. Medication and/or side effect monitoring

d. Specific screening

   i. Assess need for birth control and education (see Chapter 13). Assess PMS.

   ii. Pap smears every 1 to 3 years beginning in early adulthood. May be more frequent if risk factors present such as prior sexually transmitted disease, prior abnormal Pap smears, and/or more than one sex partner. If the woman is not sexually active, may do single-finger bimanual assessment with cytology exam. If either is not possible, a pelvic ultrasound may be warranted every 2 to 3 years. A referral to a gynecologist with expertise with women with I/DD may be needed.

   iii. Annual breast examination should be provided by the primary care provider and education for the woman on monthly breast examinations. May need to role model self-breast examination and have individual with I/DD illustrate skill until successfully demonstrated.

   iv. Osteoporosis—Important to consider whether the person with I/DD is on many seizure or psychiatric medications that can cause osteoporosis or if the person is nonweight-bearing. May appear earlier in persons with neural tube defects. Conduct bone density screening if risk factors present: hypothyroid, long-term polypharmacy, and mobility limitations. Counsel individual with I/DD about need for prevention, to include intake of vitamin D and calcium, exercise, and to quit smoking (Massachusetts Department of Mental Retardation, University of Massachusetts Medical School's Center for Developmental Disabilities Evaluation and Research, 2003).

   v. Cardiac—Assess blood pressure on a regular basis. Re-evaluate cardiac status if individual with I/DD had congenital heart condition.

   vi. Nutrition—Assess daily diet, food allergies, and unusual cravings (see Chapter 16).

   vii. Dental—Assess wisdom teeth and/or gum disease (see Chapter 23).

    viii. Vision—Regular checkups. Assess for glaucoma every 3 to 5 years for high-risk individuals. Test for glaucoma one time during this period if no risk present (Massachusetts Department of Mental Retardation, 2003).

    ix. Hearing—Check during annual examination.

2. The middle adult (40s to 60s)

   a. History—Obtain information as listed above for the young adult. If baseline, at young adult, add information at each visit to update. Continue to be diligent about assessment of secondary or comorbid conditions.

   b. Physical examination

    i. Sensitivity to taste and smell declines, with males experiencing greater decline.

    ii. Sensitivity to touch decreases after age 45 years.

    iii. Sensitivity to pain decreases after age 50 years; also less tolerant of pain.

    iv. Tires more easily as ages.

   c. Laboratory work continues as in young adulthood.

    i. Cholesterol

    ii. Prolactin

    iii. TSH

    iv. Electrolytes

    v. HIV or HBV screening if necessary

    vi. Liver function tests—annually if Hepatitis B carrier

    vii. Medication and/or side effect monitoring

   d. X-rays

    i. Mammogram—Follow practice guidelines, but mammograms should begin every 1 to 2 years starting at age 40 years, and yearly after age 50 years.

    ii. EKG—May take baseline after age 40 years if cardiac concerns present.

   e. Specific screening

    i. Assess presence and symptoms of perimenopause and menopause and use of HRT. Average age for menopause is 51 years, but may be earlier due to specific conditions, such as Down syndrome. Follow current practice guidelines involving HRT.

    ii. Pap tests should continue throughout this period.

iii. Prostate examination beginning at age 50 years. May also consider prostate-specific antigen (PSA) or digital rectal examination. Family history and African American ethnic background are risk factors.

iv. Osteoporosis—As stated above under young adult. Additional risk factor is being a post-menopausal woman.

v. Cardiac—Assess blood pressure on a regular basis.

vi. Skin—Assess for skin cancers.

vii. Nutrition—Continue to assess daily diet in conjunction with exercise. Decreased mobility and hypotonia will likely affect weight and need to assess for secondary effects related to obesity.

viii. Dental—Continue to check on a regular basis for changes in dentition, gums, and periodontal disease.

ix. Vision—Assess for near vision, dynamic vision related to reading moving signs as in driving, light sensitivity, and speed of visual information processing. Vision problems increase after age 45 years. Assess for glaucoma every 2 to 4 years.

x. Hearing—Gradual hearing loss increases after age 50 years and is greater in males.

xi. Colon cancer screening—Beginning at age 50 years. Do fecal occult blood testing yearly. Sigmoidoscopy should be completed every 5 years or a colonoscopy every 10 years (Massachusetts Department of Mental Retardation, 2003).

3. Special considerations for specific conditions

   a. Down syndrome (American Academy of Pediatrics, Committee on Genetics, 2001; Cohen, 1999; Massachusetts Department of Mental Retardation, University of Massachusetts Medical School's Center for Developmental Disabilities Evaluation and Research, 2003; Smith, 2001)

     i. Physical examination should include thyroid function tests (T4 and TSH) and a CBC every 3 years.

     ii. Skin care should be discussed. Skin problems often require prescription medications to correct.

     iii. Audiologic evaluation is required every 1 to 2 years due to risk of sensorineural and conductive hearing loss, which is common.

     iv. A vision examination is also required every 1 to 2 years due to common eye disorders and problems, such as cataracts and keratoconus.

     v. Problems with sleep should be explored, with special attention given to signs and symptoms of sleep apnea.

     vi. Assess for decline in ability to perform activities of daily living.

      vii. Assess for changes in mental status, behavior, and mental health.

     viii. Assess for dementia, such as ataxia, seizures, decline in function, incontinence of stool and/or urine, and memory loss. Differentiate from thyroid problem and/or atlantoaxial subluxation. Alzheimer's disease should only be diagnosed after all other diagnoses are ruled out.

      ix. Assess weight. Examine diet and exercise.

      x. Cardiac—Assess for mitral valve prolapse or aortic regurgitation; may need echocardiogram. Recommend baseline echocardiogram in adulthood if there are no other cardiac records available. If cardiac condition is present, subacute bacterial endocarditis prophylaxis will be required.

      xi. Dental—Continue with biannual visits.

      xii. May want to consider a fasting blood glucose due to increased risk for diabetes. This should occur when symptoms appear.

     xiii. Males should undergo an annual testicular examination due to a higher prevalence of testicular cancer.

     xiv. Spinal cervical X-rays should be considered if signs and symptoms of atlantoaxial instability emerge or if sports participation is planned. May do baseline spinal cervical X-rays as adult. Signs may include weakness, gait disturbances, increased deep tendon reflexes, and spasticity. Symptoms may include torticollis, loss of upper or lower extremity strength, and neck pain.

      xv. Document signs and symptoms of premature aging and consider preventive guidelines for a person older than the individual with Down syndrome when conducting comprehensive health care.

     xvi. Continue language and speech therapy if warranted.

  b. Fragile X (American Academy of Pediatrics, Committee on Genetics, 1996).

      i. Levels of hyperactivity may decrease over time, but shyness and attention problems continue.

      ii. Assess recent history of seizures, which may be atypical, especially if cognitive decline is present.

     iii. Macro-orchidism may be present, but does not interfere with sexual functioning.

  c. Williams syndrome (Prober, 2004).

      i. Audiologic exam every 1 to 2 years. Common problems include moderate high frequency loss and ear wax build-up.

      ii. Thyroid function tests (e.g., TSH) should be performed every 2 years.

      iii. Complete oral glucose tolerance test to assess for diabetes.

      iv. Dental cleaning needs to take place every 3–4 months, rather than biannually.

      v. Assess for gastrointestinal problems, such as constipation, diarrhea, and diverticulitis.

      vi. Assess for mental illness problems, such as anxiety disorder and phobia.

      vii. Assess for premature aging.

4. Secondary conditions exist for many conditions that result in I/DD, such as Down syndrome and cerebral palsy. Nurses and health care professionals need to identify the possible secondary conditions for each condition and then assess for these conditions as part of the health history and physical examination. Discussion and education about secondary conditions is needed at each visit to either prevent their occurrence or limit their effect.

   a. Prevention of secondary conditions.

   b. Identification of secondary conditions.

   c. Interventions for secondary conditions.

   d. Trajectory of conditions. The trajectory of conditions resulting in I/DD across the lifespan have not been described well in the literature. Little is known about these conditions, such as Down syndrome and neural tube defects in adulthood. It is important to document findings so that further discussion and research can occur to describe the health and related secondary conditions of specific conditions throughout adulthood. As this is done, anticipatory guidance can begin in areas of future function and lifespan.

5. Portability of the medical record (An excellent example is the *Health Care Tool Kit* from the Wisconsin Council on Developmental Disabilities, P.O. Box 7851, Madison, WI 53707-7851; 608/266-7826).

   a. Referrals—It is important for the nurse and other health care professionals to identify experts in the care of persons with I/DD in all disciplines to which referrals can be made. Primary care providers need to be aware of specialized clinics and services that are available to their patients. Dentists and psychologists/mental health professionals with expertise in I/DD have been difficult to identify in many communities.

   b. Consultation between health care professionals.

   c. Managed care—Can be a part of an individual's HMO/PPO or state Medicaid/Medicare plan. The nurse and other health care professionals should be aware of the care services reimbursed in each type of plan.

      d.   Medicaid/Medicare—Should be aware of the diagnostic criteria, application requirements, and funding for Medicaid/Medicare in the state in which the nurse and other health care professionals practice.

C.   Immunizations—Recommendations are based on assumption that normal childhood immunizations were received.

    1.   TB—Repeated annually. Follow guidelines if active disease.

    2.   Tetanus-diphtheria booster every 10 years.

    3.   Influenza—Annually beginning at age 50 years or older. May need earlier if history of heart, lung, or kidney disease; cancer; or diabetes.

    4.   Pneumococcal pneumonia—Usually given around age 65 years, but may need to be given earlier if history of heart, lung, or kidney disease; cancer; HIV; or diabetes.

    5.   Hepatitis B

        a.   Three doses should be received once in lifetime (0, 1–2, 4–6 months).

    6.   Varicella/VZV—Two doses should be received once in lifetime (0, 4–8 weeks) for susceptible persons, including persons living in institutional settings or having documented history of disease.

D.   Medications

    1.   Education/appropriate dosing and safety.

    2.   Polypharmacy—Practice safe medication management, including assessing side effects and interactions with other medications.

    3.   Ensure that individuals with I/DD and/or family members are knowledgeable about their medications, their uses, times to administer, side effects, and need to take the full prescription.

II.   Age-Appropriate Lifestyle

Adults with I/DD should have the ability to live their lives as they desire. Decisions should be person-centered whenever possible. Activities should be age and developmentally appropriate.

A.   Exercise and Recreation

    1.   Exercise and recreation programs (e.g., Special Olympics, YMCA, etc.)

    2.   Prevent comorbid conditions, such as heart disease.

    3.   Assess need for adapted exercise programs if there are issues of immobility, use of wheelchair or other adapted equipment, or physical limitations due to health status.

B.   Tobacco, Alcohol, and Drug Use

    1.   Risk assessment

    2.   Education

C. Safety

   1. Personal

      a. Education

      b. First aid—Individuals with I/DD should receive instruction in common first aid practices. This includes knowledge of how to use "911," CPR if able, and how to phone for help.

   2. Environmental hazards should be assessed in each setting in which the individual with I/DD resides or visits frequently. Hazards such as asbestos, lead, smoke, radon, and pesticides can affect health and development.

      a. Living arrangements

      b. Work and/or school environment

      c. Transportation—Assess for accessibility and safety

D. Occupational Hazards

   1. Chemicals, toxins, and physical hazards

   2. Infectious disease hazards

   3. Musculoskeletal injuries

   4. Stress

E. Mental Health (see Chapter 18)

   1. Mental health promotion—Assess activities and things that make a person with I/DD happy and explore how often they are able to do them. How satisfied is the person with I/DD with their life? How would they describe their quality of life?

   2. Depression—Assess whether the depression, if present, is a result of an acute event, such as a move, or a long-term event, such as an abusive parent. Individuals with I/DD often experience the loss of a person due to death, for example, for a longer period of time than a person without I/DD.

   3. Dementia—Assess whether a secondary condition is part of a specific condition resulting in I/DD, such as Down syndrome, or a part of normal aging. In Down syndrome, screen for dementia annually after age 40 years (Massachusetts Department of Mental Retardation, 2003).

   4. Dual diagnosis in a person with I/DD may occur, but should not be diagnosed without thorough evaluation and examination.

F. Planning for a Successful Adulthood

   1. Informed consent—Individuals with I/DD have the right to be informed about decisions regarding their health in a developmentally age-appropriate manner. If English is a second language or the person is hard of hearing, then accommodation must be made so that the individual with I/DD can be assisted to understand the decision to be made so that consent is informed.

2. Guardianship—When an individual with I/DD reaches adulthood, a decision should be made as to whether a parent(s), sibling, or other adult should be made a guardian or whether the individual with I/DD is not in need of a guardian. If possible, this is a decision to be made with or by the person with I/DD.

3. Advanced directives—Should be determined by the person with I/DD after being informed about the alternatives. If needed, a support person to the individual with I/DD should be present to assist in the decision-making process. If the person with I/DD is not able to make their own decisions regarding advanced directives, the guardian may do so (see Chapter 26).

4. Living arrangements—Persons with I/DD may choose to live in a variety of settings, from fully independent to fully dependent on others for their care. An accurate assessment should be made in determining the correct setting throughout the lifespan. Choices will need to be made as to whether an adult with I/DD remains at home with their family or moves out to another setting determined by their needed supports. Nurses and other health care professionals can assist the person with I/DD and their family in making these decisions and suggesting possible locations.

5. Marriage and family—A person with I/DD should have the choice to marry and/or have a family. It is important to determine whether the person with I/DD is capable of caring for themselves and another economically, emotionally, and physically. If not, they should be counseled about the difficulty in successfully fulfilling that role. Before a decision is made to have a baby, the person with I/DD should receive genetic counseling and be counseled about their ability to care for a child in the same ways listed for marriage. The decision to marry and/or have a child is important and must be made after careful counsel and education. In many cases, the person with I/DD does not have an intimate relationship; instead, they build very close relationships with their family members, enjoying being an aunt or uncle, for example.

6. Friendships—These are important to a person's quality of life, including persons with I/DD. Opportunities to develop friendships are very important and should be provided, both for individual and group social gatherings. Often this becomes difficult after a person with I/DD finishes high school due to transportation issues.

7. Employment—Many opportunities are present for persons with I/DD to obtain employment. Staff from the Department of Rehabilitative Services or Department of Labor in each state, for example, can help a person to find a job, if needed. In many cities, social service agencies can also assist in this area.

8. Higher education—General education programs are present in many community colleges and universities for persons with I/DD. Nurses and other health care professionals should be aware of such programs in their county and/or geographical area so that they are able to suggest such programs, if desired, after the person with I/DD completes high school.

III. Summary

Adults with I/DD should receive the same quality of health care and have the same opportunities for normal development throughout their lifetime. Decisions regarding their health and life should be person-centered whenever possible. The individual with I/DD and their family should continue to be active partners in the interdisciplinary team. Preventive health guidelines should be followed except when specific guidelines for specific conditions exist. More information is needed to describe the health and life experiences of adults with specific conditions resulting in I/DD.

References

Agency for Healthcare Research and Quality. (2003). *The pocket guide to good health for adults.* Washington, DC: Author.

American Academy of Pediatrics, Committee on Children with Disabilities. (1997). General principles in the care of children and adolescents with genetic disorders and other chronic health conditions. *Pediatrics, 99,* 643–644.

American Academy of Pediatrics, Committee on Genetics. (2001). Health supervision for children with Down syndrome. *Pediatrics, 107,* 442–449.

American Academy of Pediatrics, Committee on Genetics. (1996). Health supervision for children with Fragile X syndrome. *Pediatrics, 98,* 297–300.

Anderson, L., Larson, S., Lakin, C., & Kwak, N. (2003). Health insurance coverage and health care experiences of persons with disabilities in the NHIS-D. *DD Data Brief, 5*(1), 1–19.

Centers for Disease Control and Prevention. (2004). *Recommended adult immunization schedule by age group and medical conditions. United States, 2003–2004.* Retrieved May 13, 2004 from http://www.cdc.gov

Cohen, W. I. (1999). *Health care guidelines for individuals with Down syndrome: 1999 revision.* Retrieved May 10, 2004 from http://www.denison.edu/collaborations/dsq/health99.html

Marks, B. A., & Heller, T. (2003). Bridging the equity gap: Health promotion for adults with intellectual and developmental disabilities. *Nursing Clinics of North America, 38,* 205–228.

Massachusetts Department of Mental Retardation, University of Massachusetts Medical School's Center for Developmental Disabilities Evaluation and Research. (2003). *Preventive health recommendations for adults with mental retardation.* Boston: Author.

Prober, B. R. (2004). *Adult medical issues.* Retrieved May 10, 2004 from http://www.wiliams-syndrome.org/fordoctors/adult_medical.html

Smith, D. S. (2001). Health care management of adults with Down syndrome. *American Family Physician, 64,* 1031–1038, 1039–1040.

Sexuality

Marilyn J. Krajicek, RN, EdD, FAAN, David Thomas, MA, and Dalice Hertzberg, RN, MSN, FNP-C

13

Objectives

At the completion of this chapter, the learner will be able to:

1. Discuss the implications of having intellectual and developmental disabilities (I/DD) on sexuality.

2. List the objectives of sex education for the child, adolescent, and adult with I/DD.

3. Describe the implications of consent on sexual activity for the individual with I/DD.

4. Describe the importance of social skills in creating and maintaining relationships for individuals with I/DD.

5. Discuss the risks of sexual expression for people with I/DD, including sexually transmitted infections, family planning, and potentially illegal acts.

6. List the rights of individuals with I/DD, including those who live in group homes, with regard to sexuality and expression of sexuality.

Key Points

- Services for individuals with I/DD are family/person-centered, coordinated, community-based, comprehensive, culturally sensitive, inclusive, and continuous across all levels and sites of care.

- Holistic services recognize the uniqueness of each individual with I/DD.

- Individuals with I/DD have the same rights and responsibilities as other members of the community with regard to sexual expression.

- Individuals with I/DD may require support to exercise rights and responsibilities regarding expression of sexuality.

I.   Introduction

The many concerns surrounding the sexuality of people with I/DD have been with us for decades, but we are only now beginning to address them comprehensively. This curriculum has been designed with one key notion about human sexuality in mind. This notion is that human sexuality is best learned—by those with or without I/DD—within the context of human relationships.

II.   Human Sexuality within the Context of Human Relationships

A. People with I/DD are capable of loving, marrying, and feeling sexual pleasure.

1. People with I/DD often learn about their bodies' sexual functioning later than their nondisabled peers.

2. Segregated services may further delay development of appropriate social skills.

3. "Protection against decision making"—People with I/DD are often stripped of their opportunity to practice decision making regarding sexual activity and then they are unable to make a decision when it is necessary to do so.

4. When all sexuality is denied, a person with an I/DD has no opportunity to distinguish between good and bad sexual expression.

5. Keep in mind that the notable differences between adolescents with and without I/DD are primarily in the area of learning adaptations and not in the capacity to love, desire to develop relationships, or ability to enjoy sex (Butler, 1999; Kempton, 1998).

III.   Sexual Development and the Individual with I/DD

A. The presence of I/DD may affect the development of sexuality physiologically, intellectually, and socially.

1. Genetically based conditions, such as Prader-Willi syndrome, may delay the onset of sexual maturity or may result in precocious puberty.

2. Individuals with I/DD may be more likely to develop comorbid conditions that affect sexuality and sexual behavior, such as dementia (e.g., Down syndrome), seizure disorders, attentional disorders, mood disorders, anxiety, and psychotic disorders (e.g., dual diagnosis).

3. Comorbid conditions can affect sexual desire, judgment, sexual dysfunction (such as erectile problems), and asocial behavior.

4. Individuals with I/DD may lack the usual opportunities for development of sexual identity.

5. Mental retardation affects the individual's expression of sexuality.

6. Neurological conditions, such as spina bifida or other conditions causing paresis or paralysis, affect arousal, sensation, and performance related to sexual activity.

7. Disorders of social interaction, which occur with mental retardation and autism spectrum disorders, may lead to social isolation or to misunderstanding of the individual's intentions on the part of others.

8. The changes in roles and responsibilities that come with sexual maturity may be poorly understood by the individual with an I/DD and may lead to undesirable behaviors. Examples include:

   a. Sexual acting out, such as inappropriate touching

   b. Public masturbation

   c. Anger or acting out after refusal by another person (Federoff, Federoff, & Ilic, 2001; Hays, 1999; Koller, 2000; Krajicek & Cassidy, 1997)

B. Sexual development may affect the individual with an I/DD.

1. Hormonal changes may affect the behavior of the individual with an I/DD. Examples include:

   a. Individuals with a seizure disorder may experience lowered control of seizures with puberty and the onset of menses in women.

   b. Individuals may exhibit more labile behaviors with the onset of puberty.

   c. The average age of menarche (first menstrual cycle) has dropped to about 10.5 years: Women/girls with I/DD experience PMS like anyone else, but often symptoms are attributed to other causes such as challenging behavior.

   d. Adolescence is similar for people with I/DD, but typical moodiness may be exacerbated due to fewer opportunities for sexual expression and heightened rejection among peers.

2. Mental retardation affects the individual's ability to successfully adapt to the physical changes of puberty and sexual maturity.

3. The physiologic changes that arise with the onset of puberty are often poorly understood by the adolescent with an I/DD.

4. Individuals with autism spectrum disorders may experience withdrawal or a heightened aggressive behavior in response to frightening hormonal changes, which may be misconstrued as stalking or harassment (Ailey, Marks, Crisp, & Hahn, 2003; Koller, 2000; University of Texas Southwestern Medical Center at Dallas, 2000).

C. Sexual development throughout the lifespan

1. Outline of milestones in the typical sexual development of the individual from birth through death (see Table 13.1)

D. Barriers to learning about healthy sexuality for people with I/DD

Table 13.1 Sexual Development throughout the Lifespan

Age	Physical & Developmental	Behavioral	Psychosocial
<2 Yrs	Psychosexual: Oral stage Needs warm physical contact Children with I/DD can mature typically Trust vs. mistrust Differentiates between "self" and others	Reflexive male infantile erection Self-exploration of genitals Children with I/DD: delayed cognitive development Infants with I/DD: pain, feeding problems = distrust	Gender identity/role: pink–girls, blue–boys Research shows mothers more affectionate with girls Fathers more rough with boys Emphasis on cleanliness/tidiness for girls For infants with I/DD, separation from primary caregivers can cause confusion, withdrawal, and fear of abandonment
2 Yrs	Psychosexual: Anal stage Needs hugging, kissing Gender identity, autonomy Societal expectations and limits Mastery of body, environment	Touching genitals discouraged Neuromuscular control of bowel/bladder Play includes rhythmic motor activities Immobility can inhibit body exploration Immobility can decrease sensory development	Learning giving, receiving, turn-taking All toddlers need limits set on self destructive or socially inappropriate behavior; limits build a child's esteem
3 to 5 Yrs	Increased autonomy, independence Psychosexual: Phallic stage Sense of initiative Language, motor behavior, and fantasy	Pleasure in fondling of genitals Close to opposite-sex parent Immobilization may prevent masturbation Fantasy play with peers important Encourage parent and work play Isolation can inhibit peer/sex play	Sense of privacy, pride Awareness of difference between sexes For children with I/DD, explain their disorder in simple terms Interested in physical differences of the sexes Curious about reproduction, menstruation
6 to 12 Yrs	Psychosexual: Latency period Independent, able to meet basic needs Achievement in social and academic areas Lack of information about sex, sexuality	Genital exposure or inspection of peer Separation of sexes during play Teasing about boy/girlfriends Kissing games Isolation inhibits socialization skills Same-sex friends	Preoccupied with body changes, romantic interests Children with I/DD: parents need to teach self-control and behavior limits to develop a sexual value system Male: body image & penile size stressed among peers
13 to 20 Yrs	Puberty: reproductive ability 11-13 yr: female maturation 13-17 yr: male maturation Teens with I/DD: typical or delayed puberty Unique self-identity	Male: increase in sexual activity at puberty Female: slow sexual interest, peaks at 25-30 yr Masturbation: primary sexual outlet Erotic caressing without coitus common Initial sexual intercourse usually male-initiated	Female: body image/breast size important Male: peers talk about sexual activity, "scoring" Female: peer talk about love, affection, marriage Peers start with same sex, then evolve to mixed peers Social isolation, fears, being different: impede development

Table 13.1 Sexual Development throughout the Lifespan (continued)

AGE	PHYSICAL & DEVELOPMENTAL	BEHAVIORAL	PSYCHOSOCIAL
13 to 20 Yrs (cont.)		Sexual impulse of children with I/DD is typical. Socialization with both sexes. Decision making: sexual activity, responsibility. Responsibility for teen's own disability	Teens with I/DD: sexual impulses often discouraged by adults. Teens with I/DD: often lack information regarding sexuality. Teen girls with I/DD: often increase sexual activity for attention. Self-respect and respect for others
21 to 29 Yrs	Sexual physical maturation completed. Physical attractiveness important. Intimate relationships with both sexes	Premarital coitus common. Female orgasm more common than in past. Duration of foreplay increased from past. Mild I/DD: marriage, family common. People with I/DD: isolation, increased masturbation	Intimacy vs. isolation. Female: career and home responsibilities. Male: often more focused on career and income. Marriage: increased sexual activity. Decreased sexual activity common with children & careers. Persons with I/DD: often independent through vocational program. Solidification of values through peer discussions/exposures
30 to 45 Yrs	Hair thinning, graying, weight increase. People with I/DD: morbidity of disease. Adjustment or frustration with life choices. People with I/DD: physical isolation	Marriage: may have decreased sexual activity. Divorced/widowed: new sexual relationship. Female, never married: abstains or casual sex. Sexual interest: decrease in males, increase in females. People with I/DD may need peer skills. People with I/DD may need limit setting	Generativity vs. stagnation or self-absorption. Time spent in careers, childrearing, family. Promote wellness through health/sex education
46 to 65 Yrs	Decreased hormone production. Both sexes: decrease in sexual response. Decreased strength. Physiological processes slowing. Risk of chronic illness. Sense of well-being and control	Male interest decreased. Female interest may increase without pregnancy risk	Anxiety related to sexual performance and attraction. Female: empty nest syndrome. Male: relieved at less responsibility. Renewed couple relationship and problem solving
> 65 Yrs	Decline in health status. Illness recovery can by prolonged	Female: sex dependent upon past enjoyment and available sexual partner. Male: report more sexual interest than women. May have decreased activity/mobility tolerance	Decreased self-esteem affects sexual interest. Society and media discourage an active senior sex life. Declining opportunities for sexual outlet or expression

Adapted from: Cheatham, King, & Bartz, 1993; Kempton, 1998; Kempton, McKee, Stigall-Mucigrosso, 1997; Morse & Roth, 1994; National Information Center for Children and Youth with Disabilities, 1992; Vivien, 1977.

1. People with I/DD are given many negative messages about sexuality such as:

   a. People with I/DD should not have sex, or do not have sexual feelings and desires.

   b. Disabled bodies are undesirable.

   c. People with I/DD are sexually dangerous and the innocent in society need to be protected from them; or conversely, they are sexually innocent and must be protected from a dangerous society (Ailey et al., 2003; Block, 2000; Greydanus, Rimsza, & Newhouse, 2002; Krajicek & Cassidy, 1997; McCabe, 1999; Walcott, 1997).

IV.　Teaching about Sexuality

A. Sex education is vital because:

1. The risk of abuse is considerably greater among individuals with I/DD than it is in the general population.

2. Misinformation and lack of information can lead to greater occurrence of abuse.

3. Sex education will aid in developing the skills needed to stay safe or to report victimization when it occurs.

4. Individuals with most types of I/DD can have children, so information is needed to prevent unwanted pregnancies.

5. Information about HIV/AIDS is critical as the infection rate among people with I/DD is high.

6. Sex education helps in promoting healthy sexuality and sexual expression. (Greydanus, Rimsza, & Newhouse, 2002; Kempton, 1998; Wheeler, 2001)

B. Children with I/DD may be included in generic sex education programs as long as the information is adapted to the child's unique needs.

1. Specialized sex education programs may be needed for children who require extensive adaptation or who have significant mental retardation.

2. Sex education should target the individual's developmental level as well as their unique learning needs and styles (Ailey et al., 2003; Greydanus, Rimsza, & Newhouse, 2002; Krajicek & Cassidy, 1997).

C. Sex education includes important concepts and skills.

1. Sexuality education begins in early childhood as identify formation begins.

2. Information on how to avoid sexual victimization should be included with regard to children and adults.

3. Early knowledge should include modesty, privacy, gender constancy (knowing what sex you are), and understanding sociosexual relationships like marriage.

4. Language training is essential because it demystifies the language so it can be spoken—people have to know the words to use in order to talk about subject matter. In case something happens, a child needs to have the necessary words to report it.

5. Important skills to develop include initiating and maintaining friendships.

6. Development of good self-esteem and a healthy self-concept is part of the basis for healthy sexuality.

7. Teach positive aspects of sexuality, rather than conveying that sex is something to be avoided by concentrating education on the negatives.

8. Do not punish sexual expression; rather, teach the person the appropriate time and place for it. For example, a child who is masturbating in the living room is instructed that the activity is a private one, and should be performed in a private setting (Ailey et al., 2003; Krajicek & Cassidy, 1997; Walcott, 1997; Waldman, Swerdloff, & Perlman, 1999).

D. Considerations in teaching about sexuality

1. Before you begin teaching about sexuality, determine your own comfort level, knowledge, and ability. Begin where you, the teacher, are at your highest level of comfort and ability.

2. The most effective teacher considers his or her own prejudices, and keeps sex education value-free. If you have strong prejudices, be honest about them, and try to keep them from coloring the information you give. Your students should have information to make their own informed decisions.

3. Assess where students are regarding comfort level, intellectual level, and knowledge.

4. Teach about all aspects of sexuality: the physical (what), social (when and where), and emotional (why) of sexuality.

5. It is often helpful to use slang or common sexual terminology until students begin to understand appropriate medical and technical language. Pair the slang term with the medical term (e.g., "come" or semen).

6. Be honest and direct.

7. Listen to and analyze questions: Decipher what students are asking for and the motives for questions, then offer answers that address these questions.

8. Use a variety of visual and tactile aids and methods of presentation that are appropriate to the students' learning styles and level of functioning. For example, if you are demonstrating use of a condom, use a model of a penis, not a banana, to avoid confusion in learners who may be very concrete.

9. Repeat key points frequently, and ask students to echo what is taught to ensure they grasp the concept.

10. Demonstrate behaviors being taught (modeling) and engage students in role plays when possible and as appropriate to the learner's intellectual level. For

example, if you are teaching that shaking hands is appropriate behavior between acquaintances, shake the students' hands in greeting; do not hug them!

11. Exploit "teachable moments," that is, take advantage of opportunities for teaching that occur in everyday life. For example, if students see a couple holding hands, talk about that behavior and what it means.

12. Before tackling new information, make sure students have learned as best as possible information that has been taught previously.

13. Use assessments where possible to determine students' mastery of materials (Ailey et al., 2003; Guest, 2000; Hingsburger, 1998; Kempton, 1998; Walcott, 1997).

E. Age-appropriate teaching about sexuality (see Table 13.1)

1. Teaching about sexuality to infants, toddlers, and preschool-aged children (ages birth through 5 years)

   a. Discuss sex in a matter-of-fact way, the same as you discuss anything else.

   b. Teach children social skills, beginning at an early age. To develop a healthy sexuality and awareness of self, the young child understands that he is loved and his body is good.

   c. Learning occurs during play and through asking questions.

   d. Young children do not understand adult sexual behavior or abstract concepts. Creating an open environment in which questions are answered accurately and simply is the best approach at this stage.

   e. The young child who is cared for by a few consistent caregivers learns that his or her body is private.

   f. Use correct terminology for body parts and avoid words like "PP" for penis or "bottom" for vagina.

   g. Don't worry about telling a child too much about sex. Children are likely to tune out what they do not understand.

   h. Children sometimes use objectionable language they hear others use. Instead of laughing or scolding the child, calmly explain the meaning of the word(s) and note that many people do not like it when such language is used.

   i. As children mature, they begin to learn modesty, the realization that the body belongs to the self and that others do not have access to it.

   j. Reinforce that "private" means not for seeing or for touching. To accomplish this, be a good model, offer explanations, and be persistent. Strategies include:

      i. Grooming should be done in a private place.

    ii.   Make sure the bathroom door is closed when a child is using it.

    iii.   When (not if) a child makes a mistake, address it immediately by explaining why it is a mistake.

    iv.   As they desire privacy, children should be given it.

    v.   It is very important to reinforce with the child that *private* does not mean *dirty*.

    vi.   When a child with I/DD confuses public with private behavior, she or he may not be able to accurately read social cues. It may therefore be necessary to explain to the child the reaction(s) the mistake evokes in others (for instance, the look of shock on an adult's face).

2.   Teaching about sexuality to school-aged children (ages 6 through 10 years)

    a.   Children in this age group understand more about health, disease, and sexuality.

    b.   They become interested in birth, marriage, and death.

    c.   They often have questions about sex and sexuality. It is important to respond truthfully and calmly to questions; help children to feel more comfortable in asking you about sex. Try to provide an answer to questions posed.

    d.   Avoid lecturing. Although this might alleviate your anxiety, remember that children have a short attention span and will need time to ask questions.

    e.   When you do not know the answer to a question, just say so. Then seek out the answer and share it with the child.

    f.   Children hear about AIDS from TV, friends, and adults. Teach them that people do not get AIDS from being bad. Use concrete examples, such as cuts, to explain how germs get into the bloodstream. Teach them that they should not take drugs.

    g.   Children should receive information about homosexuality, appropriate to their intellectual and developmental level.

    h.   Describe the physical changes that occur before the child reaches puberty (e.g., wet dreams, menstruation, breast development, etc.). Older children are especially interested in this, as their bodies may be beginning to change. Teach both boys and girls about menstruation and erections.

    i.   Discuss more than just biological facts. Children need to learn about values, emotions, and decision making.

    j.   All children need to know how to protect themselves from abuse. It is essential to teach children that it is okay for them to say "no" to adults who ask them to do things they find uncomfortable (see Section VII).

k. Facilitate the development of social skills. Being part of a valued social circle bolsters self-esteem.

l. Discuss friendships with children, who they would like to have as a friend, and what they would like to do with friends.

3. Teaching about sexuality to adolescents (ages 10 years through early 20s)

a. Early adolescents (ages 10–14 years) are entering puberty and become more interested in what their peers are doing, and in conforming with their peers.

b. They MUST know about prevention NOW, regardless of the activities they may or may not be involved in. They need to learn how to say "no" and to have the self-confidence to do so.

c. Teens need to know that sex can have consequences like pregnancy, sexually transmitted infections (STIs), and HIV infection. They should know why sexual intercourse is not healthy for children and that they should wait before beginning it. Protection from STIs should be included. Sources for birth control and condoms should be available.

d. Specific information about HIV and the prevention of HIV

e. Early and middle adolescents (ages 14–18 years) feel that they are invulnerable and often dismiss warnings about pregnancy and sexually transmitted infections and diseases.

f. Emphasize public versus private behavior; in some states 12 years is the age at which unwelcome sexual behavior becomes illegal, and the youth may be labeled as a sex offender.

g. Sex education should include information about sexual preference, sexual activities, birth control, and sexually transmitted diseases, including AIDS, as well as about illegal sexual acts.

h. Sex education should include development of healthy self-esteem as well as basic information on sexual development, hygiene, and behavior.

i. Include information on relationships, such as how to make and keep friends, intimate friendships versus acquaintances, and dating and appropriate behavior with family members, helpers, and strangers.

j. Communication skills are important to learn: nonverbal communication, assertiveness vs. aggression, asking for what you want, hearing and responding to "no," saying "no," and decision making.

k. Late adolescence (19–21 years) is the beginning of adulthood. Sexual identity is formed and solidified and adolescents are emancipating from home.

l. During this age period, adolescents are most like adults, and take on adult sexual responsibilities. Teaching focuses on fine tuning earlier information, with more specific information tailored to the adolescent's health conditions (Ailey et al., 2003; Brown & Jemmott, 2002;

Greydanus, Rimsza, & Newhouse, 2002; Hingsburger, 1998; Kempton, 1998; Melberg-Schweir & Hingsburger, 2000).

F. Teaching methodologies and considerations

1. Use audiovisuals such as slides or videos, coupled with role play.

2. Special curricula for teaching social skills may be helpful; however, many of these curricula are expensive. An example is the Circles curriculum by James Stanfield and Associates, Inc.

3. Social skills may be taught by problem solving specific situations in the students' daily lives.

4. Adults with I/DD who have not received any sex education may require very basic information tailored to their developmental level.

5. Recognize the typical obstacles to learning such as:

   a. Anxiety provoked by staff who are perceived as controlling and powerful

   b. Anxiety around learning due to failure at previous attempts at learning

   c. Anxiety and discomfort about the topic

   d. Anxiety about the topic provoked by the teacher's unease

6. Adjust your teaching to the learning style of the student(s). Determine if the student is:

   a. Able to sequence tasks

   b. Able to understand multistep instructions

   c. Able to tolerate interruption

   d. Able to handle disruptions and distractions

   e. Able to attend to information; can attend better in the morning or the afternoon

   f. More alert in the morning or in the afternoon

7. What has the student been able to learn in the past? What is it about those topics that facilitated learning (e.g., motivation, teaching method, experience)?

   a. Evaluate constantly. Make sure your strategies are working and that the person learning is not becoming frustrated.

   b. Understand how the individual's I/DD affects learning.

   c. Assess whether learner is a visual, psychomotor, or auditory learner (Ailey et al., 2003; Guest, 2000; Hingsburger, 1998; Walcott, 1997).

V. Family Planning

A. Choosing to become a family (this includes males and females)

1. Decision making with regard to pregnancy

   a. Physical risk of pregnancy and childbearing for women with I/DD

   i. Is the woman able to understand the changes her body will go through and the different care it requires with pregnancy?

   ii. Is the woman able to make the lifestyle changes necessary for a healthy pregnancy?

   iii. Is the woman able to keep her prenatal visits consistently?

   iv. Is adequate support available to the woman to successfully navigate these changes?

   v. Is the father of the child involved? If so, does he understand and is he able to make the lifestyle changes necessary to support her (Carty, 1998; Christian, Stinson, & Dotson, 2001; Ehlers-Flint, 2002)?

2. Some women have increased health risks with pregnancy due to their I/DD or co-occurring health conditions (e.g., obesity or diabetes).

3. Teratogenicity of medications for psychiatric or behavioral disorders and/or seizure disorders

4. Effect on the fetus of medications the woman might be taking for conditions related to her I/DD (e.g., thyroid medication for a woman with Down syndrome)

5. Genetic implications: Does the woman or man have a genetic disorder that may be passed on to the offspring? This can complicate parenting greatly and require additional support.

  a. For example, in women with Down syndrome, pregnancy is rare but may occur. One study reviewed 30 pregnancies in 26 women with Down syndrome and found that there were 10 children with Down syndrome, 18 children without it, and 3 spontaneous miscarriages (Quint, 2004; Rogers, Tuleja, Vensand, & Through the Looking Glass, 2004; Welner, 1997).

6. Prospective parents with genetic syndromes should receive preconception counseling if possible; if the prospective mother is already pregnant, the couple should receive genetic counseling. Prenatal testing appropriate to the stage of pregnancy should be performed. Subsequent counseling to aid the couple in the decision to continue or terminate the pregnancy is important. All teaching and counseling should be focused on the couple's developmental level, and inclusion of family members should be considered (DeVries, vanden Boer-van den Berg, Niermeijer, & Tibben, 1999; Ward, Howarth, & Rodgers, 2002; Welner, 1997).

7. Ability to become pregnant—Most women with I/DD will be able to conceive. Factors that may prevent or reduce the possibility of conception include:

  a. Genetic disorders such as Prader-Willi syndrome and Down syndrome

    b. Disorders that occur in the general population, such as a history of pelvic inflammatory disease or tubal pregnancy, which may make conception difficult or dangerous (life-threatening); or polycystic ovarian syndrome

  8. Parenting for the individual with an I/DD

    a. Is the individual(s) cognitively, physically, and emotionally able to provide nurturance and safe care for an infant?

    b. Is the individual(s) able to financially support a child?

    c. Is adequate support available to the individual(s) so they can safely and effectively raise a child?

    d. Is the child's father involved, and what is his understanding of and ability to provide care for the infant (Ehlers-Flint 2002; Kirshbaum & Olkin, 2002; O'Toole & Doe, 2002)?

B. Birth control

  1. Table 13.2 includes a list of birth control methods and advantages and disadvantages of each.

  2. Considerations in choosing a birth control method

    a. Some methods may work better for one individual than others.

    b. Different people prefer different methods.

    c. One should find a method she or he likes, that is easy to use, and that has no medical contraindications (e.g., a woman who has had pelvic inflammatory disease should not use an IUD because of the increased risk of infection).

    d. Some methods require a prescription while some are available without prescription.

    e. Most methods are used by the woman, but some must be used or applied by the man.

    f. Always make sure the method of birth control works or is used when having sexual intercourse.

    g. Some methods are more effective or reliable than others and should be tailored to the individual's lifestyle and physical and cognitive abilities.

    h. Some methods of birth control (e.g., natural family planning) depend on regular menses. Many women with I/DD experience irregular menses; this may be complicated by anti-epileptic and psychotropic medications.

    i. Some methods of birth control have additional preventive health advantages, e.g., the pill protects against formation of liver tumors but does not protect against HIV (Drey & Darney, 2004; Kempton, 1998; Welner, 1999; Zieman et al., 2002).

Table 13.2   Contraceptive Methods for Women with I/DD

Method	Prescription	Advantages	Disadvantages	Considerations for Women with I/DD
Oral contraceptive pill (OCP)	Yes	99% effective; ↓ risk of uterine CA; ↑ risk of breast CA; do not have to use at time of intercourse; ↓ cramps and bleeding; protective for PID, endometrial, & cervical CA; ectopic pregnancy; reversible	Not for smoker or hx of blood clots, stroke, migraines, hypertension, or gallbladder disease; must take daily without fail; ↓ effect w/ antibiotics; ↑ risk liver tumor; ↑ depression	Must remember to take daily; can regulate menses and ↓ cramps and flow; some protective effects on health; may interact with seizure medications; good for adolescents if they can remember to take it
Depo-Provera injection	Yes	97% effective; can be used by woman who cannot use OCP; reversible; lasts 3 months	Weight gain; may cause amenorrhea; delay in fertility when discontinued; may ↑ risk of osteoporosis; ↑ LDL and ↓ HDL	Can regulate menses and ↓ cramps and flow, may stop menses altogether; no pills to remember; may significantly ↑ risk of osteoporosis in women at risk and who take antipsychotics
Norplant	Yes	99% effective; ↓ cramps and flow, ↓ risk PMS; ↓ ectopic pregnancy, ↓ risk endometrial and cervical CA; lasts 5 years	Surgically placed/removed; amenorrhea or irregular bleeding; local discomfort or inflammation, ↑ ovarian cysts	May pick at site or device; can regulate menses; may be preferred over Depo-Provera
Intrauterine device	Yes	98–99.5% effective; do not have to use at time of intercourse; change once a year; ↓ risk endometrial CA; reversible	Best for women who have given birth; ↑ cramps and bleeding; not for women who have had STI or PID*; possible uterine perforation with insertion	Must check string in vagina monthly to determine placement; may increase spotting, bleeding, and cramps; most women with I/DD are often nulliparous
Diaphragm	Yes	94% effectiveness; no systemic effects; some protection from STIs	Must use at time of intercourse; use with contraceptive jelly or cream; ↑ risk UTI; messy; high failure rate	Must be able to stop progress of intimacy to place diaphragm; must have adequate coordination to place
Contraceptive foam	No	Easy to obtain; no side effects; few contraindications; protection from STI	Used at time of intercourse; may cause irritation; ↓ effectiveness	Woman must be able to stop progress of intimacy to apply foam; must have adequate coordination to apply foam vaginally
Condoms	No	97% effective if used properly; easy to obtain; no side effects; no contraindications; protects from STI	Must be used at time of intercourse by male; inspected for tears; must be cooperation between couple	Cooperation between couple to use; must be able to stop progress of intimacy to apply; must be applied correctly
Natural family planning/fertility awareness	No	75% effective; no side effects other than pregnancy	Must be used consistently; woman must be well educated in method; must be no contraindications to pregnancy; best with predictable, regular menses	Must be physically and intellectually able to learn method, take own basal temperature, plot fertile days in cycle, and schedule intimacy appropriately; often irregular menses due to condition or medications
Sterilization—tubal ligation	Yes	Permanent—100% effective after one year; no protection from STI	Requires consent, surgery, and anesthesia; may cause irregular menses; irreversible	Must be able to legally consent to procedure

STI–Sexually transmitted infection
PID–Pelvic inflammatory disease

*IUD can cause recurrence of PID, a severe illness which may cause sterility.

References: Hatcher et al., 1998; Hatcher et al., 2002–2003; Sulpizi, 1996; University of Texas Southwestern Medical Center at Dallas, 2000; Zieman et al., 2002.

3. Male-directed birth control

   a. Condom—the only nonpermanent form of birth control that can be used by the male. When used properly, condoms are 97% effective.

      i. Easy to obtain, no side effects, and protects from STI.

      ii. Males with I/DD may have difficulty planning ahead to use a condom. Males with upper extremity involvement, such as with cerebral palsy, may not be able to apply the condom correctly.

      iii. Individuals with latex allergy or sensitivity should choose nonlatex varieties.

   b. Vasectomy—permanent contraception that involves severing the vas, preventing passage of sperm into seminal fluid. Probably the most effective form of contraception. Advantages and disadvantages for men with I/DD include:

      i. A relatively quick outpatient surgical procedure that is effective and permanent.

      ii. Does not require forethought or planning prior to sexual intercourse.

      iii. Disadvantages include a possible increased risk of prostate cancer, and requirement for informed consent (Hatcher et al., 1998; Sulpizi, 1996; Welner, 1999; Zieman et al., 2002).

VI. Sexual Health

A. Women's health

   1. Adolescence

      a. Young women with I/DD may experience early or late sexual maturation, depending on their underlying medical condition. For example, early maturation, or precocious puberty, may occur in girls with hydrocephalus, obesity, or spina bifida; late maturation may occur in girls with Prader-Willi syndrome or Williams syndrome.

      b. Delayed maturation may occur in girls with Down syndrome.

      c. Menstruation and hygiene are important issues—Many young women with I/DD are inadequately prepared for menarche, and have little or no knowledge of body changes.

      d. In adolescents, menstrual periods are often irregular, making hygiene more difficult. Young women with significant cognitive delays may need assistance with hygiene during their menses.

      e. All young women should receive education on puberty and self-care during menses, as well as sex education.

     f.   Sexual exploitation/abuse is an increased risk for young women with I/DD. Young women with severe cognitive or physical disabilities who require assistance with personal care may have difficulty preventing sexual abuse.

     g.   Rebellious adolescent behavior may take the form of sexual acting out, making them vulnerable to sexual exploitation.

     h.   All women with I/DD should receive instruction on prevention of sexual abuse, and what to do if they are abused (Greydanus, Rimsza, & Newhouse, 2002; Krajicek & Cassidy, 1997; Nosek, Foley, Hughes, & Howland, 2001; Quint, 1999; Welner, 1997).

  2. Adolescent pregnancy—Young women with I/DD may be at a higher risk for pregnancy, unprotected sex, and sexually transmitted diseases.

     a.   Lack of sex education and lack of availability of contraception to young women with I/DD.

     b.   Attitudes of family and caregivers that their "child" has no sexual desires, or misconceptions about fertility.

     c.   Cognitive disability may contribute to lack of awareness of body.

     d.   In an unplanned pregnancy, abortion must be viewed with great caution as a possible option—informed consent is necessary and may be difficult to obtain.

     e.   Pregnancy may result in significant risks to the unborn child and to the mother, due to the physical and emotional immaturity of the young mother. Intellectual and developmental disability significantly complicates these factors (Greydanus, Rimsza, & Newhouse, 2002; Krajicek & Cassidy, 1997).

  3. Adult health—Women and men (see Chapter 12).

  B. Men's sexual and physical health (see Chapter 12).

VII. Sexual Abuse

  A. People with I/DD are more vulnerable to sexual abuse.

    1. Communication difficulties may result in abusers taking advantage of the individual, assuming they will not be able to accuse them.

    2. People with I/DD may have low self-esteem, and be more vulnerable to exploitation.

    3. People with I/DD who require personal physical care may be either more exposed to an abuser or physically unable to resist. This is particularly true for those individuals who live in large institutional settings who may be exposed to a number of different people daily with varying levels of safety.

    4. Lack of knowledge of accepted sexual behavior may lead to abuse.

5. Women with I/DD as likely to experience abuse as other women, and may be more likely to be abused.

B. Individuals with I/DD may not be believed when they report physical abuse, or may not be able to communicate adequately.

1. Providers must have systems set in place to investigate allegations or suspicions of sexual abuse on the part of people with I/DD.

2. In persons who have communication difficulties, or who have severe mental retardation, physical and behavioral symptoms may be detected.

    a. Unusual bruises or injuries without explanation, injury to the genital or anal area, or presence of an STI in an individual who is not known to have consensual sex are all signs of possible sexual abuse.

    b. Behavioral changes such as unusual reticence toward a specific individual or activity (e.g., a day program), fearful behavior, or agitation may suggest abuse.

C. Prevention of sexual abuse

1. Agencies should have policies in place to investigate allegations of sexual abuse.

2. Staff and providers need training in sexuality, so they are comfortable discussing the subject with individuals.

3. People with I/DD need accurate, accessible sex education that addresses staying safe, sexual abuse, and how to report it.

4. Agencies need policies and procedures on providing personal care, e.g., same-sex individuals should provide care (Aylott, 1999; Nosek, Foley, Hughes, & Howland, 2001; Quint, 2004).

VIII. Sexual Expression

A. Individuals with I/DD may require support from family, friends, caregivers, and others to express their sexuality.

1. Caregivers, health, and other service providers may hold negative attitudes toward sexual expression on the part of people with I/DD, whether in group or individual living situations.

    a. Negative attitudes on the part of caregivers may lead to individuals with I/DD experiencing punishment for sexual expression.

    b. In group home or institutional settings, people with I/DD may not have privacy in which to sexually express themselves.

2. Health care providers are responsible for supporting and providing advice and counseling to individuals with I/DD, as well as to couples, to aid them in their sexual expression.

    a. A potential method to be used in counseling individuals with I/DD about sexuality is the Permission, Limited Information, Specific Suggestions, & Intensive Therapy (PLISSIT) model of sexuality counseling

b. The PLISSIT model takes into account varying levels of knowledge and comfort on the part of the counselor, whether a professional sexuality counselor, health care provider, or other care provider.

c. Can help to address education and communication needs on the part of the individual, as well as ways to overcome functional limitations that may interfere with sexual satisfaction.

d. The model includes four levels of intervention: Permission, Limited Information, Specific Suggestions, and Intensive Therapy. The first three levels may be delivered by health or human service providers without specialized knowledge.

e. In the Permission level, the counselor "gives permission" to the individual, by bringing up the topic of sexuality.

f. In the Limited Information level, the counselor offers basic education and addresses specific sexual concerns.

g. In the Specific Suggestions, a sexual history or profile of the individual is prepared to diagnose the sexual problem, determine the cause, and formulate interventions. Interventions may include specific instructions, recommendations as to positioning to overcome functional limitations, or use of devices to enhance sexual pleasure.

h. The fourth level, Intensive Therapy, is usually performed by a professional sex educator, and includes specialized treatment for the sexual problem (Block, 2000; Christian, Stinson, & Dotson, 2001; Esmail, Esmail, & Munro, 2001; Yool, Langdon, & Garner, 2003).

B. Heterosexual relationships

1. People with I/DD experience sexual desire and excitement the same as nondisabled people. The only differences are in individuals with medical conditions affecting sensation, such as spina bifida.

2. They may be less aware of appropriate behavior due to limited opportunities for forming friendships and heterosexual relationships.

3. Opportunities for social activities with the opposite sex, in addition to appropriate support, can aid people with I/DD in developing healthy, mutually satisfactory relationships.

4. It is important for people with I/DD to have privacy for appropriate sexual activity.

5. Both partners should be able to consent to sexual activity (Ailey et al., 2003; McCabe, 1999; Shuttleworth, 2000).

C. Homosexual relationships

1. There is little data on homosexuality and people with I/DD. Some sources suggest that homosexuality is as likely to occur in individuals with I/DD as in the general population.

2. As in any sexual relationship, both partners must be able to consent to sexual activity.

3. People with I/DD who are homosexual should receive teaching about prevention of sexually transmitted diseases and health risks associated with their sexual orientation.

4. Homosexual people with I/DD deserve the same rights and respect as other people with and without I/DD in terms of expressing their sexuality (Ailey et al., 2003; Butler, 1999; Garnets, 2002; McCabe, 1999; Thompson, Bryson & deCastell, 2001).

D. Alternative forms of sexual expression.

1. Some people with I/DD may have significant difficulties with formation of relationships due to the extent or type of their disability. For example, some individuals with autism who do not develop language choose to avoid relationships.

2. Masturbation or self-stimulation may be an option for sexual expression. Masturbation is a pleasurable, releasing experience; it may also be a means for determining what one likes and does not like sexually.

    a. There exists no evidence that masturbation impairs physical health, except when abusive means are used.

    b. Some individuals may masturbate in relation to objects, or may use sex devices when masturbating, including anal masturbation.

    c. Some individuals with I/DD may need masturbation training, both to provide an outlet for sexual tension and to perform it safely.

    d. Masturbation can become a problem when:

        i.   It is done in public, or at an inappropriate time or place

        ii. It is done to excess, causing harm, or in exclusion of other activities

    e. People with I/DD who masturbate may require assistance in determining when and where it is appropriate, and how to masturbate without harm.

    f. When determining the cause of problem masturbation, the provider should consider

        i.   Medical causes, such as urinary tract infection

        ii.   Environmental considerations, such as lack of structured routine, inconsistent or inadequate interventions

        iii. Lack of appropriate education (Ailey et al., 2003; Butler, 1999; Esmail, Esmail, & Munro, 2002; Kempton, 1998; Koller, 2000; Walsh, 2000).

3. Inappropriate sexual behavior

    a. People with I/DD may become involved in sexually inappropriate behavior due to:

        i.   Victimizations by staff or other residents while in an institution

       ii.   Restrictive and punitive early experiences

      iii.   Victimization as a child or adolescent

      iv.   Lack of appropriate sex partner

       v.   Lack of knowledge about the laws and social customs—many children and adolescents without I/DD do not receive clear instruction on acceptable and unacceptable sexual behavior

      vi.   Lack of social skills, or immaturity

b. Although both sexes may be involved in sexually inappropriate behavior, males are most commonly involved.

c. Sexual behavior is inappropriate within the setting of a segregated living or employment setting if it is:

       i.   Harmful to someone, or involves nonconsent

       ii.   Interferes with others

      iii.   Upsets others

      iv.   Would be judged socially unacceptable in another setting

d. Sexual behavior is criminal if it is against the law, or if "the time, place, type of activity, the other people immediately involved with the perpetrator, the community, and the legal system" deem it so (Kempton, 1998, p. 167). Illegal sexual behavior is in part determined by state law and by the age of the perpetrator.

e. Examples of clearly illegal sexual behavior include:

       i.   Inappropriate touching of a child

       ii.   Forcing sexual attentions on another person, or causing injury through sexual activities

f. Individuals who have exhibited sexually inappropriate behavior should be clearly and consistently told that the behavior is not acceptable, and what the alternatives, if any, are. For example, a young man who masturbates in public should be consistently warned against repeating the behavior publicly, and encouraged to masturbate in private only.

g. Individuals who have been arrested for illegal sexual behavior should receive appropriate therapy, which may include counseling, intensive treatment methods, restriction of rights, and or medications (Kempton, 1998; Koller, 2000; Walsh, 2000).

E. Considerations for service providers and caregivers

1. Rules and regulations of service agencies may be restrictive and prohibit any kind of relationship or sexual activity within the service setting.

2. Changes in the rules and regulations of service agencies can better support the needs of all individuals receiving support from the agencies.

3. Staff may have personal values that affect their ability to provide self-determination in the area of sexuality to consumers.

4. Agencies may be caught in the double bind of preventing abuse and victimization of clients while providing rights regarding sexual behavior to consumers.

5. Agencies wishing to provide sexual rights to consumers may need to engage in education and values clarification exercises with staff members.

   a. Help staff to distinguish acceptable sexual behavior from inappropriate sexual behavior in accordance with the policies of the agency, and help them to understand how and when intervention is warranted.

   b. Offer staff training on how to respond to questions about sexuality or to sexual expression of clients under their care.

   c. Present definite instructions for staff on how they can help residents to report or avoid sexual abuse, and precisely what to do if sexual abuse is either suspected or discovered.

6. Policies and practices should be analyzed and implemented based on the following factors:

   a. Agency values and philosophies

   b. Staff values and training

   c. Community values

   d. Values and regulations of state agencies

   e. Values and philosophies of the advisory board of the agencies

   f. Parents' values and wishes

   g. Consumers' values and wishes

   h. Consumers' rights (Kempton, 1998)

IX. Summary

It is important to recognize that individuals with I/DD are sexual beings. Depending on a person's age and level of intelligence, education regarding, for example, sexual development, safe sex, appropriate sexual behavior, and STDs should be appropriately tailored. A variety of educational approaches and curricula have been presented.

References

Ailey, S. H., Marks, B. A., Crisp, C., & Hahn, J. E. (2003). Promoting sexuality across the life span for individuals with intellectual and developmental disabilities. *Nursing Clinics of North America, 38,* 229–252.

Aylott, J. (1999). Preventing rape and sexual assault of people with learning disabilities. *British Journal of Nursing, 8,* 871–875.

Block, P. (2000). Sexuality, fertility, and danger: Twentieth-century images of women with cognitive disabilities. *Sexuality and Disability, 18,* 239–254.

Brown, E. J., & Jemmott, L. S. (2002). HIV prevention among people with developmental disabilities. *Journal of Psychosocial Nursing & Mental Health Services, 40*(11), 14–21.

Butler, J. (1999). Sexuality. In N. Lennox & J. Diggens (Eds.), *Management guidelines. People with developmental and intellectual disabilities* (pp. 143–150). North Melbourne, Australia: Therapeutic Guidelines Limited.

Carty, E. M. (1998). Disability and childbirth: Meeting the challenges. *Canadian Medical Association Journal, 159,* 363–369.

Cheatham, D., King, E., & Bartz, A. (1993). *Childbirth education for women with disabilities and their partners.* Columbus, OH: The Ohio State University, The Nisonger Center UAP.

Christian, L., Stinson, J., & Dotson, L. A. (2001). Staff values regarding the sexual expression of women with developmental disabilities. *Sexuality and Disability, 19,* 283–291.

Dee, V. (1977). Sex education. In M. L. Siantz (Ed.), *The nurse and the developmentally disabled adolescent* (pp. 187–211). Baltimore: University Park Press.

DeVries B. B., vanden Boer-van den Berg, H. M., Niermeijer, M. F., & Tibben, A. (1999). Dilemmas in counseling females with the Fragile X syndrome. *Journal of Medical Genetics, 36,* 167–170.

Drey, E. A., & Darney, P. D. (2004). Contraceptive choices for women with disabilities. In S. L. Welner & F. Haseltine (Eds.), Welner's guide to the care of women with disabilities. (pp. 109–130). Philadelphia: Lippincott, Williams & Wilkins.

Ehlers-Flint, M. L. (2002). Parenting perceptions and social supports of mothers with cognitive disabilities. *Sexuality and Disability, 20*(1), 29–51.

Esmail, S., Esmail, Y., & Munro, B. (2001). Sexuality and disability: The role of health care professionals in providing options and alternatives for couples. *Sexuality and Disability, 19,* 267–282.

Federoff, J. P., Federoff, B. I., & Ilic, K. (2001). Sexual disorders, developmental disorders, developmental delay, and comorbid conditions. *The NADD Bulletin, 4*(2), 23–28.

Garnets, D. (2002). Sexual orientations in perspective. *Cultural Diversity & Ethnic Minority Psychology, 8*(2), 115–129.

Greydanus, D. E., Rimsza, M. E., & Newhouse, P. A. (2002). Adolescent sexuality and disability. *Adolescent Medicine: State of the Art Reviews, 13*(2), 223–247.

Guest, G. V. (2000). Sex education: A source for promoting character development in young people with physical disabilities. *Sexuality and Disability, 18,* 137–142.

Hatcher, R. A., Trussel, J., Stewart, F., Cates, W. Jr., Stewart, G. K., Guest, F., et al. (1998). *Contraceptive technology.* New York: Ardent Media.

Hays, S. R. (1999). Psychosocial health care patterns and nursing interventions. In P. A. Edwards, D. L. Hertzberg, S. R. Hays, & N. M. Youngblood (Eds.), *Pediatric rehabilitation nursing* (pp. 258–288). Philadelphia: Saunders.

Hingsburger, D. (1998). *Do? Be? Do?: What to teach and how to teach people with developmental disabilities.* Eastman, Quebec: Diverse City Press.

Kempton, W. (1998). *Socialization and sexuality: A comprehensive training guide for professionals helping people with disabilities that hinder learning.* Syracuse, NY: Program Development Associates.

Kempton, W., McKee, L., & Stigall-Mucigrosso, L. (1997). *An easy guide to loving carefully for men and women* (3rd ed.). Haverford, PA: Winifred Kemptor.

Kirshbaum, M., & Olkin, R. (2002). Parents with physical, systemic, or visual disabilities. *Sexuality and Disability, 20*(1), 65–80.

Koller, R. (2000). Sexuality and adolescents with autism. *Sexuality and Disability, 18,* 152–153.

Krajicek, M. J., & Cassidy, E. A. (1997). Sexuality. In H. M. Wallace, R. F. Biehl, J. C. MacQueen, & J. A. Blackman (Eds.), *Mosby's resource guide to children with disabilities and chronic illness,* (pp. 145–155). St. Louis: Mosby.

McCabe, M. P. (1999). Sexual knowledge, experience, and feelings among people with disability. *Sexuality and Disability, 17,* 157–170.

Melberg-Schweir, K. M., & Hingsburger, D. (2000). *Sexuality: Your sons and daughters with intellectual disabilities.* Baltimore: Paul H. Brookes.

Morse, J. S., & Roth, S. P. (1994). Sexuality: The nurse's role. In J. S. Morse & S. P. Roth (Eds.), *A life-span approach to nursing care for individuals with developmental disabilities.* Baltimore: Paul H. Brookes.

National Information Center for Children and Youth with Disabilities (NICHY). (1992). Sexuality education for children and youth with disabilities. *NICHY News Digest, 1*(3), 1–28.

Nosek, M. A., Foley, C. C., Hughes, R. B., & Howland, C. A. (2001). Vulnerabilities for abuse among women with disabilities. *Sexuality and Disability, 19,* 177–189.

O'Toole, C. J., & Doe, T. (2002). Sexuality and disabled parents with disabled children. *Sexuality and Disability, 20*(1) 89–101.

Quint, E. H. (1999). Gynecological health care for adolescents with developmental disabilities. *Adolescent Medicine State of the Art Reviews, 10,* 221–229.

Quint, E. H. (2004). Gynecological health care for women with developmental disabilities. In S. L. Welner & F. Haseltine (Eds.). *Welner's guide to the care of women with disabilities* (pp. 261–270). Philadelphia: Lippincott, Williams & Wilkins.

Rogers, J. G., Tulega, C. V., Vensand, K., & Through the Looking Glass. (2004). Baby care preparation: Pregnancy and post-partum. In S. L. Welner & F. Haseltine (Eds.), *Welner's guide to the care of women with disabilities* (pp. 169–184). Philadelphia: Lippincott, Williams & Wilkins.

Shuttleworth, R. P. (2000). The search for sexual intimacy for men with cerebral palsy. *Sexuality and Disability, 18,* 263–282.

Sulpizi, L. K. (1996). Issues in sexuality and gynecologic care of women with developmental disabilities. *JOENN, 25,* 609–614.

Thompson, S. A., Bryson, M., & de Castell, S. (2001). Prospects for identity formation for lesbian, gay, or bisexual persons with developmental disabilities. *International Journal of Disability, Development and Education, 48*(1), 53–65.

University of Texas Southwestern Medical Center at Dallas. (2000). *The patient with mental retardation: Issues in gynecologic care. A continuing education monograph.* Retrieved October 18, 2001 from http://www3.utsouthwestern.edu/cme/endurmat/gyn_ment/index.htm

Walcott, D. D. (1997). Family life education for persons with developmental disabilities. *Sexuality and Disability, 15,* 91–98.

Waldman, H. B., Swerdloff, M., & Perlman, S. P. (1999). Sexuality and youngsters with mental retardation. *Journal of Dentistry for Children, 66,* 348–352.

Walsh, A. (2000). IMPROVE and CARE: Responding to inappropriate masturbation in people with severe intellectual disabilities. *Sexuality and Disabilities, 18*(1), 27–30.

Ward L., Howarth J., & Rodgers, J. (2002). Difference and choice: Exploring prenatal testing and the use of genetic information with people with learning difficulties. *British Journal of Learning Disabilities, 30*(2), 50–55.

Welner, S. L. (1997). Gynecologic care and sexuality issues for women with disabilities. *Sexuality and Disability, 15*(1), 33–40.

Welner, S. L. (1999). Menopausal issues. *Sexuality and Disability, 17,* 259–267.

Wheeler, P. N. (2001). Sexuality: Meaning and relevance to learning disability nurses. *British Journal of Nursing, 10,* 920-927.

Yool, L., Langdon, P. E., & Garner, K. (2003). The attitudes of medium-secure unit staff toward the sexuality of adults with learning disabilities. *Sexuality and Disability, 21,* 137–150.

Zieman, M., Guillebaud, J., Weisberg, E., Shangold, G. A., Fisher, A. C., & Creasy, G. W. (2002). Contraceptive efficacy and cycle control with the Ortho Evra™/Evra™ transdermal system: The analysis of pooled date. *Fertility and Sterility, 77*(2), S13–S18.

Zieman, M., Nelson, A., Hatcher, R., Nelson, A., Darney, P., Creinin, M., et al. (2002). *A pocket guide to managing contraception.* Tiger, GA: Bridging the Gap Foundation.

Older Adults

Joan Earle Hahn, DNSc, APRN, BC, CDDN and Kathryn Pekala Service, MS, RN, FNP, CDDN

14

Objectives

At the completion of this chapter, the learner will be able to:

1. State two reasons why care needs of older individuals with intellectual and developmental disabilities (I/DD) are gaining greater recognition.

2. Describe at least six characteristics of older individuals with I/DD and their known similarities and differences to the general older population.

3. Describe unique aging challenges and potential secondary conditions for individuals with specific condition(s) that may be associated with an I/DD (e.g., Down syndrome, cerebral palsy, spina bifida, and Fragile X).

4. Identify family issues of older individuals with I/DD, the role of the family, and the services and community resources that families can access.

5. Identify the role of nurses and health care providers in providing support to older individuals with I/DD, families, and care providers, and in facilitating opportunities that encourage older individuals with I/DD to live meaningful lives.

Key Points

- The number of individuals with I/DD who are aging is expected to increase due to better medical care, improved sanitation, and greater survival rates to adulthood.

- Older individuals with I/DD are more likely to have one or more health problems associated with aging than their younger peers have.

- Older adults with I/DD are more prone to secondary conditions, the consequences of which may be minimized through preventive care interventions across the lifespan.

Key Points *(continued)*

- A diagnosis of dementia requires a change from baseline, includes change in cognitive status (by tests) and a decline in everyday functioning, and uses ICD-10 criteria; therefore, it is important to establish baseline functioning and to obtain observations from multiple sources.

- Most care provided for individuals with I/DD is by families, and as the individual with I/DD ages, the likelihood of being admitted to long-term care settings increases.

- Nurses and other health professionals have a key role to play in case finding, assessment, prevention of functional decline, health promotion, and disease prevention for aging and older persons and their families and in educating other professionals and supportive persons.

- Both disability and aging-service systems and their interfaces are key resources to be used in planning comprehensive interventions that meet the needs of older persons with I/DD and their families.

I.   Introduction and Overview

A. Increasing numbers of older persons with I/DD (Janicki, Dalton, Henderson, & Davidson, 1999)

1. Increasing numbers of older persons in the general population are due to increases in longevity because of improved medical care and sanitation.

    a. 12% of general population were over age 60 in 2004.

    b. One in four (25%) of general population will be over age 60 by 2040.

2. Persons with I/DD are experiencing increases in longevity similar to the general population—due to improved medical care and sanitation, and their greater survival to adulthood.

    a. Persons with I/DD in the U.S. age 60 or older estimated to be at 173,000 in 1995.

    b. An estimated 332,900 baby boomers were born between the years 1946 and 1964 (AAMR-IASSID Workgroup on Eipdemiology and Alzheimer's Disease, 1995).

    c. Numbers of older persons with I/DD may double or triple by 2025.

3. Number of persons with I/DD are based on estimates and may underrepresent actual numbers.

    a. Persons not known to service system for a variety of reasons: may have been hidden by family due to stigma; had little or no community services as cohort; definition of developmental disability not standardized; older adults look much like older persons without disability; and if history of etiology is unknown, it may be difficult to determine the presence of an I/DD at an older age.

b. No universal system in U.S. to tabulate number of persons with I/DD known to services.

4. Average life expectancy for persons with I/DD, with some exceptions, is approaching same age as general population (Janicki et al., 1999; Strauss & Eyman, 1996).

a. Some individuals are as healthy as individuals in the older population without lifelong I/DD.

b. "Differential mortality"—older cohorts have healthier individuals who live longer (see World Health Organization, 2001).

c. Average life expectancy for persons with Down syndrome has improved, yet is lower than persons with I/DD by 10 to 20 years (World Health Organization, 2001) and the older population without I/DD.

i. Life expectancy with Down syndrome in 1920 was age 9 years and is now reported to be from the mid-50s (Chicoine & McGuire, 1997) to 60–64 (Strauss & Eyman, 1996).

ii. Some individuals with Down syndrome live to their 80s or 90s (Chicoine & McGuire, 1997).

d. Risk factors for decreased longevity exist (see Eyman & Borthwick-Duffy, 1994; Hayden, 1998).

i. Associated health conditions more commonly found for individuals with severe degree of mental retardation (severe-profound), seizure disorder, or cerebral palsy

ii. Major medical problems (e.g., chronic upper respiratory conditions, infections, heart condition, choking)

iii. Decreased mobility, toileting, and eating skills (see Eyman & Borthwick-Duffy, 1994)

B. Greater recognition of older persons with I/DD

1. Aging families—aging caregivers

a. An estimated 60% of persons with I/DD live with family (Fujiura, 1998).

b. 25% live with caregivers ages 60 and older; 35% live with middle-aged caregivers (Braddock, 1999; Fujiura, 1998).

c. Persons with I/DD may outlive older parents (Bigby, 1997), and parental death or illness may precipitate a crisis whereby the individual with I/DD with aging needs becomes known to the service system and requires services.

    d. Sibling relationships vary across the life course, are dependent on family history, and are often the most significant relationships (Bigby, 2000).

2. Educational and vocational programs (Bigby, 1997)

    a. May outlive programs (e.g., reach retirement age in work or day program).

    b. Aging changes may precipitate need for service changes or adaptations to meet aging needs.

3. Greater number of older persons with I/DD may be seen in generic health care settings such as primary care, senior and adult day health, home health care, emergency rooms, and specialty clinics due to:

    a. Shift in number of persons residing in institutions to living in community settings (Braddock & Hemp, 1997) with increased numbers of people living in community residential settings brings more persons into generic health care settings.

    b. Increased mandated use of generic managed care for community-based Medicaid-eligible persons with I/DD (Kastner, Walsh, & Criscione, 1997).

4. Aging in place in residential settings—Survey data from a national probability sample of the noninstitutionalized population, including samples from nursing and personal care homes and facilities for people with I/DD (Altman, 1995), revealed:

    a. Over a third of people in long-term care facilities were age 50 or older.

    b. About 20% were 65 and over.

    c. One in 10 have lived at least three-quarters of their life in residential settings.

    d. Older persons were less likely to live in group or foster homes and more likely to live in nursing homes.

    e. Older persons had similar needs for assistance with ADLs as persons under age 25 with severe/profound levels of mental retardation.

5. Health professional education about I/DD has been found lacking (Hahn & Willis, 2000; U.S. Public Health Service, 2002; Walsh, Hammerman, Josephson, & Krupka, 2000).

6. A growing body of multidisciplinary research, mostly cohort studies, about aging needs of persons with I/DD began in the mid-1980s (Janicki & Wisniewski, 1984); is growing, yet still limited and in need of further study about aging changes, diseases associated with aging, barriers and facilitators to engaging in health promoting activities, measurement instruments, trajectory of healthy aging, impact of health on caregivers, prevention of secondary conditions, use of technology, and role of cost (Davidson, Heller, Janicki, & Hyer, 2004).

7. Research, mostly cohort studies, can build on previous studies using gerontological and/or geriatric medicine principles and practices (Davidson et al., 2004).

8. Although recognized as an important issue for gerontological nurses (Newbern & Hargett, 1992; Service & Hahn, 2003), research about the nursing needs of older persons is limited to a few studies that began in the late 1960s (Barnard, Collar, & Worthy, 1969); it received some attention in the late 1980s and 1990s (Hahn, 1994; McBreen, 1989; Service, 1996), and is now receiving greater attention in research that looks at the effectiveness of nursing practice interventions (Hahn & Aronow, 2003).

9. Research findings to date can guide health care professionals in care of older persons.

C. General aging and health-related characteristics of older persons with I/DD

1. Similarities to population aging without I/DD

   a. Persons with I/DD are not a homogeneous group—vary widely in abilities and levels of impairments and disabilities (Walker, Walker, & Gosling, 1999) and grow less alike as they grow older (Janicki & Ansello, 2000).

   b. At greater risk for increased functional impairments, polypharmacy, morbidity, and mortality associated with advancing age (World Health Organization, 2001) compared to younger peers (Cooper, 1998).

   c. Generally experience the same physical process of aging as individuals without lifelong disabilities (with some exceptions—e.g., persons with Down syndrome) and age-associated conditions (e.g., presbycusis or difficulty hearing high frequency sounds, presbyopia or difficulty seeing fine print or detail) (Factor, 1997; Service & Hahn, 2003), and as they age into middle years, they are functionally, socially, and, for some, genetically at risk for functional decline, similar to persons at older ages in nondisabled populations.

   d. Acquire adult or age-related conditions at similar or higher rates as older persons without I/DD, e.g., diabetes, ischemic heart disease, stroke, ulcers (see Evenhuis, Henderson, Beange, Lennox, & Chicoine, 2001).

   e. Some similarities exist in the course of dementia with the onset of select maladaptive behaviors (e.g., lack of boundaries, withdrawal) that accompany functional decline as early indicators that may prompt a concern about dementia (Urv, Zigman, & Silverman, 2003); however, functional decline warrants comprehensive evaluation to rule out other conditions.

   f. Each person ages uniquely and is impacted by lifelong health and lifestyle patterns, genetics, life experience, health habits, or external conditions similar to those without I/DD (World Health Organization, 2001).

2. Differences compared to population aging without I/DD

   a. Persons with I/DD are at greater risk for increased functional impairments, morbidity, and mortality associated with advancing age (World Health Organization, 2001) due to several risk factors including:

      i. Early onset of age-related conditions (may be increased for syndrome-specific or neurodevelopmental disorders) (Davidson et al., 2004)

      ii. Long-term progression of lifelong disability

      iii. Interaction of age-related conditions and lifelong disabilities (e.g., sensory aging changes compounded by earlier sensory pathology)

   b. Older persons with I/DD acquire health conditions at higher rates than older persons without I/DD that may be attributed to "factors related to syndromes, associated developmental disabilities, and lifestyle and environmental issues" (Evenhuis et al., 2001, p. 182). For example:

      i. Persons with Down syndrome are at greater risk for developing Alzheimer's disease (Evenhuis et al., 2001).

      ii. Conditions such as sensory impairment, thyroid disease, and non-ischemic heart disease had an increased prevalence compared to the general population in a study of persons with I/DD (Kapell et al., 1998).

   c. In some research, they may have lower rates of age-related conditions or risk factors than the general aging population (e.g., hypertension, hyperlipidemia, adult-onset diabetes) (Janicki, McCallion, & Dalton, 2002).

   d. Older persons are likely to experience conditions that have the potential to contribute to functional decline in activites of daily living (ADLs), instrumental activities of daily living (IADLs), and quality of social interaction (Henderson & Davidson, 2000).

   e. Persons with I/DD are at risk for secondary conditions (*Improving the Health and Wellness of Women with Disabilities*, 2003; Patrick, Richardson, Starks, & Rose, 1994; Pope, 1992; Pope & Tarlov, 1991; Turk, Overeyender, & Janicki, 1995) associated with the primary etiology of their disability (e.g., pain, skin breakdown, functional incontinence, depression and anxiety, osteoporosis, emotional dependence, or abuse and neglect).

   f. Persons aging with I/DD are at greater risk for medication issues, including polypharmacy (Seltzer & Lutchterhand, 1994; World Health Organization, 2001) that may be due to earlier age-related sensitivity to medications (e.g., Down syndrome); risks of adverse effects due to inability of person to communicate side effects or symptoms or ineffective reporting by informants; overmedication and inappropriately prescribed medications; or greater risks of medication interactions.

g. Health care may be restricted by a number of factors including lack of knowledge and training about the health issues of older persons with I/DD (Janicki & Breitenbach, 2000) and other barriers (e.g., less likely to have hearing aid for identified hearing loss) (Altman, 1995).

h. Psychosocial characteristics that differ from the general population (Bigby, 2000; Sutton, 1993) include living with family of origin into their later years; not being employed with a self-sustaining income; not having retirement and/or pension plan or having confusing retirement issues when employed or in disability programs; dual stigmatization related to both disability and aging; having a locus of control often with family or care staff; having social networks limited to family or paid staff; and being more likely to have a guardian or conservatorship.

i. May experience grief due to losses that might include: decline or loss in functional abilities from aging or chronic illness; loss of family, friends, or care staff or other persons who provide support; residential transitions; changes in opportunities; or lack of choice making (Ludlow, 1999; Service, Lavoie, & Herlihy, 1999).

D. Characteristics of persons aging with I/DD related to a specific syndrome or condition

1. Persons with Down syndrome (Evenhuis, 1999; Hahn, Charron, & Willis, 2003; Oliver, 1999; Seltzer & Luchterhand, 1994; Service & Willis, 1999, 2003) may exhibit precocious/premature signs of aging and/or physical signs of aging even 20 years earlier than is usual (Hawkins & Eklund, 1994) including alopecia, functional decline noticed after age 50, early menopause (Carr & Hollins, 1995; Schupf et al., 1997; Seltzer, Schupf, & Wu, 2001), age-related hearing and visual disorders, epilepsy, and Alzheimer's disease (Janicki & Breitenbach, 2000), and acquire age-associated health conditions with Down syndrome that include:

    a. cataracts

    b. thyroid disease

    c. bunions

    d. osteoarthritic changes in the spine

    e. sleep apnea

    f. presbycusis

    g. exacerbation of pre-existing cardiac condition

    h. obesity

    i. osteoporosis

    j. periodontal disease

2. Persons with cerebral palsy, a nonprogressive condition, may be affected at earlier ages by age-related changes that impact function (Overenynder, Janicki, & Turk, 1994), such as decreased muscle reserve resulting in problems with ambulation, pain, and reduced stamina at an earlier age (Janicki, 1999), and are at increased risk of developing age-related secondary conditions (Evenhuis et al., 2001; Seltzer & Luchterhand, 1994), such as increased respiratory and swallowing problems, worsening bowel and bladder function, back and hip deformities, loss of bone density with fractures, skin breakdown, increased GI problems (e.g., oral-motor and gastroenterology concerns; upper and lower GI dysmotility resulting in dysphagia, reflux, constipation, and fecal impaction; dental erosion; esophagitis; anemia; feeding problems; aspiration; and pneumonia), depression, dental concerns, and pain from untreated conditions such as "degenerative musculoskeletal conditions, constipation, reflux esophagitis, and allergic rhinitis" (Henderson & Davidson, 2000, pp. 381–382).

3. Persons with spina bifida (Lollar, 1994) with extended life expectancy are at risk for secondary conditions with aging, including increased risk for infection/sepsis, urinary tract infections, skin breakdown, and tethered cord.

4. Persons with Fragile X (World Health Organization, 2001) are at risk for secondary conditions of mitral valve prolapse, musculoskeletal disorders, early menopause, epilepsy, visual impairments, and a tremor/ataxia syndrome (FXTAS) that causes cognitive and motor dysfunction noticed in parents and grandparents of individuals with Fragile X (Jacquemont et al., 2004).

II.   Role of Health Care Providers

A. Health promotion and disease prevention

1. Persons with I/DD face barriers to receiving standard preventive health services and should receive standardized age-appropriate health promotion and preventive health interventions (see http://www.ahrq.gov/clinic/prevnew.htm for *Guide to Clinical Prevention Services* (1996) written by the U.S. Preventive Services Task Force (USPSTF)).

2. Additional recommendations may be found in condition-specific guidelines (e.g., *Health Care Guidelines for Individuals with Down Syndrome: 1999 Revision* (Cohen, 1999)).

3. Health screening is important for those conditions for which persons with I/DD may be at increased risk (e.g., persons who lived in large institutions may be at higher risk for certain conditions, such as hepatitis B, Helicobacter pylori, and tuberculosis) (Evenhuis et al., 2001).

4. Obtain baseline functional and mental status assessment in middle-aged years and screen for changes because of difficulties with diagnosis of dementia in people with I/DD (Service & Hahn, 2003).

B. Comprehensive geriatric assessment (see *Geriatric Assessment Methods for Clinical Decision Making. NIH Consensus Statement*, 1987).

1. The primary goal of comprehensive geriatric assessment is the prevention of functional and physical decline by conducting a multidimensional assessment that determines health status, age-related changes, age-related health problems, and secondary conditions associated with the primary cause of disability; assists in prioritizing health problems, and allows development of an individualized plan of care specific to the older person's needs.

2. It may take place in various settings (e.g., clinic, hospital, home) and may be conducted by one primary health care provider or by members of a multidisciplinary team.

3. Components of comprehensive geriatric assessment include: assessment of demographics and of function (ADLs and IADLs), nutrition, sleep, psychosocial history, environmental health, health maintenance, finances, past medical history, mental health, medications, family history, review of systems, and physical examination.

4. Comprehensive assessment of older persons with I/DD has the potential to identify unrecognized problems, to correctly diagnose and treat misdiagnosed problems (Henderson & Davidson, 2000; Lennox, Green, Diggens, & Ugoni, 2001) as well as to attend to overdue health maintenance activities (Hahn & Aronow, 2003; Lennox et al., 2001).

C. Prevention of secondary conditions

1. Secondary conditions, often preventable, are acquired secondary to the primary cause of the I/DD (Patrick et al., 1994; Pope, 1992; Pope & Tarlov, 1991; Turk, Overeyender, & Janicki, 1995).

2. These conditions may worsen with age, and age-related changes may compound the risk of developing a secondary condition (e.g., more fragile, less elastic age-related skin changes—compounded by immobility and need for assistance to move—increase risk for skin breakdown).

3. General strategies suggested for prevention include active prevention measures across the lifespan beginning at earlier ages, use of technologies, health promotion, increased assistance as needed when impacted by declining function, and addressing age-related concerns by health care providers (Grogan & Fryberger, 1999; Improving the Health and Wellness of Women with Disabilities, 2003; World Health Organization, 2001).

4. Select secondary conditions impacted by aging for persons with I/DD are listed below. (For more information about secondary conditions, see Grogan & Fryberger (1999)).

    a. Pain

        i. Associated with age-related conditions that have pain as a chief complaint such as arthritis or conditions common for persons with

I/DD such as gastroesophageal reflux (Henderson & Davidson, 2000).

  ii. May be difficult to assess with diminished verbal communication skills, or is often ignored, dismissed, or not validated. This empha-sizes the importance of both self-report and observational measures of nonverbal indicators of pain (Hadjistavropoulos & Craig, 2002), assessment by those who know the person or who have expert observation skills (Zwakhalen, van Dongen, Hamers, & Abu-Saad, 2004), treatment of underlying conditions with pain symptoms, and provision of adequate pain management.

  iii. Pain assessment tools specific for persons with I/DD are in need of more research.

b. Pressure sores (skin breakdown)

  i. Preventable condition with increased risk due to age-related changes in skin (less elastic, more fragile) and declining function or mobility status due to disease or poor health

  ii. Basic preventive strategies (e.g., nutrition, assistance with move-ment, avoid friction shear); early detection and treatment

c. Functional incontinence—inability to access toilet or the assistance to get to the bathroom

  i. Not a "normal" consequence of aging; however, other age-related changes may increase likelihood of incontinence (e.g., mobility changes, motivation, arthritis).

  ii. Age-related changes may compound lifelong urinary problems (e.g., infrequent urination or poor bladder management programs) (Improving the Health and Wellness of Women with Disabilities, 2003).

  iii. As function declines, environmental/physical support or cueing may be needed to maintain continence.

d. Depression and anxiety

  i. May be prompted by fears associated with aging, declining inde-pendence, or losses due to aging physical changes, disease, and other transitions or psychosocial changes.

  ii. Screen, assess, explore, and treat co-existing health issues that may be depression (e.g., pain, stress, losses or grief, lack of social sup-port, declining independence, abuse).

  iii. Treatment for depression

e. Osteoporosis—age-related bone loss, underrecognized or not assessed, may be an accelerated loss at the time of menopause and some women may experience menopause at an earlier age than is usual.

      i.   Bone loss may also occur because of chronic immobility, lack of weight-bearing activity (Turk, Overeynder, & Janicki, 1995), or long-term use of certain medications (e.g., corticosteroids, anticonvulsants).

      ii.   Most significant predictors of bone mineral density were Down syndrome, mobility status, and race in a study of adults ages 60 to 80 with I/DD with osteoporosis and osteopenia (Tyler, Snyder, & Zyzanski, 2000).

      iii. Screen with radiological procedures (dual X-ray absorptiometry) or serum markers for osteoporosis and individualize treatment (Ott, 1999).

      iv. Implement preventive measures for falls, which are the leading cause of fractures, by evaluating underlying medical conditions, environment, and need for assistive device; encourage exercise for muscle strength and gait training.

   f. Emotional dependence

      i.   Functional decline may prompt need for more assistance.

      ii.   Need for correct balance between care and support and promotion of independence, as overprotection could affect quality of life and ability to participate fully in life activities.

      iii. Implement supports that foster independence as well as meet need for assistance (Walker, Walker, & Gosling, 1999).

   g. Abuse and neglect

      i.   At higher risk (Herr & Weber, 1999).

      ii.   State adult protective service systems should be contacted when abuse is suspected or identified.

      iii. Best protection is adequate care and supervision (Ludlow, 1999).

      iv. Support for informal caregivers needed (including respite).

      v.   Regulations, policies, and programs needed to provide quality standards.

D. Health care communication and teaching strategies

  1. Difficulties in disease detection

   a. Disease may be advanced before it is recognized due to person's inability to report symptoms and/or health care providers and caregivers lack of ability to recognize symptoms (Beange & Bauman, 1990).

   b. Disease or illness in older persons can have an atypical presentation (Evenhuis, 1999) making it necessary to detect changes in health status through routine and close observation of physical or behavioral changes and other markers of change (e.g., lab results, change in functional abilities) (Moss, 1999).

2. Communication and teaching strategies

   a. Encourage use of a portable health history to share with health care providers to enhance continuity of care and communication.

   b. Employ teaching strategies that build on principles of teaching needs of both older adults (e.g., accommodating for age-related sensory changes) (see guidelines for teaching older persons in Picariello, 1986) and persons with I/DD who may require more time to teach (e.g., using language that is easy to understand, concrete examples).

E. Rehabilitation and habilitation

   1. Routine care for persons with I/DD across the life course is based on principles of habilitation, or the development of new skills not previously learned, usually throughout life.

   2. Rehabilitation is the relearning of lost skills to assist a person in regaining skills that have been lost as a result of illness or injury (e.g., learning to walk again following a stroke or hip replacement); persons with I/DD who experience such a loss should also be considered as candidates for rehabilitation (Conliffe & Walsh, 1999).

F. Dementia assessment and care

   1. Dementia screening and assessment (see Aylward, Burt, Thorpe, Lai, & Dalton, 1997)

      a. Individuals with I/DD are at similar risk for Alzheimer's disease as persons without I/DD (The Arc, 1995).

      b. Risks factors are increased for individuals with I/DD who have:

         i. Had some type of head injury

         ii. A family member with Alzheimer's disease

         iii. Down syndrome and are over the age of 40 (The Arc, 1995)

      c. Without a proper assessment, persons with I/DD are at risk for overdiagnosis when a change in functional status is noticed.

      d. Need to rule out other conditions that mimic dementia such as depression, hypothyroidism, sensory impairments, undiagnosed infection, adverse effects of medication, sleep apnea, and heart condition or anemia.

      e. The same six criteria as outlined according to ICD-10 should be assessed:

         i. Decline in memory (may be more difficult to detect in individuals with more severe cognitive impairment at baseline)

         ii. Decline in other cognitive abilities

         iii. Awareness of environment

      iv.   Decline in emotional control or motivation, or change in social behavior

      v.   Duration (at least six months)

      vi.   Onset and progression (gradual onset and continued decline)

  f. Obtaining a baseline functional assessment by the age of 35 can assist with later documentation of a progression of changes.

  g. A probable diagnosis of dementia requires a well-documented progression of symptoms using the ICD-10 criteria that for persons with Down syndrome may include: change in personality, long periods of activity or apathy, hyperreflexivity, loss of ADLs, visual retention deficits, loss of speech, disorientation, stereotypic behavior, abnormal neurological signs, and development of seizures (Janicki, Heller, Seltzer, & Hogg, 1995).

  h. I/DD-specific tools for assessing dementia are being developed and tested (Shultz et al., 2004).

  2. Caring for a person with I/DD who has dementia

    a. The "ECEPS" Model for Care of Persons with Dementia (Janicki, McCallion, & Dalton, 2002) is one model of care for guidance to use in planning care.

      i.   E = Early screening and diagnosis—Diagnosis and treatment of underlying disorders

      ii.   C = Clinical supports—Implement supports; dementia care professionals

      iii.   E = Environmental modification—Enhance safety, use existing skills to minimize "excess disability"

      iv.   P = Program adaptations—Staff training on dementia care

      v.   S = Specialized care—Dementia care, end of life care, and support for changing needs

    b. Practice guidelines specific to persons with I/DD are available.

G. Environmental modifications and assistive technology

  1. Assistive technology benefits older adults (see Hammel, Heller, & Ying, 1998; Heller, 1999).

  2. Environments should be evaluated for safety and for need for modification.

    a. Promote and maintain independence (e.g., hand rails on stairs, good lighting, nonskid surfaces, grab bars).

H. Providing family-centered and person-centered approaches to care

  1. Families provide the majority of care (Fujiura, 1998).

  2. Family or support networks should be acknowledged as knowing the person best.

3. Person's values and preferences should be assessed and included in planning care.

I. Health care advocacy

1. Access to health care may have been a lifelong issue with denied preventive health care, lack of teaching about preventive health practices, and some lack of control over their lives.

2. Older individuals may face stereotypes associated with both aging and I/DD (called "double jeopardy").

3. Lack of understanding by health care professionals of aging and/or I/DD.

4. Self-advocacy is a growing movement, although older individuals may not have experienced this role in their early years.

5. Not receiving needed adequate medical care may jeopardize health.

6. Need assistance with medical vocabulary to describe health problems.

7. May act as if they understand to avoid embarrassment.

8. Need assistance to understand medical prescriptions and treatment plans (Edgerton, 1994).

9. Health care providers should "speak more plainly and effectively" (Edgerton, 1994).

10. Historically, people have been protected from normal lifespan experiences, such as dealing with death and bereavement; in addition there is a lack of, or little planning for, end of life care (Botsford & Force, 2000) which should be acknowledged and addressed.

J. Inclusion and social support

1. Different pattern of social support

a. Few marry and have children or grandchildren—if spouse does not have I/DD, question arises as to which service system to access as both face aging changes.

b. Friends may include caregivers and staff who work in their residences; these relationships may be transitory in nature.

c. Some may have lacked opportunities for social interaction to develop friendships.

d. Some may have poor social skills that inhibit development of friendship.

e. Grief may not be acknowledged, allowed, or recognized (see Seltzer & Luchterhand, 1994).

2. Assess social support

a. Key persons (family, paid help, friends, and naturally occurring supports such as neighbors or church members)

b. Opportunities for social interaction

    c. Conflicts—need for counseling

    d. Abusive physical or emotional relationships

    e. Grief and bereavement

  3. Consider needed supports and opportunities to develop significant supports when planning interventions (e.g., use generic senior centers with individual vs. group attendance).

  4. Consider lifelong friendships (with peers) when evaluating residential transitions.

K. Case management for older persons

  1. Helpful when older individuals with I/DD no longer have family members (parent, sibling, child, or spouse) to depend upon for guidance and support (Natvig, 1994)

  2. May be provided by disability or aging-service system to navigate complex systems and access to services or support

L. Fostering retirement and leisure activities

  1. Individuals with I/DD typically have not held regular employment and may attend a disability service system program (day program, adult activity center); individual may not want to retire, may not understand the concept of retirement (knows no other alternative than going to a day program/has friends there), or may not be given the option to "retire." The option for retirement may be a conflict for a residential program or full-time daytime/vocational activity program (all or no attendance; no staff at facility during the day or not encouraging of retirement).

  2. Consultation with recreation or occupational therapist may be indicated to facilitate the transition to retirement using leisure activities (Seltzer & Luchterhand, 1994).

  3. Tools/programs for assisting individuals with leisure/retirement/later-life planning include: *Preretirement Education Person-Centered Later Life Planning Project*—Heller, Sterns, Sutton, & Factor, 1996); Kivnick's (1991) *Inventory of Life Strengths*; and Rinck's (1991) pictorial booklet of activities.

M. Choosing appropriate residential options

  1. 25% of persons with I/DD live with caregivers 60 and older and 35% live with middle-aged caregivers (Braddock, 1999; Fujiura, 1998).

  2. Persons with I/DD who reside in community residential settings may wish to "age in place" (LePore & Janicki, 1997) in the same living environment (family or other residence) in spite of physical or mental decline that may occur with the process of aging. However, to enable this to occur, necessary services may need to be increased, added, and/or adjusted to compensate for these changes.

3. An underlying principle in deciding the "best" residential care option is looking at a person's ability to "age with dignity," often depending on the availability of and the ability to put in place proper supports.

4. Options that may assist a person to "age in place" may include:

    a. Medicaid Home and Community Based Services (HCBS) waiver program, which includes supports for individuals only in community settings including family home, apartments, small homes, and foster homes (Braddock & Hemp, 1997)

    b. Home of his/her own concept—consumer-controlled housing (see Heller, 1999)

    c. Supportive living/independent living arrangements where the home is owned, leased, or rented by individuals with paid support personnel to provide assistance or oversight

    d. Family support programs (Braddock & Hemp, 1997) that include cash subsidies, respite care, counseling, and other in-home (family home) services to the family

5. Some individuals will move from parents' home or move from facility to facility as the supports may be lacking or regulations push toward a different type of placement (Russell, Grant, Joseph, & Fee, 1994). Options might include:

    a. Foster care (adult family or foster care) with room, board, and personal care in a family or family-like setting.

    b. Licensed Intermediate Care Facility for Persons with Mental Retardation (ICF/MR), which are community residences funded by the Medicaid Title XIX that typically serve individuals who are more dependent and need greater care. Many residents are not in need of such costly and restrictive services (Lavin & Doka, 1999). This facility necessitates compliance with regulations that are reportedly more institutional than community based.

    c. Group home or small residences with support staff that supervise living in a home that is leased or rented by agency or state department with some state limits on size.

    d. Congregate living facility, an independent noninstitutional group-living environment that integrates shelter and service needs of functionally impaired or socially isolated elders who do not require the constant supervision or level of health care provided by an institution.

    e. Nursing home only when specific admission criteria are met.

6. Crisis-driven care decisions (such as death of a family caregiver) are made as a result of lack of planning and may conflict with individual's self-determination and independence (Davidson et al., 1999; McCallion, 1993).

7. Factors to consider when planning residential options include sources of caregiving (family vs. formal service network) and individual's needs, strengths, preferences, finances, and health status; yet many older families have not planned with and for their adult child (Seltzer & Krauss, 1994). This includes formation of advanced directives (Friedman, 1998).

8. Nursing homes are no longer options for residential care for persons with I/DD unless there is the need for skilled nursing care or the person meets exclusion criteria per PASARR (Pre-Admission Screening and Annual Resident Review) regulations of the Omnibus Budget Reconciliation Act of 1987 (OBRA-87). In addition, following an annual resident review, a person who is inappropriately placed in a nursing home should be discharged; those who remain in nursing homes are to receive specialized services to address the needs as a result of the disability to maximize function and prevent decline (see Service & Willis, 2003). One study noted that less than 20% of residents with I/DD residing in nursing homes needed skilled nursing care based on reviews as mandated by OBRA-87 conducted in 1990 (Hahn, 1994).

9. Because of waiting lists (over 80,000 people—see Braddock, 1999), advance assessment and planning is needed to find the most preferred setting in which to live before a crisis occurs in the person's or caregiver's health that forces a move into a less appropriate or preferred setting

III.   Role of Community Supports

A. Navigating the service delivery systems (disability and/or aging)

1. Two sets of service systems are available to older persons with I/DD—aging and I/DD service systems.

2. Amendments to the Older Americans Act in 1987 allowed persons with I/DD to access the same services; amendments in 1992 funded collaborative models between disabilities and aging service system to foster outreach and service delivery to older persons with I/DD (LePore & Janicki, 1997).

3. Difficulties or challenges in navigating the two systems lie in the dichotomies or differences of the two service systems (Hacker, McCallion, & Janicki, 2000).

4. Barriers to accessing community care include attitudinal barriers (e.g., fear, reluctance to access systems, negative stereotypes), information and communication gaps; financial constraints (e.g., funding from different sources; competition for limited funds), lack of coordination among agencies, programmatic barriers, and lack of education and training about aging and disabilities.

5. New models continue to be developed (Janicki & Ansello, 2000; LePore & Janicki, 1997), yet needs of older persons with I/DD continue to be unmet due to lack of public or privately organized systems that adequately address the service needs of older adults with I/DD and their families.

B. Resources and services in the community for older persons/families—aging sector

 1. Access to aging services can be done through an Area Agency on Aging (AAA).

 2. Senior centers—provide information, referral support, and a variety of social service, educational, and social programs.

 3. Home health agencies are public or private agencies providing coordinated health care to individuals in their homes as referred by the physician based on qualification (e.g., home bound, in need of PT/OT/speech, or skilled nursing services).

 4. Congregate meals are provided in programs authorized by Title III-C (Older Americans Act); one meal a day.

 5. Day programs include social day care, which provides individualized program of social activity, and adult day health services, which provide similar services but focus on health-related issues.

C. Resources and services in the community for older persons/families—disability sector

 1. State Developmental Disabilities Planning Council is a state-appointed council to address issues for individuals with I/DD and may provide funding for aging initiatives (check with each state for exact title and content information).

 2. Special disability and aging programs (check each state or local area for availability).

IV. Summary—Principles for Health Care Providers to Promote Successful Aging

A. Use a lifespan, inclusive approach

 1. Begin preventive interventions early (e.g., young and middle age adults) and promote health promotion and disease prevention strategies.

 2. Establish baseline level of functional status, assess functional decline, and use comprehensive geriatric assessment to assist in identification of health issues and to formulate a plan of care.

 3. Apply similar principles of care that are used for all older persons in concert with knowledge of condition-specific aspects of care and secondary conditions noted for persons with I/DD.

 4. Aim to put in place preventive as well as protective factors to assist individuals to "age in place" in an environment that fosters his or her growth and quality of life.

B. Use person-centered and family-centered principles that foster respect and dignity.

 1. Preserve personal identity (see Herr & Weber, 1999) and adapt care principles for older persons to the needs of aging persons with I/DD.

2. Use the person's array of social support from both the family/staff and service system support networks creatively to develop needed resources.

3. Assist the older individual to understand issues, actively engage in their lives and health care, and implement needed resources related to retirement, grief, death and dying, and end-of-life decision making.

4. Assist families with middle-aged or older caregivers to address future planning issues.

C. Advocate, advocate, advocate

1. Foster family and self-advocacy when possible.

2. Assist agencies and the general public in policy development and creative solutions that include older persons with I/DD and recognize growing needs of all older persons, regardless of the nature of the I/DD.

References

AAMR-IASSID Workgroup on Epidemiology and Alzheimer's Disease. (1995). *Epidemiology of Alzheimer's disease and mental retardation.* Washington, DC: AAMR.

Altman, B. (1995). Elderly persons with developmental disabilities in long-term care facilities. *National medical expenditure survey research findings, 25* (AHCPR Pub. No. 95-0084). Rockville, MD: Public Health Service, Agency for Health Care Policy and Research.

Aylward, E. H., Burt, D. B., Thorpe, L. U., Lai, F., & Dalton, A. (1997). Diagnosis of dementia of individuals with intellectual disability. *Journal of Intellectual Disability Research, 41,* 152–164.

Barnard, K. E., Collar, B., & Worthy, E. (1969). Study of the living needs of a group of severely physically involved adult cerebral palsy individuals. Unpublished manuscript. Seattle: University of Washington, School of Nursing. Cited in Barnard, K. E. (1973). Nursing. In J. Wortis (Ed.), *Mental retardation and developmental disabilities: An annual review* (Vol. V, pp. 72–84). New York: Brunner/Mazel.

Beange, H., & Bauman, A. (1990). Caring for the developmentally disabled in the community. *Australian Family Physician, 19,* 1558–1563.

Bigby, C. (1997). Later life for adults with intellectual disability: A time of opportunity and vulnerability. *Journal of Intellectual and Developmental Disabilities, 22,* 97–108.

Bigby, C. (2000). Informal support networks of older adults. In M. P. Janicki & E. F. Ansello (Eds.), *Community supports for aging adults with lifelong disabilities* (pp. 55–70). Baltimore: Paul H. Brookes.

Botsford, A. L., & Force, L. T. (2000). *End-of-life care: A guide for supporting older persons with intellectual disabilities and their families.* Albany, NY: NYSARC.

Braddock, D., (1999). Aging and developmental disabilities: Demographic and policy issues affecting American families. *Mental Retardation, 37,* 155–161.

Braddock, D. & Hemp, R. (1997). Toward family and community: Mental retardation services in Massachusetts, New England, and the United States, *Mental Retardation, 35,* 241–256.

Carr, J., & Hollins, J. (1995). Menopause in women with learning disabilities. *Journal of Intellectual Deficiency Research, 39,* 137–139.

Chicoine, B., & McGuire, D. (1997). Longevity of a woman with Down syndrome: A case study. *Mental Retardation, 35,* 477–479.

Cohen, W., (1999). Health care guidelines for individuals with Down syndrome: 1999 revision. *Down Syndrome Quarterly*. Retrieved May 26, 2004 from http://www.denison.edu/collaborations/dsq/health99.html

Conliffe, C., & Walsh, P. N. (1999). An international perspective on quality. In S. S. Herr & G. Weber (Eds.), *Aging rights and quality of life: Prospects for older people with developmental disabilities* (pp. 237–252). Baltimore: Paul H. Brookes.

Cooper, S. (1998). Clinical study of the effects of age on the physical health of adults with mental retardation. *American Journal of Mental Retardation, 102*, 582–589.

Davidson, P. W., Heller, T., Janicki, M. P., & Hyer, K. (2004). Defining a national health research and practice agenda for older adults with intellectual disabilities. *Journal of Policy and Practice in Intellectual Disabilities, 1*, 2–9.

Davidson, P. W., Houser, K. D., Cain, N. N., Sloane-Reeves, J., Quijano, L., & Matons, L. (1999). Characteristics of older adults with intellectual disabilities referred for crisis intervention. *Journal of Intellectual Disabilities, 43*, 38–46.

Edgerton, R. B. (1994). Quality of life issues: Some people know how to be old. In M. M. Seltzer, M. W. Krauss, & M. P. Janicki (Eds.), *Life course perspectives on adulthood and old age* (pp. 53–66). Washington, DC: American Association on Mental Retardation.

Evenhuis, H. (1999). Associated medical aspects. In M. P. Janicki & A. J. Dalton (Eds.), *Dementia, aging, and intellectual disabilities: A handbook* (pp. 103–122). Philadelphia: Brunner/Mazel.

Evenhuis, H., Henderson, C. M., Beange, H., Lennox, N., & Chicoine, B. (2001). Healthy aging—adults with intellectual disabilities: Physical health issues. *Journal of Applied Research in Intellectual Disabilities, 14*, 175–194.

Eyman, R. K., & Borthwick-Duffy, S. A. (1994). Trends in mortality rates and predictors of mortality. In M. M. Seltzer, M. W. Krauss, & M. P. Janicki (Eds.), *Life course perspectives on adulthood and old age* (pp. 93–105). Washington, DC: American Association on Mental Retardation.

Factor, A. R. (1997). *Growing older with a developmental disability: Physical and cognitive changes and their implications.* Chicago, IL: Rehabilitation Research and Training Center on Aging with Mental Retardation, The University of Illinois.

Friedman, R. I. (1998). Use of advanced directives: Facilitating health care decisions by adults with mental retardation and their families. *Mental Retardation, 36*, 444–456.

Fujiura, G. T. (1998). The demography of family households. *American Journal of Mental Retardation, 103*, 225–235.

Geriatric assessment methods for clinical decision-making. NIH consensus statement. (1987). Retrieved April 8, 2004 from http://consensus.nih.gov/cons/065/065_statement.htm

Grogan, K. D., & Fryberger, Y. B. (1999). *Secondary conditions experienced by adults with developmental disabilities: Identification, prevention & management—A reference manual for physicians, nurses, allied health professionals and students serving adults with developmental disabilities.* Cincinnati, OH: University Affiliated Cincinnati Center for Developmental Disorders.

Hacker, K. S., McCallion, P., & Janicki, M. P. (2000). Outreach and assistance using Area Agencies on Aging. In M. P. Janicki & E. F. Ansello (Eds.), *Community supports for aging adults with lifelong disabilities* (pp. 439–455). Baltimore: Paul H. Brookes.

Hadjistavropoulos, T., & Craig, K. D. (2002). A theoretical framework for understanding self-report and observational measures of pain: A communications model. *Behavioral Research Therapies, 40*, 551–570.

Hahn, J. E. (1994). *Characteristics of nursing home residents with mental retardation and developmental disabilities: Nursing implications of the OBRA '87 determination of need for a nursing facility.* Unpublished dissertation. Chicago, IL: Rush University.

Hahn, J. E., & Aronow, H. U. (November 2003). *Promoting healthy aging with intellectual and developmental disability: A gerontological advanced practice nurse intervention.* Paper presented at the meeting of The Gerontological Society of America, San Diego, CA.

Hahn, J. E., Charron, K., & Willis, M. A. (2003) *James Russell, a MI/DDle-aged man with Down syndrome.* Orlando, FL: HealthSoft, Inc. Retrieved May 26, 2004 from www.health softonline.com

Hahn, J. E., & Willis, M. A. (2000). Addressing the need for nursing education about intellectual disabilities with interactive multimedia instruction: An effective choice (Abstract no. 452). *Journal of Intellectual Disability Research, 44,* 305–306.

Hammel, J., Heller, T., & Ying, G. S. (1998). Outcomes of assistive technology services and use by adults with developmental disabilities. *ADDvantage: A Newsletter about Aging and Developmental Disabilities, 10*(1), 3, 8–9.

Hawkins, B. A., & Eklund, S. J. (1994). *Aging-related changes in adults with mental retardation: Final report.* Bloomington, IN: Indiana University, Institute for the Study of Developmental Disabilities.

Hayden, M. F. (1998). Mortality among people with mental retardation living in the United States: Research review and policy applications. *Mental Retardation, 36,* 345–359.

Heller, T. (1999). Emerging models. In S. S. Herr & G. Weber (Eds.), *Aging rights and quality of life: Prospects for older people with developmental disabilities* (pp. 149–165). Baltimore: Paul H. Brookes.

Heller, T., Sterns, H., Sutton, E., & Factor, A. R. (1996). Impact of person-centered later life planning training program for older adults with mental retardation. *Journal of Rehabilitation, 62,* 77–83.

Henderson, C. M., & Davidson, P. W. (2000). Comprehensive adult and geriatric assessment. In M. P. Janicki & E. F. Ansello (Eds.), *Community supports for aging adults with lifelong disabilities* (pp. 373–386). Baltimore: Paul H. Brookes.

Herr, S. S., & Weber, G. (1999). Prospects for ensuring rights, quality supports, and a good old age. In S. S. Herr & G. Weber (Eds.), *Aging rights and quality of life: Prospects for older people with developmental disabilities* (pp. 343–370). Baltimore: Paul H. Brookes.

Improving the health and wellness of women with disabilities: A symposium to establish a research agenda (Section 4: Secondary Conditions). (2003). A Project of the Center for Research on Women with Disabilities Baylor College of Medicine. Supported by the Center for Disease Control and Prevention. Retrieved May 21, 2004 from http://www.crowdbcm.net/index.htm

Jacquemont, S., Farzin, F., Hall, D., Leehey, M., Tassone, F., Gane, L., et al. (2004). Aging in individuals with the *FMR1* mutation. *American Journal on Mental Retardation, 109,* 154–164.

Janicki, M. P. (1999). Public policy and service design. In S. S. Herr & G. Weber (Eds.), *Aging rights and quality of life: Prospects for older people with developmental disabilities* (pp. 289–310). Baltimore: Paul H. Brookes.

Janicki, M. P., & Ansello, E. F. (Eds.). (2000). *Community supports for aging adults with lifelong disabilities.* Baltimore: Paul H. Brookes.

Janicki, M. P., & Breitenbach, N. (2000). *Aging and intellectual disabilities—Improving longevity and promoting health aging: Summative report.* Geneva, Switzerland: World Health Organization.

Janicki, M. P., Dalton, A.J., Henderson, C. M., & Davidson, P. W. (1999). Mortality and morbidity among older adults with intellectual disability: Health services considerations. *Disability and Rehabilitation, 21,* 284–294.

Janicki, M. P., Heller, T., Seltzer, G., & Hogg, J. (1995). *Practice guidelines for the clinical assessment and care management of Alzheimer and other dementia among adults with mental retardation.* Washington, DC: American Association on Mental Retardation.

Janicki, M. P., McCallion, P., & Dalton, A. J. (2002). Dementia-related care decision-making in group homes for persons with intellectual disabilities. *Journal of Gerontological Social Work, 38,* 179–195.

Kapell, D., Nightingale, B., Rodriguez, A., Lee, J. H., Zigman, W. B., & Schupf, N. (1998). Prevalence of chronic medical conditions in adult with mental retardation: Comparison with the general population. *Mental Retardation, 36,* 269–279.

Kastner, T. A., Walsh, K. K., & Criscione, T. (1997). Overview and implications of Medicaid managed care for people with developmental disabilities, *Mental Retardation, 35,* 257–269.

Kivnick, H. Q. (1991). *Living with care, caring for life: The inventory of life strengths (Assessment Update).* Minneapolis: University of Minnesota, Long-Term Care DECISIONS Resource Center.

Lavin, C. M., & Doka, K. J. (1999). *Older adults with developmental disabilities.* Amityville, NY: Baywood.

Lennox, N. G., Green, M., Diggens, J., & Ugoni, A. (2001). Audit and comprehensive health assessment programme in the primary healthcare of adults with intellectual disability: A pilot study. *Journal of Intellectual Disability Research, 45,* 226–232.

LePore, P., & Janicki, M. P. (1997). *The wit to win: How to integrate older persons with developmental disabilities into community aging programs* (3rd ed.). Albany, NY: New York State Office for the Aging.

Lollar, D. J. (1994). *Preventing secondary conditions associated with spina bifida or cerebral palsy: Proceedings and recommendations of a symposium.* Washington, DC: Spina Bifida Association of America.

Ludlow, B. L. (1999). Life after loss: Legal, ethical and practical issues. In S. S. Herr & G. Weber (Eds.), *Aging rights and quality of life: Prospects for older people with developmental disabilities* (pp. 189–221). Baltimore: Paul H. Brookes.

McBreen, W. J. (1989). Elderly mentally retarded in nursing homes: Analysis of health care needs and critical nursing interventions. *Dissertation Abstracts International, 51*(9), 3922B.

McCallion, P. (1993). *Social worker orientations to permanency planning with older parents caring at home for family members with developmental disabilities.* Unpublished dissertation, SUNY at Albany.

Moss, S. (1999). Mental health: Access and quality of life. In S. S. Herr & G. Weber (Eds.), *Aging rights and quality of life: Prospects for older people with developmental disabilities* (pp. 167–187). Baltimore: Paul H. Brookes.

Natvig, D. A. (1994). The role of the nurse as a case manager/qualified mental retardation professional. In S. P. Roth & J. S. Morse (Eds.), *A life-span approach to nursing care for individuals with developmental disabilities* (pp. 385–400). Baltimore: Paul H. Brookes.

Newbern, V. B., & Hargett, M. V. (1992). The gerontological nursing and developmental disabilities. *Holistic Nurse Practitioner, 7,* 70–77.

Oliver, C. (1999). Perspectives on assessment and evaluation. In M. P. Janicki & A. J. Dalton (Eds.), *Dementia, aging, and intellectual disabilities: A handbook* (pp. 123–140). Philadelphia: Brunner/Mazel.

Omnibus Budget Reconciliation Act of 1987, Pub. L. No. 100–203, §§1819, 101 Stat. 1330 (1987).

Ott, S. M. (1999). Osteoporosis and osteomalacia. In W. R. Hazzard, J. P. Blass, W. H. Ettinger, J. B. Halter, & J. G. Ouslander (Eds.), *Principles of geriatric medicine and gerontology* (4th ed., pp. 1057–1084). New York: McGraw-Hill.

Overenynder, J. C., Janicki, M. P., & Turk, M. (Eds.) (1994*). Aging and cerebral palsy: Pathways to successful aging: A national action plan.* Albany, NY: New York State Developmental Disabilities Planning Council.

Patrick, D. L., Richardson, M., Starks, H. E., & Rose, M. A. (1994). A framework for promoting the health of people with disabilities. In D. J. Lollar (Ed.), *Preventing secondary conditions associated with spina bifida or cerebral palsy: Proceedings and recommendations of a symposium* (pp. 3–16). Washington, DC: Spina Bifida Association of America

Pope, A. M. (1992). Preventing secondary conditions. *Mental Retardation, 30,* 347–354.

Pope, A. M., & Tarlov, A. R. (1991). *Disability in America: Toward a national agenda for prevention.* Washington, DC: National Academy Press.

Rinck, C. (1991). *What do you like to do? A selection book of activities.* Kansas City, MO: UMKC Institute for Human Development, University Affiliated Program for Developmental Disabilities.

Russell, L. M., Grant, A. E., Joseph, S. M., & Fee, R. W. (1994). *Planning for the future: Providing a meaningful life for a child with a disability after your death.* Evanston, IL: American.

Schupf, N., Zigman, W., Kapell, D., Lee, J. H., Kline, J., & Levin, B. (1997). Early menopause in women with Down's syndrome. *Journal of Intellectual Deficiency Research, 41,* 264–267.

Seltzer, G. B., & Luchterhand, C. (1994). Health and well-being of older persons with developmental disabilities: A clinical review. In M. M. Seltzer, M. W. Krauss, & M. P. Janicki (Eds.), *Life course perspectives on adulthood and old age* (pp. 109–142). Washington, DC: American Association on Mental Retardation.

Seltzer, G. B., Schupf, N., & Wu, H.-S. (2001). A prospective study of menopause in women with Down syndrome. *Journal of Intellectual Disability Research, 45*(1), 1–7.

Seltzer, M. M., & Krauss, M. W. (1994). Aging parents with coresident adult children: The impact of lifelong caregiving. In M. M. Seltzer, M. W. Krauss, & M. P. Janicki (Eds.), *Life course perspectives on adulthood and old age* (pp. 3–18). Washington, DC: American Association on Mental Retardation.

Service, K. P. (May, 1996). *Social networks of elder parents of adult children with mental retardation.* Unpublished master's thesis. University of Massachusetts, Amherst, MA.

Service, K. P., & Hahn, J. E. (2003). Issues in aging: The role of the nurse in care of older people with intellectual and developmental disabilities. *Nursing Clinics of North America, 38,* 291–312.

Service, K. P., Lavoie, D., & Herlihy, J. E. (1999). Coping with losses, death, and grieving. In M. P. Janicki & A. J. Dalton (Eds.), *Dementia, aging, and intellectual disabilities: A handbook* (pp. 330–351). Philadelphia: Brunner/Mazel.

Service, K. P., & Willis, M. A. (1999). *Down syndrome: Care of the older adult* (computer-assisted instruction). Orlando, FL: HealthSoft, Inc.

Service, K. P., & Willis, M. A. (2003). *The older adult with mental retardation in a long term care setting.* Orlando, FL: HealthSoft, Inc. Retrieved May 26, 2004 from www.healthsoftonline.com

Shultz, J., Aman, M., Kelbley, T., Wallace, C. L., Burt, D. B., & Primeaux-Hart, S. (2004). Evaluation of a screening tool for dementia in older adults with mental retardation. *American Journal of Mental Retardation, 109,* 98–110.

Strauss, D., & Eyman, R. K. (1996). Mortality of people with mental retardation in California with and without Down syndrome, 1986–1991. *American Journal on Mental Retardation, 100,* 643–653.

Sutton, E. (1993). *Resource guide for specialists in developmental disabilities and aging* (revised). Akron, OH: RRTC Consortium on Aging and Developmental Disabilities.

The Arc. (1995). *Q & A: Alzheimer's disease and people with mental retardation. A fact sheet.* Arlington, TX: Author.

Turk, M. A., Overeynder, J. C., & Janicki, M. P. (1995). *Uncertain future—Aging and cerebral palsy: Clinical concerns.* Albany, NY: New York State Developmental Disabilities Planning Council.

Tyler, C. V., Snyder, C. W., & Zyzanski, S. (2000) Screening for osteoporosis in community-dwelling adults with mental retardation. *Mental Retardation, 38,* 316–21.

Urv, T. K., Zigman, W. B., & Silverman, W. (2003). Maladaptive behaviors related to adaptive decline in aging adults with mental retardation. *American Journal on Mental Retardation, 108,* 327–339.

U.S. Preventive Services Task Force. (1996). *Guide to clinical prevention services* (2nd ed.). AHCPR Publication No. OM97-0001. Washington, DC: U.S. Department of Health and Human Services, Public Health Service Agency for Healthcare Policy and Research.

U.S. Public Health Service. (2002). *Closing the gap: A national blueprint for improving the health of individuals with mental retardation. Report of the Surgeon General's Conference on Health Disparities and Mental Retardation.* Washington, DC: Author.

Walker, A., Walker, C., & Gosling, V. (1999). Quality of life as a matter of human rights. In S. S. Herr & G. Weber (Eds.), *Aging rights and quality of life: Prospects for older people with developmental disabilities* (pp. 109–132). Baltimore: Paul H. Brookes.

Walsh, K. K., Hammerman, S., Josephson, F., & Krupka, P. (2000). Caring for people with developmental disabilities: Survey of nurses about education and experience. *Mental Retardation, 38,* 33–41.

World Health Organization. (2001). *Ageing and intellectual disabilities—Improving longevity and promoting healthy aging: Summative report.* Geneva, Switzerland: Author.

Zwakhalen, S. M., van Dongen, K. A., Hamers, J. P., & Abu-Saad, H. H. (2004). Pain assessment in intellectually disabled people: Nonverbal indicators. *Journal of Advanced Nursing, 45,* 236–245.

Seizure Disorders

Jean Nelson Farley, MSN, RNC, PNP, CRRN

Objectives

At the completion of this chapter, the learner will be able to:

1. Define and explain the difference between the terms *seizure, epilepsy,* and *epilepsy syndrome.*

2. Describe the incidence and prevalence of seizure disorders in the general population and in those with intellectual and developmental disabilities (I/DD).

3. State the causes of seizure disorders.

4. Outline the categories of seizure disorders based on the International Classification System.

5. List the components of the assessment process for an individual with new onset of seizures.

6. Describe the variety of management options available for the treatment of seizures.

7. Use principles of family-centered care for individuals with a seizure disorder.

8. Apply knowledge about seizure disorders to enhance the quality of life of individuals with seizure disorders.

9. Promote self-care in individuals with seizure disorders.

Key Points

- The health care professional working with an individual with I/DD and epilepsy must be knowledgeable about the management of seizure disorders to prepare for best practice.

- Preparation for an advocacy role requires knowledge about a family's milieu, current seizure management practices, and resources available for support.

Key Points *(continued)*

- Family-centered care of an individual with a seizure disorder is crucial to optimal management, care, and quality of life.

- Systematic and appropriate application of critical thinking skills and collaboration with an interdisciplinary team can significantly enhance the quality of life of affected individuals and their families.

I. Definitions

A *seizure* is an abrupt change in behavior caused by an abnormal electrical discharge in the brain that is accompanied by a sudden alteration in motor and/or sensory functions and/or consciousness (Shafer, 1999). *Epilepsy* refers to a chronic condition in which an individual experiences recurrent seizures. Epilepsy is not a single disease, but rather a sign of underlying brain dysfunction. *Epileptic syndromes* are seizure disorders characterized by a cluster of signs and symptoms customarily occurring together accompanied by characteristic EEG findings (Weinstein, 2002).

A. Incidence and prevalence of seizures

1. Nine percent of the general population will experience a seizure at some time in life.

2. Approximately one third of this 9% lifetime rate are children with uncomplicated, febrile seizures who have no further episodes.

3. Approximately 2.3 million Americans are affected by epilepsy and seizures, with highest incidence in children and elderly persons.

4. Approximately 50% of children with a seizure disorder have some degree of mental retardation (Browne & Holmes, 2004; Ozuna, 2000; Shafer, 1999).

5. Prevalence of seizure disorders in various I/DD:

   a. Mental retardation: 20% (Airaksinen et al., 2000)

   b. Spina bifida/hydrocephalus: 15% (Noetzel, 1989)

   c. Cerebral palsy: 40–50% (Delgado, Riela, Mills, Pitt, & Browne, 1996)

6. Risk of death in epilepsy:

   a. Evidence supports that risk of death is greater in I/DD population with epilepsy (Perry, 2003).

   b. Individuals with epilepsy without other functional neurological deficits have similar death rate to the general population (Perry, 2003).

B. Etiology

1. Symptomatic:
   a. No immediate cause, but prior insult to brain has been identified:
      i. asphyxia
      ii. severe electrolyte or metabolic disturbance
      iii. stroke
      iv. trauma
      v. vascular lesion
      vi. degenerative CNS disease
      vii. static encephalopathy (cerebral palsy, mental retardation)
      viii. CNS infection
2. Idiopathic:
   a. Generally a benign course
   b. Presumed genetic origin; first gene for idiopathic epilepsy discovered in 1995
      i. benign rolandic epilepsy
      ii. childhood absence epilepsy
      iii. Recent genetic research points to a genetic defect in which the flow of potassium, sodium, and calcium into ion channels of nerve cells becomes disrupted (Carroll, 2003).
3. Cryptogenic:
   a. No cause is identified; approximately 70% of epilepsies have no known cause
   b. Presumed to be an underlying pathological cause that could be detected with improved diagnostic technology (Blair & Selekman, 2004; Lanfear, 2002; Ozuna, 2000; Shafer, 1999)
C. International Classification of Epileptic Seizures (ICES) (Commission on Classification and Terminology of the International League Against Epilepsy, 1989).
   1. First developed in 1969 by the International League Against Epilepsy, revised in 1981 and again in 1989 to add epileptic syndromes.
   2. Assists with:
      a. Assessing clinical progression
      b. Identifying appropriate treatment
      c. Evaluating response to therapy
   3. ICES Classification (Commission on Classification and Terminology of the International League Against Epilepsy, 1981):
      a. Partial (focal, local) seizures: Initial EEG changes indicate that original activation of seizure is limited to part of one hemisphere. May progress

to generalized motor seizures. Impaired consciousness defined as inability to respond normally to exogenous stimuli.

    i.   Simple partial seizures (consciousness not impaired)

        a.   with motor symptoms

        b.   with somato-sensory or special sensory symptoms

        c.   with autonomic symptoms or signs

        d.   with psychic symptoms

    ii.   Complex partial seizures (impairment of consciousness)

        a.   simple partial onset that progresses to impairment of consciousness

        b.   with impairment of consciousness at onset

    iii.   Partial seizures that are secondarily generalized (tonic-clonic, clonic, or tonic)

        a.   simple partial evolving to generalized

        b.   complex partial evolving to generalized

        c.   simple partial evolving to complex, evolving to generalized

b.   Generalized (convulsive or nonconvulsive) seizures: Involve initial involvement of both hemispheres, bilateral motor and EEG involvement.

    i.   absence

        a.   typical

        b.   atypical

    ii.   myoclonic seizures

    iii.   clonic seizures

    iv.   tonic seizures

    v.   tonic-clonic seizures

    vi.   atonic seizures

c.   Unclassified seizures: Include all seizures that cannot be classified because of inadequate data and some that defy classification in previous categories (e.g., some types of neonatal seizures).

d.   Epilepsy syndromes (Weinstein, 2002): Seizure disorders characterized by specific clinical features and a constellation of information, including:

    i.   age

    ii.   neurological signs and symptoms

    iii.   clinical course

    iv.   EEG findings

    v.   categories:

      a.   benign partial seizures (e.g., rolandic epilepsy)

      b.   infantile spasms (West syndrome) and myoclonic epilepsy

      c.   juvenile myoclonic epilepsy

      d.   atypical absence epilepsy syndromes

      e.   childhood epileptic degeneration with prominent nocturnal EEG abnormality (e.g., Lennox Gastaut syndrome and Landau Kleffner syndrome)

II. Assessment

A. History

    1. Health history (Lanfear, 2002)

      a.   Significant adverse prenatal, perinatal, and neonatal events

      b.   Significant infections, febrile illnesses, febrile seizures, head trauma, surgeries, and hospitalizations

      c.   Immunization status/untoward postvaccine side effects, especially post-DTP

      d.   Developmental milestones, school performance

      e.   Medication history/drug allergies/use of illicit drugs

      f.   History of lead or mercury poisoning

      g.   Review of systems, with careful attention to conditions that can mimic seizures: fainting, breath holding, hyperventilation, hypoglycemia, GER, sleep disturbances, bruxism, tics, migraines, TIAs, tardive dyskinesia, pseudo-seizures, rage reactions, panic attacks, ADHD, self-stimulatory behavior, and self-injurious behavior

      h.   History of prodrome or aura if diagnosis of seizure disorder already established

      i.   History of metabolic or genetic disorders

    2. Family medical history (Celano, 1998)

      a.   Seizures

          i.   mental retardation, genetic disorders

          ii.   metabolic disorders

          iii.   cerebral palsy

      b.   Family system

          i.   family constellation/birth order

          ii.   home environment

          iii.   primary/secondary caregiver

          iv.   stage of family development

          v.   response to diagnosis of seizure disorder

vi. patterns of family coping

vii. cultural beliefs, customs that may affect understanding and coping with epilepsy (Dean, 1996)

viii. spiritual beliefs that may affect coping with diagnosis

ix. socio-economic level

B. Physical assessment (Celano, 1998)

1. Growth patterns (height, weight, head circumference, and percentiles)

2. Neurological exam (primitive reflexes; DTRs; balance; RAMs; cognitive level; LOC; fundi; neurodevelopmental skills; tics; pupillary responses; strength; memory; orientation to time, place, and person; ability to follow commands)

3. Skin: cafe au lait spots, adenoma sebaceum, port wine stains, shagreen patches

4. Musculoskeletal: signs of trauma, injury

5. Sensory: visual and auditory acuity/processing, olfactory, proprioceptive

6. Major and minor congenital anomalies

7. Unusual body or body fluid odors, unusual qualities of body fluids

8. Cardiovascular: bruits, murmurs, arrhythmias

9. Abdomen: organomegaly

C. Diagnostic procedures (Weinstein, 2002)

1. Electroencephalogram (EEG)—Approximately 80% of individuals with seizure disorders have an abnormal EEG

a. Perform as soon as possible after occurrence of initial seizure

b. Assess for presence and characteristics of spike and wave pattern

c. Variety of stimuli used to provoke seizures during EEG:

i. photic (strobe light)

ii. hyperventilation

iii. sleep induction

iv. sleep deprivation

2. Ambulatory EEG monitoring

3. CCTV-EEG—Simultaneous closed-circuit TV observation of clinical behavior and EEG pattern that is useful in determining seizure type or presence of pseudo-seizures

4. Brain imaging techniques—Help to identify specific location of brain abnormality that may be focus of seizure

a. Computerized tomography (CT scan)

b. Magnetic resonance imaging (MRI scan)

     c. Positron emission tomography (PET scan)

     d. Single photon emission computed tomography (SPECT scan)

5. Laboratory studies—help to identify metabolic, toxic, and/or infectious problems that can cause seizures

     a. Glucose level

     b. CBC, blood cultures

     c. Lumbar puncture, CSF analysis

     d. Liver and renal function tests

     e. Calcium level

     f. Electrolytes

     g. Drug toxicity screens, lead level

     h. Urinalysis

     i. Metabolic screen, if warranted

     j. Chromosome analysis, if warranted

6. Psychometric evaluation

     a. May document presence of specific areas of brain abnormalities

     b. May be serially conducted to document cognitive deterioration or improvement after initiation of anticonvulsant therapy

III. Management of Seizures

A. Intraseizure care

1. Remain calm

2. Assess responsiveness:

     a. To verbal stimuli—use developmentally appropriate cues

     b. To proprioceptive stimuli (e.g., tickling)

3. Assess cardio-respiratory functioning and intervene if necessary (CPR)

4. Protect from injury (Pena, 2003; Pullen, 2003)

     a. Protect and maintain airway.

         i. Turn to side (recovery position) to allow secretions to drain and prevent aspiration.

     b. Place on bed or floor; do not lift from floor to bed while seizure is in progress.

     c. Clear immediate area of sharp or hard objects that could be a source of trauma.

     d. Do not force anything into mouth—may cause injury.

     e. Loosen clothing around neck and waist.

f.   Allow individual having partial seizure to move freely, but accompany to protect if needed.

g.   If hospitalized:

i.   Keep bed in low position.

ii.   Keep side rails up and padded.

iii.   Remove restraints if placed for another reason.

iv.   Do not try to move from floor to bed until seizure is over.

h.   Perform intraseizure and postseizure assessment

i.   Do assessment out loud to help recall events for later documentation.

a.   Note time of seizure onset and conclusion.

b.   Describe clinical appearance.

c.   Describe body parts involved and sequence of involvement.

d.   Describe postseizure behavior.

e.   Document seizure observations and any injury incurred on seizure record.

i.   Monitor for development of status epilepticus (SE). Refers to a seizure that lasts longer than 10 minutes or repeated seizures that occur over a period of 30 minutes, during which the individual does not recover or regain consciousness (Shafer, 1999). SE is a neurological emergency that may lead to transient or permanent brain injury and/or death (Gilbert, 2000).

i.   types of SE

a.   partial (e.g., Jacksonian)

b.   generalized (e.g., absence or tonic-clonic)

c.   localized (epilepticus partialis continua)

ii.   intervention

a.   Call rescue squad if seizure(s) have not subsided after 5 minutes, or follow agency protocol.

b.   Initiate safety measures for acute seizure management as outlined above.

B.   Postseizure care

1.   Continue to maintain and protect adequacy of airway/place in recovery position.

2.   Assess for return to baseline level of functioning.

3.   Allow rest period.

4.   Provide comfort measures.

a.   Change soiled clothing/bedding if incontinent.

b.   Offer analgesia if ordered for postseizure headache.

   c. Provide quiet, calm environment for recovery.

C. Postseizure assessment and management

   1. Review client level of compliance with anticonvulsant regimen.

   2. Assess for factors that may have precipitated seizure (Blair & Selekman, 2004; Lanfear, 2002).

      a. Physiological

         i.   recent illness, fever, trauma

         ii. sleep deprivation

         iii. change in exercise pattern

         iv. hormonal changes

         v.   weight gain

         vi. addition of another anti-epileptic drug (AED) or drug that could alter/lower present AED concentration

         vii. most recent serum AED drug level results

      b. Psychological

         i.   recent stress, depression, anxiety

      c. Exposure to potential seizure "triggers"

         i.   illicit drug or alcohol use

         ii. therapeutic drugs

            a. anesthetics

            b. sedative-hypnotics, especially withdrawal

            c. opiates, especially meperidine

            d. tricyclic antidepressants (dose dependent)

            e. neuroleptics, especially clozapine

            f. stimulants, especially methylphenidate, amphetamines, and cocaine

            g. antibiotics, especially quinolones and macrolides

         iii. photic stimuli (poorly adjusted TV, flashing lights)

         iv. auditory stimuli (certain sound frequencies in music, loud noises)

         v.   certain dietary triggers may lower seizure threshold

            a. excessive intake of chocolate, artificial sweeteners, caffeine

            b. hypoglycemia

         vi. olfactory stimuli (certain odors)

D. Pharmacologic management: The goal is to use the least number of medications (preferably monotherapy), while maintaining the maximum level of alertness with fewest seizures and medication side effects. However, individuals with I/DD often have multiple neurological problems, which contributes to the complexity of seizure management (Cole, 2002; Ozuna, 2000).

1. General principles in pharmacologic management of seizures (Leppik, 2002; Marks & Garcia, 1998; Weinstein, 2002)

    a. Anti-epileptic drugs (AED) generally act by stabilizing the flow of ions (calcium, sodium, and potassium) into and out of nerve cell membranes and preventing the spread of epileptic discharge.

    b. These channels are opened and closed by excitatory and inhibitory neurotransmitters that are released from nearby cells.

    c. Strive to attain a balance between seizure control and alertness when AEDs are needed to control seizures.

    d. Epilepsy is controlled by medication in approximately 70–90% of patients (Browne & Holmes, 2004).

    e. Monotherapy remains the treatment method of choice for new-onset epilepsy and is effective in preventing further seizures about 50% of the time (Browne & Bergey, 2004; Leppik, 2000).

    f. Most common cause of AED treatment failure is noncompliance (Dilorio et al., 2003).

    g. *Rational polypharmacy* may be needed for individuals with mixed or difficult to control seizure types (Ozuna, 2000).

        i.   If seizure control is not achieved with a single drug, a different single drug is tried; if unsuccessful, a second drug is added.

        ii. Choice of second drug is determined by adverse effects, drug interactions, dosing interval, cost, and mechanism of action.

    h. Selection of AED determined by

        i.   type of seizure classification

        ii.   age and sex of client

        iii. cost

        iv.   side effects (generally dose-related)

        v.   interactions with other drugs being used by client

        vi.   health and neurological status of client

        vii. overmedication with AEDs in the I/DD community has been well documented (Cole, 2002; Rutecki & Gidal, 2002)

    i. Advisable to obtain baseline hematologic profiles prior to initiating AED medications, based on their known hematologic side effects.

        i.   Health care professional should be familiar with the following characteristics of AEDs:

a.   pharmacokinetics

b.   side effects/signs of toxicity; most AEDs have potential to cause drowsiness, nausea, visual disturbances, blood dyscrasias, anorexia, and headache

c.   half-life/time needed to achieve steady state of drug in bloodstream

d.   safe dosage range

e.   safe routes/forms of administration

f.   therapeutic blood level

g.   significant drug-to-drug interactions (both AED-to-AED and AED to other concurrent medications

j.   Knowledge of AED drug half-life is critical to AED use (Callanan, 1997)

i.   Half-life is the time it takes for half of the AED drug dose to be eliminated from the body.

ii.   Takes about 4–5 half-lives for a steady-state AED blood level to be achieved.

iii.   Individual may need a single, large "loading dose" of AED medication to achieve a more rapid steady state.

iv.   Serum AED drug levels usually measured 4–5 half-lives after start of therapy.

k.   AED plasma levels (Brown, 1997)

i.   Indications for monitoring plasma AED levels:

a.   to determine if serum level is at a steady state after initiation of therapy and thereafter several times per year, as necessary

b.   following addition of another AED

c.   when interaction with non-AED is suspected

d.   when elimination may be altered by illness or disease

e.   when therapeutic effect is not achieved or symptoms of toxicity are observed

f.   when noncompliance is suspected

g.   when suspected maturational changes occur

h.   when significant weight loss or gain occurs

ii.   AED plasma determinations (Pena, 2003; Shirrell, Gibbar, Dooley, & Free, 1999):

a.   should be determined at the same time relative to a dose

b.   usually indicated whenever an AED has a narrow therapeutic range, if multiple doses are given, and/or other drugs are co-administered, which can alter drug metabolism and clearance

    i.   therapeutic range: signifies limits of drug concentration in serum that will yield desired pharmacological effect of drug without toxicity or failure

    ii.   trough level: lowest concentration of a drug in the blood serum; usually determined if there is concern that AED level is subtherapeutic

    iii.   peak level: highest concentration of drug in the blood serum; usually determined if there is concern about drug toxicity

l.   There can be differing bio-availability among AED drug forms (e.g., suspension vs. capsules, capsules vs. chewable tabs)

m.   There can be differing bio-availability between generic and trade forms of AED medications.

    i.   may lead to variable drug levels

n.   Allergic reactions to AED medications may be immediate (anaphylaxis) or take as long as 2–4 weeks to develop; often manifested by the appearance of a fine red rash.

o.   Stevens-Johnson Syndrome, a rare, but serious cutaneous reaction, may develop after initiation of AEDs (Shafer, 1999).

p.   Individuals with epilepsy should be considered for AED withdrawal if certain criteria are met (Browne & Holmes, 2004).

    i.   Predictors of successful AED withdrawal

        a.   seizure free for several years

        b.   few documented seizures over lifetime

        c.   no gross neurological abnormalities

        d.   subtherapeutic AED levels at time of discontinuance

        e.   persistently normal EEGs before and after discontinuance

    ii.   AEDs should always be withdrawn slowly, usually tapered off over 3–6 months. Abrupt withdrawal may precipitate seizures.

        a.   Children with idiopathic seizures, normal EEG, and no neurological dysfunction have a 90–95% chance of remaining seizure free without medication (Freeman, 2002).

        b.   Children with nonprogressive brain damage have a 40–60% chance of remaining seizure free, even if their EEGs are moderately abnormal (Freeman, 2002).

    iii.   Established AEDs (Fischer, 1997)

        a.   Barbiturates: phenobarbital, primidone

    b.   Hydantoins: phenytoin, fosphenytoin, mephenytoin

    c.   Benzodiazapines: diazepam, clonazepam, clorazepate, lorazepam, midazolam

    d.   Succinimides: ethosuximide, methsuximide

    e.   Miscellaneous: valproic acid, carbemazepine, paraldehyde

    f.   ACTH

iv.   Newer AEDs

    a.   Gabapentin (Neurontin)

    b.   Lamotrigine (Lamictal) (over age 16 years); high frequency of rash

    c.   Felbamate (Browne & Bergey, 2004; Freeman, 2002)

        1.   *used with caution* only for severe, refractory seizures; usually requires decrease in other AEDs

        2.   risk of aplastic anemia and hepatotoxicity

    d.   Topiramate (Topimax)

    e.   Tiagabine (Gabitril)

    f.   Levetiracetam (Keppra)

    g.   Oxcarbazine (Trileptal)

    h.   Zonisamide (Zonegran)

        1.   Vigabatrin (Sabril): not marketed in U.S. because of potential for producing myelin abnormalities in animal models and retinal toxicity seen in humans

v.   Numerous AEDs are currently in clinical development (Blum, 1998; Browne & Holmes, 2004).

vi.   Special considerations with use of AED therapy

    a.   phenytoin (Dilantin)

        1.   Absorption of oral form can be impaired if given in close proximity to or with enteral tube feedings.

        2.   IV form only compatible with normal saline; IV tubing used for administration must be fitted with a 0.22 micron filter.

        3.   IV form must be given slowly to prevent "purple glove syndrome," a delayed soft tissue injury that can occur with or without drug extravasation (Snelson & Dieckman, 2000).

        4.   Chewable and capsule forms have different half-lives (chewable has shorter half-life).

5. Suspension form should be used with caution due to risk of variable dosing (needs to be shaken well).

6. Often causes gingival hypertrophy with concomitant need for careful dental/oral hygiene.

7. Development of hirsutism with use may be objectionable to adolescents and adults.

b. Valproic Acid (Depakene, Depakote, Depacon)

1. Give with food to prevent GI disturbance.

2. Enteric-coated form helps decrease GI disturbance.

3. "Sprinkle" form should not be crushed.

4. May cause carnitine deficiency (DeVivo, 2002).

5. May cause lethargy associated with hyperammonemia.

c. Carbamazepine

1. AED level may increase if used concurrently with erythromycin, cimetidine, isoniazid, or propoxyphene.

2. Use may lower effectiveness of oral contraceptives.

d. Diazepam

1. Rectal gel form (Diastat) now available for home management of acute, repetitive ("breakthrough") seizures (Dreifuss, 1998).

e. Midazolam: intranasal route under investigation for use in febrile seizures.

f. Long-term use of AEDs and AED polypharmacy are associated with increased risk of bone density loss and osteoporosis.

E. Dietary management

1. Ketogenic diet: Attempts to put individual with seizures in state of ketosis with use of high fat, low protein, low carbohydrate diet (Blair & Selekman, 2004; Casey et al., 1999; Freeman, 2002)

a. Considered for treatment of intractable seizures; usually children with multiple handicaps or those having intolerable AED side effects.

b. Mechanism of action thought to involve stimulation of the seizure inhibition neurotransmitter, GABA (Browne & Holmes, 2004).

c. 4:1 ratio of fats to carbohydrates and protein; lack of palatability hinders compliance.

d. Requires initial hospitalization; rigid, complex protocols; and careful monitoring by professional team with expertise in this type of therapy.

e. Diet maintained for an average of 2 years; gradually discontinued if not effective after 3 months.

  f. Used primarily in children aged 1–10 years; not generally recommended for children with metabolic or mitochondrial disorders.

  g. May be effective with all seizure types, but particularly with idiopathic epilepsies and symptomatic, generalized seizure types

  h. Supplementation of calcium, B vitamins, and trace minerals needed.

  i. Side effects may include constipation, poor growth and weight gain, renal stones, optic nerve dysfunction, and dyslipidemia.

  j. Careful adherence to diet is associated with an approximate 40–50% reduction of seizures.

F. Surgical management: Removes epileptic focus from the brain while preserving normal function (Shafer, 1999; Weinstein, 2002)

 1. Criteria for selection:

  a. Clear diagnosis of seizure type and syndrome with elimination of nonepileptic etiology, such as metabolic or structural causes.

  b. Patient is truly refractory to AEDs that are appropriate to seizure type.

  c. Burdens of poorly controlled epilepsy or AED side effects are *significantly* limiting quality of life.

  d. Seizures must all arise from same portion (focus) of the brain.

  e. Excision of seizure focus will not cause unacceptable adverse effects in speech, movement, or proprioception.

 2. Preoperative assessment—Complex, presurgical investigation by epileptologist and neuropsychologist required to pinpoint seizure focus for resection or disconnection by neurosurgeon.

  a. Neurological exam, psychosocial evaluation, neuropsychological exam

  b. Imaging studies (MRI, SPECT, PET scans), CCTV-EEG monitoring

  c. Intracranial studies: depth, subdural grid mapping, epidural electrodes, Wada test

 3. Operative procedures

  a. Focal excision:

   i. removes seizure focus that can be localized to one area of the brain; most common is excision of temporal lobe focus

    a. Up to 90% of temporal lobectomies result in significant improvement of seizure control, with 68% becoming seizure free.

  b. Corpus callosotomy:

   i. to prevent spread of seizure discharges to other cerebral hemisphere

ii. may be indicated for intractable akinetic (drop) seizures or Lennox Gastaut syndrome

iii. does not stop seizures, but may limit severity and frequency

c. Hemispherectomy:

i. removes the majority of one cerebral hemisphere; occipital lobe and frontal lobe are disconnected

d. Postoperative complications:

i. depend on area of resection and may include:

a. contralateral superior quadrant anopsia

b. infection

c. hemiparesis

d. hemorrhage

e. aphasia

f. memory loss

G. Medical devices: vagus nerve stimulator (Morris & Mueller, 1999; Shafer, 1999)

1. Vagus nerve stimulation therapy—Pacemaker-like device surgically implanted in the chest with a lead tunneled from the generator to left cervical vagus nerve in the neck.

a. Uses the *NeuroCybernetic Prosthesis System* approved by FDA for use in U.S. in 1997.

b. Programmed for a dosage of stimulation that is delivered in continuous cycles 24 hours a day, regardless of seizure activity.

c. Small, hand-held magnet also given to patient or trained individual; when swiped over generator, an extra cycle of stimulation can be delivered at onset of aura or prodromal symptoms.

d. Theories of action

i. sends signal that interrupts seizures in areas of brain important for epileptogenesis

ii. produces increased blood flow to brain

iii. reduces metabolic activity of certain regions of brain

e. Candidates for device include those who:

i. are over age 12 years

ii. have diagnosis of refractory partial seizures with or without secondary generalization

iii. are poor responders to reasonable trials of AEDs

iv. are poor responders to, or candidates for, epilepsy surgery

    f. Does not eliminate need for AEDs, but when successful, allows for simplification of AED regimen; may take up to 18 months to determine effectiveness.

    g. MRI contraindicated while device in place; device not affected by microwaves, electronic devices, or computers.

    h. Extensive teaching and support required to maximize compliance and effectiveness.

    i. Possible side effects:

        i.   hoarseness

        ii. throat and neck vibrations or tingling when activated

        iii. coughing, gagging

H. Complementary and alternative therapies (CAT) in seizure management

Interventions that focus on body-mind-spirit connection to evoke healing and may be used as complements to conventional medical treatments (Freeman, 2002; Shafer, Sierzant, & Dean, 1997).

    1. Health care providers need to assess how they feel about use of complementary and alternative therapies (CATs).

    2. Health care provider must be knowledgeable about CATs to counsel regarding risks/benefits/costs.

    3. Differences in attitudes and behavior about health, illness, seizures, and therapies must be assessed in the context of the individual's culture and belief systems.

    4. Essential to assess use of CATs when taking health history of individuals with epilepsy.

    5. Types of CATs that may be used by individuals with epilepsy:

        a. Distraction techniques

        b. Behavioral techniques/biofeedback

        c. Stress management techniques (meditation, massage, aromatherapy)

        d. Physical therapies: chiropractic, osteopathy, cranio-sacral manipulation

        e. Biofeedback

        f. Nutritional therapies

            i. Vitamin B6 deficiency can produce seizures.

               a. may be added to AED regimen if seizures are difficult to control to evaluate for any beneficial effect

            ii. Low levels of calcium and magnesium are the only trace elements and minerals known to contribute to seizure activity.

            iii. Addition of other vitamin or mineral supplements to a balanced diet is of no documented benefit in seizure control.

iv. Mega-doses of vitamins, especially fat soluble vitamins and other nutritional supplements, are not indicated for the typical individual with epilepsy (Weinstein, 2002).

g. Homeopathic and herbal therapy

h. Acupuncture

i. Others: magnetic therapy, hyperbaric oxygen therapy, therapeutic touch

IV. Family-Centered Care for Individuals with Seizure Disorders

A. Utilize crisis management and grief resolution techniques with families confronted with diagnosis of a new seizure disorder.

B. Assess the family for factors that may affect their ability to adapt to having a member with a seizure disorder (Dean, 1996; Hausman et al., 1996):

1. Cognitive abilities

2. Cultural values

3. Coping skills

4. Family dynamics

5. Financial concerns

6. Lifestyle patterns

7. Health problems of other family members

8. Personality characteristics

9. Preconceived attitudes and beliefs

10. Support systems available

C. Use clear and understandable terminology when discussing diagnoses and management options to account for differing levels of health literacy.

D. Actively involve patient and family in decisions surrounding care and treatment; provide choices whenever feasible and reasonable.

E. Encourage and support families' efforts at information seeking.

F. Utilize knowledge of principles of human growth and development in developing care strategies for patients and families.

G. Seek knowledge and information to become culturally competent in providing health care.

H. Review and evaluate research findings to determine best practice with families.

I. Collaborate with other team members.

J. View the individual and family as *equal* members of the health care delivery team.

V.   Safety Promotion in Individuals with Seizure Disorders (Santilli, 1998; Shafer, 1998, 1999; Shafer, Austin, Callahan, & Clerico, 1996):

A. Factors associated with injury in individuals with seizure disorders

   1. Seizure frequency positively correlates with increase risk of injury.

   2. Seizures that alter awareness or consciousness or lead to a fall pose the greatest risks to safety.

   3. Side effects of certain AEDs (e.g., sedation, visual impairments, poor coordination, imbalance, ataxia)

   4. Majority of seizure-related injuries are minor and happen at home.

B. Accidental injuries:

   1. Are usually the primary concern of individuals with seizure disorders and their families

   2. Are a major cause of morbidity and mortality among individuals with seizure disorders

C. Prevention of accidental injury

   1. Assess workplace, home, and school to determine risks to safety and develop a management plan to *prevent injury*.

   2. Assess how important it is for the individual to participate in a risky activity.

   3. Assess benefits of participating.

   4. Assess costs (personal, financial) of safety measures.

   5. Primary prevention strategies

      a. Submersion and drowning accidents:

         i. Take showers instead of baths, use tub or shower bench, or sit in tub and use shower nozzle. Shower only when someone else is at home.

         ii. Install automatic water shut-off so that shower will shut off if drain becomes blocked.

         iii. Use "Occupied" sign on bathroom instead of locking door.

         iv. Install hand grips and nonskid strips in tub or shower stall.

         v. Parent who has seizures should sponge-bathe infant if alone.

         vi. Never leave child unattended in bathroom.

         vii. Do not use electrical appliances near water.

         viii. Keep sinks empty and toilet lids down.

         ix. Swim with a buddy who knows CPR and how to respond to a seizure.

         x. Alert lifeguards to seizure condition.

         xi. Wear a life jacket while swimming or boating.

      b. Burns:

      i.   Use microwave oven and microwave-safe dishes (dishware stays cool).

      ii.   Use back burners of stove and long oven mitts.

      iii.   Place stationary shields around fireplaces and wood-burning stoves.

      iv.   Consider installing safety devices that adjust water temperature.

      v.   Cover exposed heating units such as radiators and space heaters.

      vi.   Drink heated drinks from a thermal, covered mug.

      vii.   Do not smoke alone; avoid sources of open flame when alone.

  c. Falls and injuries:

      i.   Avoid scatter rugs; keep hallways and stairs clear of obstacles.

      ii.   Store frequently used items at easy-to-reach height.

      iii.   Use side rails for beds and chairs with sidcarms.

      iv.   Use food processors and choppers instead of knives.

      v.   Use hygiene products in plastic bottles in shower.

      vi.   Use infant sponge seat that supports infant in tub with shallow water.

      vii.   Use shatterproof safety glass for shower doors, sliding doors, and mirrors.

      viii.   Use elevators instead of stairs and escalators.

      ix.   Use protective headgear/helmet if indicated in situations involving risk of head injury; best head protection offered by hockey helmets and Danmar helmets.

      x.   Store AEDs safely away from children, preferably in a locked cabinet.

6. Secondary prevention measures:

  a. Protect personal safety:

      i.   Make sure that family members, friends, and coworkers know CPR, seizure first aid, and first aid for choking.

      ii.   Carry an emergency medical card in wallet; consider wearing Medic-alert jewelry.

      iii.   Alert local police, rescue squad, and neighbors about seizure diagnosis.

      iv.   Use auras or prodromes to take action to reduce risk of injury from seizures.

      v.   Avoid activities that are known to increase individual risk for seizures.

      vi.   Have family learn what to do by having "seizure drills" that review first aid steps and how to call for help.

VI. **Epilepsy and Its Effect on Quality of Life** (Austin & Dunn, 2000; Freeman, 2002; Ozuna, 2000)

    A. Physiological problems

        1. Poor seizure control

        2. Medication side effects

        3. Lack of control during seizures

        4. Memory loss

        5. Sleep disorders

        6. Difficulties with clear thinking and concentration

        7. Drowsiness

    B. Psychosocial issues

        1. Perceived and real social stigma, social isolation, and discrimination in workplace and school

        2. Depression

        3. Limitations on home, school, workplace, or recreational activities

            a. Drinking alcoholic beverages

            b. Employment opportunities

            c. Participation in sports

            d. Exercising

            e. Driving

                i. Restrictions on license issuance vary from state to state.

            f. Risk of seizure and risk of driving must be assessed individually by primary health care provider or neurologist.

            g. Some states may require health care provider to report the name of an individual whom they feel is driving against medical advice.

            h. Estimated that, of accidents involving an individual with epilepsy, only one of five accidents was a direct result of a seizure.

VII. **Women's Health Issues in Seizure Disorder Management** (Browne & Holmes, 2004; Callanen & Stallard, 1996; Freeman, 2002; Guberman, 1999; Klein, Passel-Clark, & Pezullo, 2003; Leppik, 2002; Shafer, 1997)

    A. Hormone-sensitive seizures

        1. Seen in both men and women, but more easily identifiable in women

        2. Catamenial epilepsy—Seizures occur in relation to the menstrual cycle:

            a. Menarchal, ovulatory, premenstrual, menstrual

            b. May be due to changes in plasma AED levels in response to hormones

c. May be due to fluctuations in estrogen and progesterone levels, which influence specific mechanisms that alter cell metabolism and neural transmission

d. Peri-menarche may be a risk for the development or worsening of epilepsy

e. Management

   i.   careful documentation of seizures with respect to cyclic changes

   ii. monitor AED dosages and levels

   iii. may need cyclical AED dose adjustment or hormone therapy

B. Reproductive dysfunction

1. Common in women with epilepsy.

2. Fertility may be as low as 2/3 of that expected in general population.

3. Sexual dysfunction may be disorders of desire or physiologic arousal.

C. Pregnancy

1. Approximately 30% of women with epilepsy have an increase in seizures during pregnancy.

2. Infants of mothers with epilepsy are about twice as likely to have an adverse pregnancy outcome or medical problems (e.g., stillbirth, neonatal death, intrauterine growth retardation, prematurity, learning disability, mental retardation, and/or epilepsy).

3. Genetic counseling is recommended preconceptually for women with epilepsy who are considering pregnancy.

D. Birth defects and epilepsy

1. Risk for fetal malformations in any individual pregnancy in a woman with epilepsy using a single, established AED is estimated at 4–6%; risk in the general population is estimated at 2–3%.

2. Defects most commonly observed include cleft lip/palate, neural tube defects, uro-genital defects, and minor congenital anomalies.

3. Registries have been developed to monitor teratogenic effects of AEDs.

E. Labor and delivery: Increased tendency for bleeding in neonate due to induction of hepatic enzymes by AEDs

1. Vitamin K used to treat this

F. Breastfeeding

1. Mothers on AEDs can breastfeed.

2. All AEDs will appear in breastmilk, but in very low concentrations that seldom affect the infant; concentration in breast milk determined by protein-binding capacity of AED.

3. Benefits of breast feeding have to be weighed with known and unknown risks of exposure of infant to AEDs.

4. Clinical symptoms of increased plasma concentration of AEDs in infants being breast fed by women on AEDs generally include lethargy, poor suck, and irritability; most often seen with phenobarbital and phenytoin.

5. If symptoms noticed, AED blood level should be checked in infant; if too high, breastfeeding may have to be stopped for a few days.

G. Contraception: Contraceptive dosages may need adjustment in women taking AEDs.

1. Evidence exists that contraception may fail when combined with AEDs, which have inducing effects on endogenous estrogen and progesterone.

H. Menopause:

1. Seizure frequency increases by approximately 30%, remains the same in 30%, and decreases in 30% of women during menopause.

2. Initial onset of seizures may occur at or after menopause in some women.

3. Effect of HRT for menopausal women with epilepsy has not been evaluated.

I. Osteoporosis

1. Link between chronic use of AEDs in females and osteoporosis.

2. Females who are nonambulatory or sedentary are at highest risk.

2. Vitamin D supplementation and controlled sun exposure recommended to offset effects of phenytoin on bone loss.

4. No guidelines have been established regarding initiation and frequency of bone density measurement in women taking AEDs.

VIII. Role of Health Care Providers in Self-Management of Seizure Disorders (Buelow, 2000; Dilorio & Henry, 1995; Hausman et al., 1996; Shafer, 1994):

A. Assessment

1. Factors that influence learning and self-management (Dilorio et al., 2003)

    a. Learning needs/readiness for learning

    b. Level of adaptation

    c. Functional level

    d. Neuro-cognitive status/developmental level

    e. Social/emotional functioning

    f. Resources and support systems

    g. Individual and family adjustment to diagnosis

2. Key education topics

    a. Description and explanation of seizure type

    b. Medications

        i. actions

        ii. side effects/signs of toxicity

        iii. importance of correct dosing and timing of medications

    c. Use of lifestyle modifications to minimize seizure precipitants

        i. Minimize exposure to auditory stimuli.

            a. Use earphones in noisy or crowded areas.

        ii. Minimize exposure to photic stimuli.

            a. Use polarized or tinted glasses.

            b. Avoid exposure to flashing or strobe lights.

            c. Focus on distant objects while in car.

            d. Use filter on computer screen to decrease contrast and flickering.

        iii. Regulate sleeping habits to ensure adequate sleep.

        iv. Plan regular exercise.

            a. Pace exercises and avoid sports that induce hyperventilation.

        v. Maintain balanced diet and regular meal patterns.

            a. Regulate meals around sleep, activity, and medications.

            b. Take frequent, small meals if appetite is poor.

            c. Avoid foods that may trigger seizures.

        vi. Avoid use of alcohol/drugs.

            a. Avoid all recreational drugs.

            b. Discuss alcohol use with primary health care provider or neurologist.

        vii. Monitor hormonal changes.

            a. Both men and women may notice cyclical patterns to seizures.

            b. Modify lifestyle to limit identified seizure triggers during high-risk cyclical phases.

        viii. Minimize stress.

        ix. Notify health care provider if experiencing significant illness, fever, or trauma.

            a. Limit other seizure triggers as much as possible during periods of illness.

    d. Safety issues

        i. first aid techniques for intra- and postictal state

ii.   how to summon emergency help

iii.   use of Medic-alert jewelry

e.   Maintenance of seizure calendar/record

f.   Driving restrictions pertinent to state of residency

g.   Recognition of seizure aura or prodrome

h.   Employment safety issues

i.   Resources for management and adaptation to seizure disorder

IX.   Summary

Seizure disorders are discussed in terms of definitions, classifications, etiologies, physical assessment, and management. Principles of family-centered care and the promotion of self-care are further covered. Health care professionals specializing in I/DD should be knowledgeable about seizure disorders and their management.

References

Airaksinen, E. M., Matalainen, R., Mononen, T., Mustonen, K., Partanen, J., & Jokela, V. (2000). A population based study on epilepsy in mentally retarded children. *Epilepsia, 41,* 1214–1220.

Austin, J., & Dunn, D. (2000). Children with epilepsy: Quality of life and psychosocial needs. *Annual Review of Nursing Research,* 1826–1847.

Blair, J., & Selekman, J. (2004). Epilepsy. In P. J. Allen & J. A. Vessey (Eds.), *Primary care of the child with a chronic condition* (pp. 469–497). St. Louis, MO: Mosby.

Blum, D. (1998). New drugs for persons with epilepsy. *Advances in Neurology, 76,* 57–87.

Brown, L. (1997). Seizure disorders. In M. L. Batshaw (Ed.). *Children with developmental disabilities* (4th ed., pp. 553–593). Baltimore: Paul H. Brookes.

Browne, G., & Bergey, G. (2004). Recent advances in the treatment of epilepsy: Live web conference. Retrieved March 26, 2004 from http://www.medscape.com

Browne, T., & Holmes, G. (2004). *Handbook of epilepsy* (3rd ed.). Philadelphia: Lippincott, Williams & Wilkins.

Buelow, J. (2000). Self-management of epilepsy: A review of the concept and its outcomes. *Disease Management & Health Outcomes, 8,* 327–336.

Callanan, M. (1997). Health education for medical therapies. *Clinical Nursing Practice in Epilepsy, 4,* 8–9.

Callanen, M., & Stallard, N. (1996). Issues for women with epilepsy. In N. Santilli (Ed.). *Managing seizure disorders: A handbook for healthcare professionals* (pp. 113–118). Philadelphia: Lippincott-Raven.

Carroll, L., (2003, February 18). Mounting data on epilepsy points to dangers of repeated seizures. *New York Times,* p. D5.

Casey, J., McGrogan, J., Pillas, J., Pyzik, J., Freeman, J., & Vining, E. (1999). Implementation of the ketogenic diet in children. *Journal of Neuroscience Nursing, 31,* 294–302.

Celano, R. (1998). Diagnosing pediatric epilepsy: An update for the primary care clinician. *The Nurse Practitioner, 23,* 69–96.

Cole, A. (2002). Evaluation and treatment of epilepsy in multiply handicapped individuals. *Epilepsy and Behavior, 3*(6, Supplement 2), S2–S6.

Commission on Classification and Terminology of the International League Against Epilepsy. (1989). Proposal for revised classification of epilepsies and epileptic syndromes. *Epilepsia, 30,* 389–399.

Commission on Classification and Terminology of the International League Against Epilepsy. (1981). Proposal for revised clinical and electroencephalographic classification of epileptic seizures. *Epilepsia, 20,* 489–501.

Dean, P. (1996). Cultural issues and epilepsy. In N. Santilli (Ed.), *Managing seizure disorders: A handbook for health professionals* (pp. 229–236). Philadelphia: Lippincott.

Delgado, M., Riela, A., Mills, J., Pitt, A., & Browne, R. (1996). Discontinuation of anti-epileptic drug treatment after two seizure-free years in children with cerebral palsy. *Pediatrics, 97,* 192–197.

DeVivo, D. (2002). Effectiveness of L-carnitine treatment for valproate-induced hepatotoxicity. *Neurology, 58,* 507.

Dilorio, C., & Henry, M. (1995). Self-management in persons with epilepsy. *Journal of Neuroscience Nursing, 27,* 338–343.

Dilorio, C., Yeager, K., Shafer, P., Letz, R., Henry, T., Schomer, D., et al. (2003). The epilepsy medication and treatment complexity index: Reliability and validity testing. *Journal of Neuroscience Nursing, 35,* 155–162.

Dreifuss, F. (1998). A comparison of rectal diazepam gel and placebo for acute repetitive seizures. *New England Journal of Medicine, 338,* 1869–1875.

Fischer, P. (1997). Guidelines for fosphenytoin administration. *Clinical Nursing Practice in Epilepsy, 4,* 13.

Freeman, J. (2002). *Seizures in epilepsy and childhood: A guide.* Baltimore: Johns Hopkins Press.

Gilbert, M. (2000). Evaluation of an algorithm for treatment of status epilepticus in adult patients undergoing video-EEG monitoring. *Journal of Neuroscience Nursing, 32*(2), 101–107.

Guberman, A. (1999). Hormonal contraception and epilepsy. *Neurology, 53*(Suppl 1), S38–S40.

Hausman, S., Luckstein, R., Zwygart, A., Cicora, K., Shroeder, V., & Weinhold, O. (1996). Epilepsy education: A nursing perspective. *Mayo Clinic Proceedings, 71,* 1114–1117.

Klein, P., Passel-Clark, L., & Pezullo, J. (2003). Onset of epilepsy at the time of menarche. *Neurology, 60,* 495–497.

Lanfear, J. (2002). The individual with epilepsy. *Nursing Standard, 16*(46), 43–55.

Leppik, I. (2000). Monotherapy and polypharmacy. *Neurology, 55*(Suppl 3), S25–S29.

Leppik, I. (2002). *Contemporary diagnosis and management of the patient with epilepsy* (5th ed.). Newtown, PA: Handbooks in Health Care.

Marks, W., & Garcia, P. (1998). Management of seizures and epilepsy. *American Family Physician, 57,* 1590–2000.

Morris, G., & Mueller, W. (1999). Long-term treatment with vagus nerve stimulation in patients with refractory epilepsy. *Neurology, 53,* 1731–1735.

Noetzel, M. (1989). Meningomyelocele: Current concepts of management. *Clinics in Perinatology, 16,* 311–329.

Ozuna, J. (2000). Seizure disorders and epilepsy. *Lippincott's Primary Care Practice, 4,* 608–618.

Pena, C. (2003). Seizure: A calm response and careful observation are crucial. *American Journal of Nursing, 103*(11), 73–81.

Perry, L. (2003). Functional neurological deficit increases the risk of death in childhood epilepsy. *Evidenced Based Nursing, 6*(1), 25.

Pullen, R. (2003). Protecting your patient during a seizure. *Nursing, 33*(4), 78.

Rutecki, P., & Gidal, B. (2002). Anti-epileptic drug treatment in the developmentally disabled: Treatment considerations with the newer anti-epileptic drugs. *Epilepsy and Behavior, 3*(6), S24–S31.

Santilli, N. (1998). Preventing accidental injury in people with epilepsy. *Clinical Nursing Practice in Epilepsy, 5,* 11–13.

Shafer, P. (1999). Epilepsy and seizures. *Nursing Clinics of North America, 34,* 743–759.

Shafer, P. O. (1997). Hormone sensitive seizures in women with epilepsy. *Clinical Nursing Practice in Epilepsy, 4,* 8–10.

Shafer, P. O. (1994). Nursing support of epilepsy self management. *Clinical Nursing Practice in Epilepsy, 2,* 11–14.

Shafer, P., Austin, D., Callahan, M., & Clerico, C. (1996). Safety and activities of daily living for people with epilepsy. In N. Santilli (Ed.). *Managing seizure disorders: A handbook for health care professionals* (pp. 171–187). Philadelphia: Lippincott-Raven.

Shafer, P. O., Sierzant, T., & Dean, P. (1997). Alternative and complementary therapies: Focus on epilepsy. *Clinical Nursing Practice in Epilepsy, 4,* 4–8.

Shafer, R. (1998). Counseling women with epilepsy. *Epilepsia, 39*(Suppl 8), S38–S44.

Shirrell, D., Gibbar, T., Dooley, R., & Free, C. (1999). Understanding therapeutic drug monitoring. *American Journal of Nursing, 99*(1), 42–44.

Snelson, C., & Dieckman, B. (2000). Recognizing and managing purple glove syndrome. *Critical Care Nurse, 20*(3), 54.

Weinstein, S. (2002). Epilepsy. In M. L. Batshaw (Ed.), *Children with disabilities* (pp. 493–523). Baltimore: Paul A. Brooks.

Nutrition

Judith Amundson, MS, RD/LD

16

Objectives

At the completion of this chapter, the learner will be able to:

1. Identify the importance of primary and secondary nutrition conditions from birth to old age, including conditions commonly found in persons with intellectual and developmental disabilities (I/DD).

2. Discuss the seriousness of nutrition disorders for quality of life and life expectancy; in particular, for persons with I/DD.

3. Analyze the necessary tools to screen for nutrition problems when a dietitian is unavailable.

4. Collaborate with a variety of professional organizations and agencies to expand the availability, access, and awareness of nutrition services, especially for persons with I/DD.

Key Points

- If people with I/DD are to meet and maintain their optimal potential, nutritional health is essential.

- People with I/DD are subject to the same nutritional disorders as the general population and may be prone to additional problems.

- Nutrition health is an often overlooked aspect in the lives of people with I/DD.

- Interdisciplinary intervention for nutritional disorders is recommended for best results.

- Person- and family-centered care is essential for optimal success.

I.   Background

The provision of sound nutritional information, assessment, and treatment plans is a vital link in caring for special populations. Until recently, however, nutrition services have been the missing link.

A. Normal nutrition for the life cycle (American Dietetic Association, 2000)

1. Full-term infants

a. Require adequate nutrition for growth and development.

b. Use the feeding experience to bond with caregivers and begin the socialization process.

c. Develop eating skills by trying a variety of flavors and textures in accordance with the infant's development stage.

d. Develop positive attitudes toward food and healthful eating habits for a lifetime.

2. Toddlers and preschool children

a. Require adequate nutrition for growth and development.

b. Develop sense of taste-acceptance of a variety of foods and enjoyment of eating.

c. Develop life-long positive eating habits.

3. School-aged children

a. Develop life-long positive eating habits.

b. Put down adequate nutrient stores to meet the demands of the adolescent growth spurt.

c. Learn the appropriate eating habits needed to prevent nutrition-related chronic health disorders.

4. Adolescents

a. Provide adequate nutrition for the growth and developmental demands of puberty.

b. Maintain nutritional state that prevents nutritional diseases and promotes health for adulthood.

5. Older adults

a. Provide nutritional adequacy to enhance quality of life.

b. Prevent nutrition-related problems associated with aging.

c. Provide treatment for age-related nutrition conditions.

B. Screening and assessment (Hammond, 2000)

1. All persons should have a basic nutrition screening.

a. Anthropometrics including height or recumbent length and weight

b. Clinical review of medical and dental records

    c.   General biochemical review

    d.   Dietary history

    e.   Developmental feeding skills

2.   Several conditions resulting in I/DD will require in-depth assessment by a registered dietitian.

    a.   Persons with cerebral palsy usually have altered energy needs leading to being underweight or overweight, and may have drug–nutrient interactions, constipation or diarrhea, feeding problems, and nutrient deficiencies.

    b.   Persons with Down syndrome also may have the above special nutritional needs and also be prone to gum disease.

    c.   Persons with mental retardation should be assessed for the above issues and additionally assessed for pica.

    d.   Persons with inborn errors of metabolism need to be followed closely for growth, altered nutritional needs, and special formula needs.

    e.   Persons with Prader-Willi Syndrome require close supervision of their weight, altered energy needs, and feeding problems.

    f.   Persons with spina bifida may have altered energy needs, altered growth, constipation, urinary tract infections, and drug–nutrient interactions.

II. Common Nutritional Issues

Obesity, drug–nutrient interactions, and feeding disorders are common to many of the above I/DDs.

A. Obesity

    1.   Definition and measurement (Goran, 1998)

        a.   Excess adipose tissue

        b.   Weight for length/height ratio for children

        c.   Skinfold thickness

        d.   Body Mass Index

    2.   Occurrence

        a.   Epidemic proportions of 20–30% in general population

        b.   May be higher in several special populations such as Down syndrome, Prader-Willi, spina bifida, and cerebral palsy

    3.   Secondary conditions and associated complications (Dietz, 1998)

        a.   Hypercholesterolemia

        b.   Hypertension

        c.   Type II diabetes

        d.   Stroke or kidney failure

      e. Coronary heart disease, congestive heart failure

      f. Sleep apnea due to upper-airway obstruction

      g. Osteoarthritis, impaired mobility

      h. Low self-esteem and other psychosocial issues, including social isolation

      i. Poor female reproductive health

4. Causes

      a. Single gene disorders (rare) (e.g., Prader-Willi syndrome)

      b. Gene-mediated propensity for weight gain

      c. Energy intake vs. energy output

      d. Endogenous chemicals (e.g., medications)

      e. Environmental influences

      f. Immobility

5. Treatment (Snetslaar, 2000)

      a. Early intervention

      b. Multidisciplinary to include medicine, nutrition, psychology, physical therapy

      c. Family participation/cooperation

      d. Increased regular physical activity

      e. Small gradual dietary changes (young children usually do not need to lose weight but grow into their weight)

      f. Therapist must be familiar with the stages of change (Sigman-Grant, 1996):

          i.   precompensation

          ii. contemplation

          iii. preparation

          iv. action

          v. maintenance

          vi. relapse

B. Failure to thrive (Kelsey, 1992)

    1. Identification

        a. Organic vs. inorganic

           i.   Organic failure-to-thrive requires a diagnosable disease, generally gastrointestinal, cardiac or pulmonary, endocrine, or central nervous system disorders (approximately 20%).

          ii. Inorganic (nonorganic) generally requires family and environmental evaluation.

          iii. Evaluation and dietary treatment require a thorough multidisciplinary team and may require hospitalization.

C. Feeding and eating disorders (Isaacs et al., 1997)

   1. Identification of feeding problems

      a. Poor suck and/or swallow

      b. Tonic bite reflex

      c. Hypersensitive gag reflex

      d. Hypersensitivity to touch or temperature

      e. Tongue thrust

      f. Anatomical abnormalities (e.g., cleft lip or palate)

      g. Severe dental caries and/or gum disease

      h. Repeated upper respiratory infections or pneumonia

      i. Frequent coughing or choking during meals

      j. Delayed feeding skill development

      k. Nasal regurgitation

   2. Diagnoses frequently related to feeding problems

      a. Down syndrome

      b. Rett syndrome

      c. Spina bifida

      d. Chronic constipation

      e. Heart disease

      f. Williams syndrome

      g. Pulmonary disease

      h. Mental retardation

      i. Seizure disorders

      j. Prader-Willi syndrome

      k. Fetal alcohol syndrome

      l. Autism

      m. Prematurity

   3. Consequences of feeding problems

      a. Inadequate weight gain

      b. Extended feeding times

      c. Choking

      d. Pneumonia

   4. Treatment

      a. Treatment may be simple or complicated and will depend on the causes of the basis of the problem: developmental, behavioral, or medical.

b. Treatment may involve input from medicine, nutrition, speech therapy, occupational therapy, psychology, and physical therapy.

c. If gastrointestinal reflux, choking, or pneumonia is present treatment may include gastrostomy tube placement.

D. Drug–nutrient interactions (Brizee, 1992; Haken, 2000; Springer & Shlafer, 1992)

1. The chemical agents used to prevent or treat disease interact with foods and nutrition in several ways

    a. Appetite

    b. Nutrient digestion, absorption, metabolism, or excretion

2. Nutritional status and diet affect the action of drugs by

    a. Altering metabolism

    b. Altering functions

    c. Some dietary components may have pharmacologic activity under certain circumstances

3. The most common interactions include:

    a. Antibiotics causing gastrointestinal problems

    b. Anticonvulsants causing deficiencies of vitamin D, folate, or carnitine

4. Stimulant medications

    a. Decreased appetite

    b. Decreased linear growth in children

    c. Decreased weight gain or weight loss in all ages

5. Corticosteroids

    a. Hypernatremia

    b. Hypokalemia

    c. Increased protein catabolism

    d. Potential deficiencies of vitamins B, B_6, C, and D, and folate

(For an extensive, detailed list of drug–nutrient interactions, see Springer and Shlafer, 1992.)

III. I/DDs with Significant Nutritional Issues

Many I/DDs either cause nutritional problems or are caused by nutritional problems. It is important to consult with registered dietitians who have experience in working with people with these conditions.

A. Inborn errors of metabolism known to cause I/DD and treatable by nutritional means (Berry, Hull, Scribanu, & Hunt, 1992)

1. Homocystinuria, a deficiency of cystathionine beta synthase causing mental retardation, ectopia lentis, and thromboembolic and cardiovascular disease. Treatment with a methionine-restricted diet started in early infancy can prevent mental retardation.

2. Phenylketonuria (PKU), a deficiency of phenylalanine hydroxylase causing high blood concentrations of the amino acid phenylalanine is routinely screened for in newborns. If treatment is begun at once, mental retardation will be avoided. Dietary treatment must determine the minimum amount of this essential amino acid and develop the appropriate intake of all protein-containing foods.

3. Galactocemia, a deficiency of galactokinase, if left untreated may cause mental and physical retardation, liver disorders, and cataracts. All dairy products must be avoided as well as many processed foods.

4. Maple syrup urine disease involves a defect in the metabolism of branched-chain (valine, isoleucine, and lycine) amino acids. Dietary restriction, as well as the possibility of peritoneal dialysis, are treatment measures. Can be fatal if not treated.

B. Wilson's disease (Stevens, 1992)

1. Wilson's disease may cause liver, kidney, brain, and cornea damage. Identification usually does not occur until the elementary school–age years.

2. Several nutritional deficiencies may exist and require treatment, including iron, zinc, pyridoxine, and manganese.

3. Feeding problems also may be present and require treatment.

C. Cerebral palsy (Bandini, Patterson, & Ekvall, 1992)

1. Anthropometric measures for persons with CP may be very difficult depending on the type of CP and the degree of ambulation and spasticity. Total body water, body cell mass, body mass index, arm span, leg length, and skinfold thicknesses are some methods that may be used. People with CP tend to be shorter than the norm and, due to lack of ambulation, may appear to have excess fat.

2. If the person with CP has a seizure disorder, certain medications may result in deficiencies of vitamin D, folate, biotin, and B_{12}.

3. If persons with CP have difficulty with feeding skills, chewing, and swallowing, other nutrient deficiencies may exist. This condition may result in gastrostomy placement.

4. Constipation and dental problems also may occur and need to be treated nutritionally.

D. Myelomeningocele/spina bifida (Ekvall, 1992)

1. Prenatal nutrition has been the focus in the prevention of SB, especially adequate intakes of folic acid.

2. Infants with spina bifida have mean weights and lengths/heights significantly lower than the norm. Lower limb atrophy leads to lower heights in children and adults. Decreased mobility and short stature tend to lead to being overweight. Ongoing calorie intake and weight management are critical aspects of dietary care.

3. Urinary infections may be treated temporarily with an acid ash diet to help prevent bacterial growth, but a lack of fruits and vegetables makes this diet unsatisfactory for the long term.

4. High fiber and high fluid diets are necessary to prevent the constipation that accompanies decreased muscle activity below the waist.

E. Prader-Willi syndrome (PWS) (Pipes, 1992)

1. Infants with Prader-Willi present with central hypotonia leading to a poor suck and swallow and possible failure to thrive.

2. Rapid weight gain begins in the toddler stage. Energy expenditures are low, fat-free body mass is low, and people with PWS have no appetite control.

3. Access to food and edible nonfood items must be strictly controlled.

4. Calorie needs of people with PWS are lower than the norm and obesity control is a life-long battle.

IV. Nutrition Services: Community and Tertiary

The field of I/DD has seen many changes in the last three decades. Not only is the lifespan for people with I/DD increasing, but also more and more people are moving into the community. This has resulted in the need for more community-based services. "It is the position of The American Dietetic Association that program planning for persons with developmental disabilities should include comprehensive nutrition services as part of health, vocational, and educational services" (Lucas & Blyler, 1997, p. 189).

A. Resources for all services, and especially nutrition services, vary from community to community.

1. Federal services available for assistance:

a. University Centers of Excellence in Disability (UCEDs) provide multidisciplinary training and services.

b. Maternal and Child Health Bureau's Children with Special Health Care Needs Programs (CSHCN) provide state and community services for infants, children, and youth to age 21 years.

c. United States Department of Agriculture's (USDA) National School Lunch Program includes community-based programs for adults as well as Head Start and school systems providing nutritious meals.

d. USDA sponsors the Women, Infants, and Children (WIC) programs for income-eligible pregnant women and children under the age of 5.

e. USDA sponsors the Food Stamp program for eligible families.

f. Title VII of the Social Security Act serves the nutrition needs of elderly citizens.

g. Early periodic screening, diagnosis, and treatment (EPSDT) is sponsored by the Medicaid program and may include nutrition services.

2. Community/regional services are inconsistent.

a. School districts may have dietitians on staff or they may have access to a consultant dietitian.

b. County health departments may have dietitians on staff.

c. WIC programs will have nutritionists on staff.

d. The county or region may have access to CSHCN programs with dietitians.

3. Recommendations from the ADA position paper (Lucas & Blyler, 1997). To meet the multiple needs of persons with I/DD, the American Dietetic Association recommends the following measures:

a. Provide nutrition services, including ongoing nutrition monitoring, as an essential component of health care programs.

b. Include a registered dietitian who has experience in the nutrition needs of persons with I/DD in agencies developing policy in the areas of education, vocation, and health services at the federal and state levels.

c. Collaborate with providers to ensure that there are policies in place that promote family-centered, interdisciplinary, coordinated, community-based, and culturally competent services.

d. Encourage participation of qualified dietetic professionals on primary and specialty care teams and in vocational, educational, and residential programs that serve this population throughout the life cycle.

e. Provide the opportunity for increasing the level of nutrition knowledge among all health care and human service providers.

f. Obtain reimbursement for medical nutrition therapy (MNT), enteral/oral nutrition products, and feeding equipment as part of comprehensive health care for persons with I/DD, regardless of diagnosis or living environment.

g. Develop improved referral mechanisms between tertiary care centers and community-based providers and programs.

h. Develop and implement content and/or field experience that addresses the nutrition needs of persons with I/DD in undergraduate and graduate nutrition programs, and provide specialized interdisciplinary nutrition training for practicing dietitians.

i. Encourage a climate of health and wellness for persons with I/DD throughout the life span.

j. Promote nutrition research in an effort to continuously improve the quality of care provided to those with I/DD.

V. Summary

Good dietary habits are necessary for good health and quality of life. These habits are particularly important for people of all ages with I/DD. It is important that health professionals conduct appropriate health assessments incorporating the assessment of nutritional status and dietary habits, comprehensive management, and adequate health education, including knowledge of nutrient/drug interactions.

References

American Dietetic Association. (2000). *Manual of clinical nutrition* (6th ed.). Chicago: Author.

Bandini, L., Patterson, B., & Ekvall, S. W. (1992). Cerebral palsy. In S. W. Ekvall (Ed.) *Pediatric nutrition in chronic diseases and developmental disorders: Prevention, assessment, and treatment* (pp. 93–98). New York: Oxford University Press.

Berry, H., Hull, A., Scribanu, N., & Hunt, M. (1992). Hereditary metabolic disorders. In S. W. Ekvall (Ed.). *Pediatric nutrition in chronic diseases and developmental disorders: Prevention, assessment, and treatment* (pp. 311–368). New York: Oxford University Press.

Brizee, L. (1992). Drug–nutrient interactions—Concerns for children with special health care needs. *Nutrition FOCUS for Children with Special Health Care Needs, 7*(6), 1–5.

Dietz, W. H. (1998). Health consequences of obesity in youth: Childhood predictors of adult disease. *Pediatrics, 101,* 518–525.

Ekvall, S. W. (1992). Myelomeningocele. In S. W. Ekvall (Ed.). *Pediatric nutrition in chronic diseases and developmental disorders: Prevention, assessment, and treatment* (pp. 107–113). New York: Oxford University Press.

Goran, M. I. (1998). Measurement issues related to studies of childhood obesity: Assessment of body composition, body fat distribution, physical activity, and food intake. *Pediatrics, 101,* 505–518.

Haken, V. A. (2000). Interactions between drugs and nutrients. In L. K. Mahan & S. Escott–Stump (Eds.). *Krause's food, nutrition, & dietary therapy* (pp. 399–414). Philadelphia: W. B. Saunders.

Hammond, K. A. (2000). Dietary and clinical assessment. In L. K. Mahan & S. Escott–Stump (Eds.). *Krause's food, nutrition, & dietary therapy* (pp. 353–380). Philadelphia: W. B. Saunders.

Isaacs, J. S., Cialone, J., Horsley, J. W., Holland, M., Murray, P., & Nardella, M. (1997). Feeding and eating. In Dietetics in Developmental Disabilities and the Pediatric Nutrition Practice Group of the American Dietetics Association (Ed.). *Children with special health care needs: A community nutrition pocket guide* (pp. 31–48). Chicago: American Dietetic Association.

Kelsey, K. (1992). Failure to thrive. In S. W. Ekvall (Ed.). *Pediatric nutrition in chronic diseases and developmental disorders: Prevention, assessment, and treatment* (pp. 183–188). New York: Oxford University Press.

Lucas, B. L., & Blyler, E. (1997). Position paper of the American Dietetic Association: Nutrition in comprehensive program planning for persons with developmental disabilities. *Journal of the American Dietetic Association, 97,* 189–194.

Pipes, P. (1992). Prader-Willi syndrome. In S. W. Ekvall (Ed.). *Pediatric nutrition in chronic diseases and developmental disorders: Prevention, assessment, and treatment* (pp. 157–159). New York: Oxford University Press.

Sigman-Grant, M. (1996). Stages of change: A framework for nutrition interventions. *Nutrition Today, 31,* 162.

Snetslaar, L. (2000). Counseling for change. In L. K. Mahan & S. Escott–Stump (Eds.). *Krause's food, nutrition, & dietary therapy* (pp. 451–453). Philadelphia: W.B. Saunders.

Springer, N. S., & Shlafer, M. (1992). Drug-induced malnutrition. In S. W. Ekvall (Ed.). *Pediatric nutrition in chronic diseases and developmental disorders: Prevention, assessment, and treatment* (pp. 229–242). New York: Oxford University Press.

Stevens, F. (1992). Failure to thrive. In S. W. Ekvall (Ed.). *Pediatric nutrition in chronic diseases and developmental disorders: Prevention, assessment, and treatment* (pp. 183–188). New York: Oxford University Press.

Eating and Swallowing Disorders (Dysphagia) in Adults and Children

17

Lee S. Barks, RN, ARNP, PhD(c), CDDN, FAAMR
and Justine Joan Sheppard, CCC-SLP, PhD, BRS-S

Objectives

At the completion of this chapter, the learner will be able to:

1. Define feeding and swallowing disorders (dysphagia).
2. Identify signs and potential outcomes of dysphagia.
3. Identify individuals at risk for dysphagia and those at risk for complications from dysphagia.
4. Identify the components of the dysphagia evaluation and identify possible influences on evaluation results.
5. Describe the clinical and advocacy roles health professionals play in the person-centered interdisciplinary approach to evaluation and treatment.
6. Identify management strategies for activities that involve swallowing, eating, drinking, taking oral medications, and oral hygiene.

Key Points

- Dysphagia is most simply defined as "difficulty in swallowing" (Dark, 1997). It may occur to a greater or lesser degree, with varying degrees of difficulty/distress for the individual and greater or lesser impact on social participation.
- There is a high prevalence of dysphagia in adults and children with intellectual and developmental disabilities (I/DD).
- Dysphagia confers health risk on persons with I/DD chiefly for three reasons: a) it may result in aspiration into the airway and respiratory compromise; b) it often confers nutritional risk, including fluid and electrolyte imbalance and lowered immunity, when insufficient intake of food and/or fluids occurs, and may culminate in malnutrition (Best Practice, 2000b); and c) it predisposes to choking and its associated morbidity and mortality (Bazemore, Tonkonogy, & Ananth, 1991).

Key Points *(continued)*

- Goals of assessment and treatment include safety and quality of life. The nurse and interdisciplinary team provide and interpret information to family members, advocates, and those with dysphagia so they can participate effectively in making treatment decisions.

I. Physiology of Normal Swallowing

A. Swallowing is the continuous movement of the bolus from lips to stomach in four stages:

1. Oral preparation—Rate of eating and size of bolus are regulated, the bolus is mixed with saliva and masticated as needed for ease of transport to the stomach, and the bolus is collected and moved into position for initiating the reflexive coordinations of swallowing

2. Oral initiation—The bolus is propelled toward the pharynx to initiate the swallowing reflex. Sensory-motor coordinations of the swallowing reflex direct the bolus toward the esophagus, preventing reflux back into the mouth and into the naso-pharynx, and penetration and aspiration into the lower airway.

3. Pharyngeal—The bolus is propelled through the pharynx into the esophagus.

4. Esophageal—Timely and sufficient relaxation of the cricopharyngeal and cardiac (lower esophageal, or LE) sphincters and resumption of their tonic closure coordinated with esophageal transport of the bolus into the stomach. Effective function prevents retrograde movement of the bolus from the esophagus into the pharynx (nonacid reflux) and of stomach contents into the esophagus and pharynx (acid reflux).

B. Behaviors in which swallowing is a significant functional component are: saliva control, eating, taking oral medications, and controlling the oral hygiene bolus.

C. Neuromuscular control of swallowing is complex.

1. Primary centers are in the cortex and brain stem, with primary reflexive control mediated in the brain stem by six cranial nerves (CN): 5th (Trigeminal), 7th (Facial), 9th (Glossopharyngeal), 10th (Vagus), 11th (Accessory), and 12th (Hypoglossal).

2. Cortical and subcortical regions modify and integrate with the CN regions to control muscles participating in oral, pharyngeal, and esophageal swallowing (Perlman & Schulze-Delrieu, 1997). Any interruption of innervation or mechanical obstruction can result in dysphagia.

3. Coordination of facial, oral, pharyngeal, laryngeal, esophageal, gastrointestinal, respiratory, and postural motor subsystems are required in this process, in addition to autonomic regulation of hunger and thirst (Bass, 1997).

II. Feeding and Swallowing Disorders

A. Dysphagia is sufficient disruption of the feeding and swallowing process to result in functional, behavioral, and/or social/personal consequences or probable risk to health and safety of the individual during one or more of these behaviors that involve swallowing. It is the complex of a "feeding and swallowing" disorder, the complex of physiological, functional, and behavioral signs and symptoms, rather than a primary medical diagnosis (American Association of Speech-Language Hearing, 2001).

1. Most common etiologies for dysphagia in I/DDs are neurological, anatomical, gastrointestinal, psychiatric; also cognitive medication usage that impacts swallowing function (Crary & Groher, 2000; Murry & Carrau, 2001).

2. Severity ranges from mild, requiring only diet modifications or selected strategies, to profound, requiring enteral feeding, and in the most severe, tracheostomy for pulmonary toilet (Groher, 1997).

3. Dysphagia may include aspiration, difficulties with oral preparation of the bolus, gastroesophageal reflux disease (GERD), and/or esophageal dysmotility disorders (Crary, 2003).

4. Medical consequences include, but are not limited to:

   a. Pulmonary disorders, including pneumonia and gastric asthma (asthma triggered by gastroesophageal reflux (GER)). Prevalence of GER in asthmatics is estimated at 34% to 80% (Makkar & Sachdev, 2003).

   b. Dehydration, malnutrition, failure to thrive.

   c. Esophageal dysplasia, vomiting, rumination, food refusal.

   d. Failure to advance eating skills, traumatically conditioned dysphagia/feeding phobia (Bohmer, Klinkenberg-Knol, Niezen-de Boer, & Meuwissn, 2000; Ekvall, 1993; Johnson & Hirsch, 2003; Rogers, Stratton, Msall, & Andres, 1994; Rosenthal, Sheppard, & Lotze, 1995; Sheppard, Liou, Hochman, Laroia, & Langlois, 1988; Zarate, Mearin, Hidalgo, & Malagelada, 2001).

   e. In I/DD, aspiration, as it occurs during videofluoroscopic assessment, is generally "silent" (Rogers et al., 1994).

5. Onset may be congenital, interfering with acquisition of developmental feeding and swallowing skills, then resolving or persisting into adulthood. Adult onset disorders occur with acquired medical conditions and physiological changes of aging.

6. At particular risk of dysphagia are those:

    a. With multiple disabilities, cerebral palsy, traumatic head injury, genetic or metabolic disorders (such as Down syndrome or the mucopolysaccharidoses), cerebral infarcts, or hydroencephaly

    b. With upper motor impairments affecting ability to control head and neck position

    c. Who take routine medications such as anti-epileptic medications, muscle relaxants for spasticity, or anticholinergics for drooling, possibly experiencing reduced alertness and coordination and strength of muscles during the swallow

    d. With dystonia, dyskinesia, or hypotonia, experiencing difficulty chewing and moving food about in the mouth and pharynx

    e. With inappropriate and disruptive mealtime behaviors such as laughing or rapidly stuffing large amounts of food

    f. With psychiatric disorders, such as autism and bipolar disorder (Siktberg & Bantz, 1999)

    g. With adult onset neurological disorders, such as tardive dyskinesia and Parkinsonism (Best Practice, 2000a, 2000b)

7. Some neurologically normal infants with wheeze and stridor experience swallowing dysfunction and silent aspiration (Sheikh et al., 2001).

8. Adult onset issues include stroke, dementias, Parkinson's disease, myasthenia gravis, multiple sclerosis, and dental and periodontal disorders.

9. Natural aging of people with I/DD is associated with deterioration of feeding and swallowing capabilities, with onset of dysphagia, or increasing severity. These changes may begin in the fourth decade in more severely involved individuals (Sheppard, 2002).

B. Aversive behavior during mealtime (may be referred to as oral hypersensitivity or oral sensory defensiveness) may occur in children and adults. These behaviors interfere with nutrition and hydration, and, in children, with advancing eating skills. Oral hypersensitivity may result from pain of gastrointestinal disorder, particularly GERD; dental and periodontal disease; or autism, among other causes.

C. In rumination, there is laryngo-pharyngeal reflux and a period of voluntary reorganization of the bolus before reswallowing. In most instances it is associated with GERD, although it may occur without diagnostic signs of GERD (Gravestock, 2000).

D. Pica is a feeding and swallowing disorder in which there is ingestion of nonfood boluses (Asgarali, Nandapalan, Phillips, & Osunug, 1996; Burke & Smith, 1999; Dallal, Odum, & Ahluwalia, 1996).

E. Choking is an acute aspiration event or upper airway obstruction, varying in appearance from prolonged coughing to asphyxiation.

F. GERD is experienced by many people with or without I/DD. Stomach contents flow from the stomach into the esophagus and may enter the pharynx, with reflux aspiration into the trachea and lungs sometimes occurring (Dark, 1997).

    1. This may happen at night, with the individual in supine position (Koufman, 2002) or awake and upright.

    2. Emesis may be aspirated into the lungs prior to, during, or after swallowing (Bohmer et al., 2000); GERD occurs because of abnormality in the lower esophageal sphincter.

    3. GERD may result in epigastric pain (heartburn) due to irritation of the esophagus by stomach acid. Repeated exposure results in ulceration, scarring, and stricture (Dark, 1997).

    4. Most seriously, over time and in the presence of stomach acid, the squamous epithelium of the esophagus transforms to columnar epithelium (Barrett's esophagus), a precursor of esophageal adenocarcinoma (Leslie, Carding, & Wilson, 2003). Approximately 10% of those with GERD develop Barrett's esophagus. Approximately 80% have a hiatal hernia (Dark, 1997). A high prevalence of GERD is associated with I/DD, and nonverbal individuals may be unable to communicate adequately their symptoms.

    5. Koufman (2002) distinguishes between GER, which can occur up to 50 times a day physiologically, and GERD, in which tissue damage results. Bohmer and colleagues (2000) state that GERD is considered when recurrent vomiting, food refusal, or hematemesis occurs. Predisposing factors for GERD include:

        a. Anti-epileptic drugs, constipation, cerebral palsy, scoliosis, feeding gastrostomy, convulsions, and IQ <35.

        b. Slow stomach emptying enables GERD by allowing stomach contents to be available for reflux long after they should leave the stomach. Supine positioning allows stomach contents to pool in the fundus, rather than moving into the pylorus and resulting in precluding pyloric distention, stimulation of peristalsis, and outflow into the duodenum.

        c. Other predisposing factors are: diabetes mellitus, cerebral palsy, many medications, and high stomach pH (insufficient acidity).

III. Effect of Dysphagia on Daily Living Activities

Difficulties with saliva management, eating and drinking, taking oral medications, and managing the oral hygiene bolus limit participation of people with I/DD and increase need for support.

A. Saliva management—Impairments that affect saliva swallowing may result in tracheal aspiration, choking/coughing on saliva, chronic airway congestion, and drooling. Secondary effects on hydration, respiratory health, and skin integrity are common.

B. Managing the oral hygiene bolus—Difficulties with control of the oral hygiene bolus reduce effectiveness of oral hygiene routines due to primary distress and secondary behavioral resistance. Portions of the oral hygiene bolus may be aspirated.

C. Factors that tend to increase bacterial density in the mouth elevate risk of pneumonia in aging individuals (Langmore et al., 1998; Langmore, Skarupski, Park, & Fries, 2002).

D. Taking oral medications. Special needs for medications preparation, bolus size, special utensils, prescribed "feeding" techniques, and head-neck and body positioning during ingestion complicate medication administration and provision of adequate "wash-down" to clear the esophagus. Secondary effects include behavioral resistance, medications esophagitis, and failure to adequately medicate.

E. Eating and drinking.

1. Associated disabilities include, but are not limited to, poorly developed or absent skills for self-feeding and oral management of liquids, nonchewable solids (e.g., puréed, ground, or finely chopped foods), or chewable solids. Disabilities may also include distress and difficulty on initiating and completing the swallow, high prevalence of "choking" during eating, odynophagia (painful swallowing), and reflux and regurgitation. These problems are complicated by the high prevalence of primary audition, communication, and psychiatric disorders.

2. Secondary effects may be malnutrition, dehydration, respiratory illness, and oxygen desaturation during eating. Reduced independence and behavioral eating disorders are apparent (Rosenthal et al., 1995). These effects tend to worsen with age (Sheppard, 2002).

IV. Signs and Symptoms of Dysphagia

(See Table 17.1.)

V. Outcomes/Complications of Dysphagia

A. Aspiration is the most serious outcome of dysphagia. It is defined as the passage of food, fluid, medication, or saliva below the vocal cords into the trachea, and can result in resolution without residual pathology, complete airway obstruction, or pneumonitis. The physiological response to aspiration depends on host resistance, the toxicity of the aspirate, and the frequency and amount of aspiration.

1. Pneumonitis entails fibrin formation in the lung, local pooling of fluid, bacterial pneumonia, and pulmonary fibrosis, or scarring.

2. In persons with I/DD and dysphagia, aspiration or microaspiration is silent in most instances (Rogers et al., 1994) and may go undetected until wheezing is heard or signs of pneumonia (fever, chills, sweating, delirium,

Table 17.1	Signs of Dysphagia in Children and Adults (Best Practice, 2000a, 2000b)

- drooling or coughing on saliva accumulations
- lack of progression in eating skills, such as chewing and drinking from a cup
- spillage of food from the mouth
- food or meal refusal
- prolonged mealtimes (i.e., longer than 30 minutes)
- effort, fatigue, reduced alertness, discomfort, or anxiety with mealtimes
- respiratory distress associated with oral intake, i.e., increased rate of breathing, cyanosis, congested breath sounds
- gagging, coughing, or choking associated with oral intake
- recurrent respiratory infections
- aversive behaviors during activities involving swallowing
- absence or weakness of voluntary cough or swallow
- changes in voice quality (hoarse, moist) directly associated with eating
- difficulty with oral management of food, medication, or oral hygiene bolus
- frequent throat clearing or coughing
- sudden change in eating behavior
- gradual or sudden weight loss, chronically low body weight, or failure to thrive
- dehydration
- delayed initiation of swallowing
- more than two swallows for each bite-sized mouthful
- oral or nasal regurgitation
- coughing or sneezing following intake

shortness of breath, malaise, grossly moist breath sounds, adventitious lung sounds) are apparent. This occurs in approximately half of all dysphagia patients who aspirate (Galvan, 2001).

B. Dehydration and malnutrition are serious outcomes of dysphagia (Galvan, 2001). Difficulties in communicating thirst and hunger and inability to access food and liquids independently complicate this problem.

C. Chronically low body weight is associated with dysphagia. In a study of adults with I/DD, there was a significant negative relationship between body mass index and severity of dysphagia (Sheppard et al., 1988). In children, if failure to thrive continues over a long period without reversal, it may result in delayed puberty (Amundson et al., 1994).

D. Enteral nutrition may also be an outcome of dysphagia. Although oral care and social opportunities suffer, nutritional intake, hydration, and vitamin levels may all improve (Ekvall, 1993; Leibovitz, 2002).

VI. Management of Complications of Dysphagia

A. Disorders of the esophagus and stomach may complicate both identification and treatment.

   1. Achalasia, a disorder of the esophagus, is "an idiopathic neuromuscular disorder of the esophagus which is associated with incomplete relaxation of the upper or lower esophageal sphincter (LES)" (da Silveira & Rogers, 2002, p. 157).

      a. Achalasia may be evidenced by inability to ingest more than small quantities of food and fluid, due to stasis of food/fluid in the pharynx or at the aperistaltic segment in the esophagus. In immobile people, following a meal, achalasia may also appear as GERD when the person reclines and regurgitation without force is seen, with appearance of undigested, uncurdled food and fluid that flows up the esophagus and dribbles out (nonacid reflux).

   2. GERD may be treated with surgical fundoplication.

   3. Thoracic stomach, in which the stomach lies above the diaphragm and GERD is severe, is difficult to manage. Positioning at an incline becomes critical, and usually continuous infusion feeding is employed at a small hourly rate.

B. Constipation is a dysphagia complication when there is

   1. Insufficient intake to stimulate peristalsis, the person is immobile and intake of dietary fiber and fluid is insufficient (Folder et al., 2002).

   2. Management entails increases in fluid, dietary fiber, judicious use of laxatives in a stepwise approach, positioning with gravity, and movement, even passive movement.

C. Medication side effects may complicate dysphagia.

D. Pulmonary disorders should be evaluated medically.

   1. All "asthma" should be evaluated by the interdisciplinary team (IDT) and physician, to identify occult aspiration with subsequent wheezing.

   2. When anxiety, sweating, and air hunger are seen, they should be evaluated by a pulmonologist to identify respiratory insufficiency associated with pulmonary fibrosis or peribronchial infiltration, secondary to aspiration.

   3. The most serious complication of dsyphagia is aspiration pneumonia, or aspiration pneumonitis.

   4. Pulmonary syndromes may occur after aspiration, depending on the amount and nature of the aspirated material, the frequency of aspiration, and the host's response to the aspirated material.

      a. Persons with compromised respiratory function may be more likely to aspirate, due to their inability to sustain a normal pause in breathing throughout the swallow and their tendency to swallow air, increasing likelihood of gastric distention, reflux, and aspiration.

E. Musculo-skeletal disorders

1. Infantile cortical hyperostosis (Caffey's disease) in children causes pain and swelling, particularly in mandibular and thoracic regions, that affect oral preparatory and oral initiation stages of swallowing and breath support for swallowing (Sheppard & Pressman, 1988).

2. In adults, diffuse idiopathic skeletal hyperostosis (Forestier's disease) has been associated with dysphagia (Deutsch, Schild, & Mafee, 1985; Eviatar & Harrell, 1987; Hirano et al., 1982).

3. Temporomandibular joint dysfunction may occur in children or adults (Honig, 1993).

4. Subluxation of the corniculate cartilage, although a rarer occurrence, causes difficulty in swallowing solid food and should be considered in differential diagnosis when skeletal issues are suspected.

5. Skeletal changes associated with cerebral palsy include high palatal arch, open-bite, dental malocclusion, and spinal deformities, such as kyphosis and scoliosis (Sheppard, 1994).

6. Spinal deformities interfere with sitting for eating, making it more difficult to control bolus motility in the oral and pharyngeal stages of swallowing and to protect the airway, tending to increase intra-abdominal pressure—thus disrupting esophageal motility (Woods, 1994).

VII. Dysphagia Identification and Clinical Assessment by the Interdisciplinary Team

A. The nursing role

1. The nursing assessment—May include screening assessments that have been developed specifically for children and adults with I/DD, such as the Dysphagia Disorders Survey (Sheppard & Hochman, 1988) and the Screening Tool of Feeding Problems (Kuhn & Matson, 2002).

2. The nurse identifies dysphagia through observations and history from family or residential providers and refers to the primary medical provider or requesting clinical and/or instrumented evaluations.

3. The nurse conducts a review of neurologic factors predisposing to dysphagia, such as degenerative nervous system disease, shunt malfunction, and epilepsy classification and management (see Chapter 15).

4. The nurse evaluates the drug regimen for:

a. Medication administration practices that place the person at risk by use of techniques such as allowing neck extension to occur in oral intake, or other improper positioning.

b. Use of forms of oral medication that do not correspond to recommended texture/consistency.

    c. Oral presentation in amounts that are too large to be managed, and insufficient or inappropriate form of "wash-down" (liquid or solid that follows oral medications to clear the medication through the esophagus).

    d. Administration of any medications that may contribute to dysphagia.

    e. Any medications that must be given whole but are not given so and may contribute to esophageal irritation. Karch and Karch (2000) provide such a list of medications.

    f. Any medications in use that may decrease level of consciousness or affect GI tract function.

5. Feeding mode status—When the mode of intake is enteral nutrition, the nurse should assess how the feeding method affects physiologic function.

6. Gastrointestinal (GI) status—May include a history of *Helicobacter pylori* infection (Chi et al., 2003; Levine et al., 2004), constipation, esophageal erosion, bleeding, GERD, and presence of hiatal hernia, gastroparesis, or thoracic stomach.

7. Diagnostic tests—Radiologic reports showing peribronchial or lower lobe infiltrates, fibrosis, or chronic pneumonia, and other laboratory tests should be reviewed for history of blood or urine abnormalities related to nutritional deficiencies, infection, or metabolic dysfunction that may influence eating difficulty and require resolution.

8. Surgical procedures—History should be reviewed for surgical procedures that may relate to swallowing capabilities or be associated with traumatically conditioned aversions to eating. These would include maxillofacial and dental surgeries, and those that involve the respiratory and digestive systems.

9. Musculoskeletal status and tone—High tone may predispose to increased intra-abdominal pressure, placing abdominal contents under pressure and resulting in vomiting or GERD. Low tone predisposes to poor coordination of the swallow. Presence of skeletal deformity may limit positioning for oral intake.

10. Respiratory status—Including evidence of active pulmonary disease, presence of rales, rhonchi, and history of choking or pneumonia.

11. Skin integrity.

12. Orofacial conditions and periodontal disease.

13. Communication—Including communication difficulties and special communication modalities used by the individual and the caregivers.

14. Vision and hearing.

15. Oversight by the nurse is often needed in the home environment to collect pertinent data, in preparation for medical and other allied health assessments.

B. The speech-language pathologist's (SLP) role

    1. Typically serves as the dysphagia specialist on the interdisciplinary team, performs the clinical dysphagia evaluation (CDE), and makes recommenda-

tions for any instrumented, medical assessments that are needed to complete the dysphagia evaluation.

2. The CDE includes a physical assessment of anatomy and physiology of the motor systems that support feeding and swallowing and a detailed observation of the functional capabilities for controlling saliva, eating, drinking, taking oral medications, and controlling the oral hygiene bolus. It also includes an assessment of issues that influence functional adequacy, such as environment, feeding strategies, and diet consistencies and textures (Sheppard, 1987).

3. Instrumented examination of swallowing

   a. *Videofluoroscopic swallowing study/modified barium swallow (MBS)*—A real-time, videotaped radiograph of the individual swallowing radiopaque substances that may include food or fluid mixed with barium or barium simulation of different food viscosities and textures. Varying liquidity of the test material, bolus size, texture, and swallowing conditions will reveal any difficulty in the four phases of swallowing.

      i. It is important to ascertain in advance that the radiology equipment will accommodate any special seating equipment that is used for feeding, or that comparable equipment is available for positioning the person and that an SLP will participate

   b. *Esophagram*—This is a fluoroscopy study that examines in detail esophageal structure and motility. Part of the test, drinking while reclining, may not be advisable for the individual with dysphagia. Alternately, the study may be performed by infusing the test liquid into the esophagus by NG tube (Marquis & Pressman, 1994).

   c. *Upper GI series (UGIS)*—A fluoroscopy study that examines the esophagus, the stomach, and the upper intestine as the barium bolus is swallowed and as the stomach fills and empties. The study may reveal hiatal hernia, thoracic stomach, achalasia, and structural abnormalities that may predispose to aspiration, obstruction to gastric outflow, or GERD (Marquis & Pressman, 1994).

   d. *Fiberoptic endoscopic evaluation of swallowing (FEES)*—An endoscope is passed through the nostril into the oral pharynx. Structures in the pharynx are viewed during swallowing of saliva and typical diet foods. Oral initiation and pharyngeal phases of swallowing are examined for aspiration, delayed initiation of swallowing, and stasis of the bolus in the pharynx (Migliore, Scoopo, Robey, 1999).

   e. *Fiberoptic endoscopy of the esophagus, stomach, and upper duodenum (EGD)*—A fiberoptic endoscope is passed into the individual's esophagus to view the esophagus and stomach for structural abnormalities, ulceration, or erosion. Tissue may also be biopsied or examined for evidence of GERD, Barrett's esophagus, or other abnormalities that reflect dysphagia.

    f.   *Esophageal manometry*—Measures intra-esophageal pressures during the swallow, including pressures within the upper and lower esophageal sphincters.

    g.   *24-hour pH probe*—A probe is placed into the esophagus to sense reductions in pH (increased acidity) that may occur as stomach acid moves upward in the esophagus. This procedure may be done with a nasogastric probe in place or with a wireless system (Pandolfino et al., 2003). The remote system may be tolerated better by the individual with I/DD.

    h.   *Gastric emptying time (GET)*—A test for gastroparesis (delayed stomach emptying).

C. The occupational therapist's role

    1. The occupational therapist (OT) typically serves on the team as the specialist in sensory assessment and self-feeding, and sometimes seating. Assessment and recommendations may include physiological and behavioral impairments that may interfere with independence and participation, optimum body postural alignments and supports, and specialized equipment for supporting ingestion capabilities, independence, and participation.

D. The physical therapist's role

    1. The physical therapist (PT) serves on the team as the specialist in body postural alignment and supports and mobility issues that may interfere with activities that involve swallowing (Bray, Beckman, & Barks, 1987). Assessment and recommendations may include orthopedic status and behavioral impairments that may interfere with seating and mobility, seating equipment, optimum body postural alignments, and supports and special strategies for safe handling of the individual and for facilitating mobility.

E. The dietitian's role

    1. The dietitian (RD) assesses nutritional and hydration status and factors influencing nutrition and hydration for both oral and enteral nutrition (Brody, 1999; Brody, Touger-Decker, VonHagen, & Maillet, 2000; Logemann & Martin-Harris, 2001). The assessment includes anthropometrics; nutritional status; general nutritional requirements and special nutritional needs for individual diagnoses; intake issues, such as personal preferences, meal and food refusal, and variability in intake; and medication-nutrition interactions.

F. Other allied health, educational, and medical specialists—May include respiratory therapists, psychologists, social workers, special educators, and appropriate medical specialists for conducting specialty evaluations and recommending management plans.

VIII. Management Strategies for Treatment of Dysphagia: Implementation of Team Recommendations

Treatment of dysphagia involves two distinct elements.

A. The *individual management plan* assures use of optimum strategies to promote health and safety during activities that involve swallowing, while being considerate of the personal, family, or individual preferences that are central to an acceptable quality of life.

B. The *individual mealtime management plan (IMMP)* includes consideration of a group of interventions that promote health, safety, independence, and enjoyment of eating. Recommendations from the IDT for strategies that meet the specific needs of the individual are incorporated into the IMMP. These strategies may be solely compensatory, such as diet modifications, or they may be therapeutic in that they improve underlying competency or advance skill (Sheppard, 1994), such as oral exercises by the OT or SLP, outside mealtimes. The components of the plan are:

   1. Premeal interventions—Included are prescriptive activities, such as rest, positioning, and readiness routines that promote optimum alertness and receptiveness for the meal.

   2. Positioning—Correct body postural and head-neck alignment reduce aspiration (Logemann, 1998) and improve capabilities for eating (Sheppard, 1994).

   3. Diet—The prescriptive dysphagia diet includes instructions for specially prepared textures, viscosities, temperature, and taste enhancements to facilitate safe, comfortable, and efficient swallowing; calorie regulation for increasing, maintaining, or reducing weight; and regulation of amounts of solids and liquids for weight considerations and for management of GERD.

   4. Utensils—Adaptive utensils include specially designed eating implements, plates, cups, and straws.

   5. Supervision

   6. Feeding techniques—Includes assistance for maintaining postural alignment during eating, assistance for self-feeding, special spooning and cup techniques for dependent eaters, and cueing, feedback, and reinforcement strategies.

   7. Communication—Communication modalities include speech, nonverbal signals, and augmentative systems.

   8. After-eating interventions—Include positioning constraints in persons with GERD to avoid exacerbating reflux or vomiting, and oral hygiene to clear residuals from the mouth.

   9. Eating environment—Care should be taken in regulating the visual and acoustic environments with the goal of minimizing the stresses associated with noise, disorganization, and excessive tension.

10. Infection control (see Chapter 21)

C. Monitoring all nutritional intake by nurses (see Table 17.2), dietitians, and family or residential staff should include a comparison of those amounts to daily minimum requirements provided by the dietitian or physician, and alerting the physician and IDT to failure of the person to take in these amounts.

    1. Enteral nutrition—For some individuals, continued oral intake poses unacceptable risk of respiratory and nutritional disorders. In these cases, the risks of oral intake outweigh the benefits.

        a. The nutritional intake method selected may be either:

            i. Total nonoral (enteral nutrition, or EN, with no oral intake)

            ii. Combined oral and enteral nutrition, often used when the individual needs supplementation only of food or fluids

            iii. Total oral nutrition with only medications given by tube

---

Table 17.2   Ongoing Dysphagia Nurse Monitoring Responsibilities

- mealtime capillary oxygen saturation measured by pulse oximetry whenever the person is identified as possibly at risk
- gagging, coughing, or choking at times of oral intake
- wheezing
- "wet" sounding respirations
- pooling of food in the mouth
- taking more than three swallows to clear the mouth
- swallowing large mouthfuls rapidly
- vomiting
- bleeding gums
- smell of formula on breath after meals
- persistent drooling
- pain/heartburn at tip of breastbone
- agitation during or after oral intake
- throwing head back or other maladaptive head-neck or body posture during eating
- mealtime eating lasting longer than 30 minutes
- consistent meal refusal or refusal of liquids or solids
- loss of alertness, increased sleeping
- loss of skills
- eating nonedible objects (due to potential for intestinal obstruction)
- tooth grinding (bruxism)
- rumination

b. Change to a total liquid diet may increase risk of GERD. Additional nursing interventions are then needed, such as postprandial positioning to facilitate expedient stomach emptying and prevent GERD (Brody, 1999; Gustafsson & Tibbling, 1994).

d. The individual should be positioned (Brody, 1999) sitting upright during feeding and for at least 90 minutes following oral intake (Best Practice, 2000b), or in inclined sidelying at a sufficient incline against gravity to result in movement of chyme from left to right in the stomach and into the pylorus, to stimulate gastric emptying.

d. Of paramount importance in the decision-making process regarding the placement of any type of feeding tube is the understanding that tube feeding is not a panacea and is not always permanent. There is an ongoing need for re-evaluation of ability for oral intake at least annually, as factors leading to tube placement can change.

    i. Finally, the individual may still aspirate, due to GERD and/or saliva (Best Practice, 2000b). When tube feedings are infused, it is important for those administering to take care not to infuse with manual pressure or to conduct postural drainage while stomach contents are present, due to the high incidence of GERD in nonambulatory persons with I/DD.

    ii. Nursing care in EN has included both testing for elevated glucose in tracheal aspirates and placement of blue food dye into infusion bags to mark refluxate. The evidence base shows these practices should be abandoned with adoption of nonrecumbent positioning (Maloney & Ryan, 2004).

2. Enteral tubes—There are four basic types of tubes used in enteral nutrition, with which all nurses are familiar (Potter & Perry, 2001).

a. A nasogastric (NG) tube is for short-term use only (30 days or less). NG tubes are flexible and small-bore due to the undesirable consequence of holding the lower esophageal sphincter (LES) open when the tube is in place, which can lead to GERD.

b. A gastrostomy tube (G-tube) or percutaneous endoscopic gastronomy (PEG) tube is inserted surgically. Placement of a PEG is a simpler procedure, usually entailing less risk than abdominal surgery, but complications in people with I/DD have included perforation of internal organs, when scoliosis is so severe that bony landmarks are misleading. The most common complication is infection at the insertion site, occurring within a few days of placement (Perlman & Shulze-Delrieu, 1997).

c. The third type of enteral tube is a jejunostomy tube (J-tube), placed surgically into the jejunum, or gastro-jejunostomy tube (G-J tube), placed through a gastrostomy into the stomach and threaded by an interventional radiologist through the pylorus into the jejunum. Jejunal tube placement is generally confirmed radiographically and is used to infuse liquid below the stomach, when GERD or vomiting are a problem.

d. The fourth type, "a transgastric jejunal (G-J) tube is an alternative when antireflux surgery (fundoplication) fails, or is hazardous or inappropriate" (Godbole et al., 2002, p. 135). Morbidity associated with jejunal feeding can be quite high.

e. A variety of tubes and appliances including "buttons" are used for infusion of tube feedings.

f. Wearing of the J-tube and infusion pump may limit freedom of movement, especially in children.

g. Although home re-insertion of G- and J-tubes by parents or other caregivers is usually prescribed to prevent rapid stoma closure, subsequent feeding by J-tube without checking tube placement on X-ray is not recommended.

h. Frequency of tube fallout must be monitored by the nurse and reported frequently to the surgeon who placed it and oversees its use (Guenter & Silkrowski, 2001; Smith & Soucy, 1996).

IX. Training Caregivers

Training caregivers for children and adults with I/DD is an essential part of the dysphagia management plan.

A. Caregiver education/training content includes basic knowledge of swallowing, swallowing disorders, management of nutrition and hydration, oral hygiene, medication administration, techniques and strategies for managing saliva control, and behavioral training strategies for improving skills (Chadwick, Jolliffe, & Goldbart, 2002).

B. Education for families should be culturally sensitive and individualized for the family member.

C. Education/training for residential and program staff and personal assistants should be more comprehensive. A high level of staff knowledge and skills is critical in caring for individuals who are known to be at risk for aspiration and/or choking.

D. Staff turnover and inadequate staffing patterns are of concern and should be accommodated in training programs and the training and retraining cycles.

X. Summary

Eating and swallowing disorders in children and adults with I/DD are serious and potentially fatal. Knowledge of the pathophysiology of chewing and swallowing mechanisms, assessment and management of dysphagia, and appro-

priate education of the individual with I/DD who has an eating and swallowing disorder along with family members and/or caregivers are essential for nurses and health care professionals caring for this population.

References

American Association of Speech-Language-Hearing. (2001). *Roles of speech-language pathologists in swallowing and feeding disorders: Position statement.* Rockville, MD: Author.

Amundson, J., Sherbondy, A., Van Dyke, D., Alexander, R., da Silveira, E., & Rogers, A. (1994). Early identification and treatment necessary to prevent malnutrition in children and adolescents with severe disabilities. *Journal of the American Dietetic Association, 94,* 880–883.

Asgarali, S., Nandapalan, V., Phillips, D., & Osunug, O. (1996). Aspiration pneumonia in a mentally handicapped patient due to a foreign body impacted in the pharynx: A near fatal outcome. *Journal of Accident and Emergency Medicine, 13,* 291.

Bass, N. (1997). The neurology of swallowing. In M. Groher (Ed.). *Dysphagia* (pp. 7–35). Boston: Butterworth-Heineman.

Bazemore, P., Tonkonogy, J., & Ananth, R. (1991). Dysphagia in psychiatric patients: Clinical and videofluoroscopic study. *Dysphagia, 6,* 2–5.

Best Practice. (2000a). Identification and management of dysphagia in children with neurological impairment. *Best Practice 2000, 4*(3), 1–6.

Best Practice. (2000b). Identification and nursing management of dysphagia in adults with neurological impairment. *Best Practice 2000, 4*(2), 1–6.

Bohmer, C., Klinkenberg-Knol, E., Niezen-de Boer, M., & Meuwissn, S. (2000). Gastroesophageal reflux disease in intellectually disabled individuals: How often, how serious, how manageable. *The American Journal of Gastroenterology, 95,* 1868–1872.

Bray, M., Beckman, D., & Barks, L. (1987). Crisis intervention for persons with severe eating difficulty. Rockville, MD: American Occupational Therapy Association. Chapter Nine.

Brody, R. (1999). Nutrition issues in dysphagia: Identification, management, and the role of the dietitian. Proceedings of the fourth annual Ross medical nutrition and device roundtable, Charleston, SC., April 1999. *Nutrition in Clinical Practice, 14*(5), 47–51.

Brody, R., Touger-Decker, R., VonHagen, S., & Maillet, J. (2000). Role of registered dietitians in dysphagia screening. *Journal of the American Dietetic Association, 100,* 1029–1037.

Burke, L., & Smith, S. (1999). Treatment of pica: Considering least intrusive options when working with individuals who have a developmental handicap and live in a community setting. *Developmental Disabilities Bulletin, 27*(1). Retrieved November 16, 2004 from http://www.ualberta.ca/~jpdasddc/bulletin/articles/burke1999.html

Chadwick, D., Jolliffe, J., & Goldbart, J. (2002). Carer knowledge of dysphagia management strategies. *International Journal of Language & Communication Disorders, 37,* 345–357.

Chi, C.-H., Lin, C.-Y., Sheu, B.-S., Yang, H.-B., Huang, A.-H., & Wu, J.-J. (2003). Quadruple therapy containing Amoxicillin and Tetracycline is an effective regimen to rescue failed triple therapy by overcoming the antimicrobial resistance of *Helicobactor pylori. Alimentary Pharmacology & Therapeutics, 18,* 347–353.

Crary, M. (2003). *Introduction to adult swallowing disorders.* St. Louis, MO: Butterworth-Heineman.

Crary, M., & Groher, M. (2000). Basic concepts of surface electromyographic biofeedback in the treatment of dysphagia: A tutorial. *American Journal of Speech-Language Pathology, 9,* 116–125.

Dallal, H., Odum, J., & Ahluwalia, N. (1996). Covert dysphagia in the mentally handicapped: Two case reports and a review of published literature. *Dysphagia, 11*, 194–197.

Dark, G. (1997). *Online medical dictionary*. University of Newcastle upon Tyne. Laboratory Cancer Research Trust. Retrieved May 18, 2004 from http://cancerweb.ncl.ac.uk/cgi-bin/omd?dysphagia

da Silveira, E., & Rogers, A. (2002). Treatment of achalasia with botulinum A toxin. *American Journal of Therapeutics, 9*, 157–161.

Deutsch, E., Schild, J., & Mafee, M. (1985). Dysphagia and Forestier's disease. *Archives of Otolaryngology, 111*, 400–402.

Ekvall, S. (1993). *Pediatric nutrition in chronic diseases and developmental disorders: Prevention, assessment, and treatment*. New York: Oxford University Press.

Eviatar, E., & Harrell, M. (1987). Diffuse idiopathic skeletal hyperostosis with dysphagia (a review). *The Journal of Laryngology and Otology, 101*, 627–632.

Folder, S., Maynard, F., Stevens, K., Gilbride, J., Pires, M., & Jones, K. (2002). *Association of Rehabilitation Nurses practice guidelines for the management of constipation in adults*. Retrieved May 19, 2004 from www.rehabnurse.org/professionalresources

Galvan, T. (2001). Dysphagia: Going down and staying down. *American Journal of Nursing, 101*(1), 37–43.

Godbole, P., Margabanthu, G., Crabbe, D., Thomas, A., Puntis, J., & Abel, G. (2002). Limitations and uses of gastrojejunal feeding tubes. *Archives of Diseases in Childhood, 86*, 134–137.

Gravestock, S. (2000). Eating disorders in adults with intellectual disability. *Journal of Intellectual Disability Research, 44*, 625–637.

Groher, M. (1997). *Dysphagia: Diagnosis and management* (3rd ed.). Boston: Butterworth-Heinemann.

Guenter, P., & Silkroski, M. (2001). *Tube feeding: Practical guidelines and nursing protocols*. Gaithersburg, MD: Aspen.

Gustafsson, P., & Tibbling, L. (1994). Gastro-oesophageal reflux and oesophageal dysfunction in children and adolescents with brain damage. *Acta Paediatrica, 83*, 1081–1085.

Hirano, H., Suzuki, H., Sakakibra, T., Higuchi, Y., Inoue, K., & Suzuki, Y. (1982). Dysphagia due to hypertrophic cervical osteophytes. *Clinical Orthopedics and Related Research, 167*, 168–172.

Honig, J. (1993). Temporomandibular joint dysfunction in children. *Pediatric Nursing, 19*(1), 34–38.

Johnson, J., & Hirsch, C. (2003). Aspiration pneumonia: Recognizing and managing a potentially growing disorder. *Postgraduate Medicine Online, 113*(3). Retrieved February 21, 2004 from http://www.postgradmed.com

Karch, A., & Karch, F. (2000). A hard pill to swallow: A handy guide to medications that must be swallowed whole. *American Journal of Nursing, 100*(4), 25.

Koufman, J. (2002). Laryngopharyngeal reflux: Position statement of the Committee on Speech, Voice, and Swallowing Disorders of the American Academy of Otolaryngology—Head and Neck Surgery. *Otolaryngology, Head and Neck Surgery, 127*(1), 32–35.

Kuhn, D., & Matson, J. (2002). A validity study of the screening tool of feeding problems (STEP). *Journal of Intellectual Disability, 27*, 161–167.

Langmore, S., & Miller, R. (1994). Behavioral treatment for adults with oropharyngeal dysphagia. *Archives of Physical Medicine and Rehabilitation, 75*, 1154–1160.

Langmore, S., Skarupski, K., Park, P., & Fries, B. (2002). Predictors of aspiration pneumonia in nursing home residents. *Dysphagia, 17*, 298–307.

Langmore, S., Terpenning, M., Schork, A., Chen, Y., Murray, J., Lopatin, D., et al. (1998). Predictors of aspiration pneumonia: How important is dysphagia? *Dysphagia, 12*, 69–81.

Leibovitz, A. (2002). Homocysteine blood level in long-term care residents with oropharyngeal dysphagia: Comparison of hand-oral and tube-enteral-fed patients. *Journal of Parenteral and Enteral Nutrition, 26*(2), 94–97.

Leslie, P., Carding, P., & Wilson, J. (2003). Investigation and management of chronic dysphagia. *British Medical Journal, 326*(7386), 433–436.

Levine, A., Milo, T., Briode, E., Wine, E., Dalal, I., Boaz, M., et al. (2004). Influence of *Helicobacter pylori* eradication on gastroesophageal reflux symptoms and epigastric pain in children and adolescents. *Pediatrics, 113*(1), 54–58.

Logemann, J. (1998). *Evaluation and treatment of swallowing disorders* (2nd ed.). Austin, TX: Pro-ed.

Logemann, J., Martin-Harris, B. (2001). Role of RDs in dysphagia screening: Concerns. *Journal of American Dietetic Association, 101,* 179–180.

Makkar, R., & Sachdev, G. (2003). Gastric asthma: A clinical update for the general practitioner. *Medscape General Medicine, 5*(3). Retrieved August 13, 2003 from http://www.medscape.com/viewpublication/122_index

Maloney, J., & Ryan, T. (2004). Detection of aspiration in enterally fed patients: A requiem for bedside monitors of aspiration. *Journal of Enteral and Parenteral Nutrition, 28*(1), 62.

Marquis, J., & Pressman, H. (1994). Radiologic assessment of pediatric swallowing. In S. Rosenthal, J. Sheppard, & M. Lotze (Eds.). *Dysphagia in the child with developmental disabilities: Medical, clinical, and family interventions.* (pp. 189–208) San Diego: Singular Publishing Group.

Migliore, L., Scoopo, F., & Robey, K. (1999). Fiberoptic examination of swallowing in children and young adults with severe developmental disability. *American Journal of Speech-Language Pathology, 8,* 303–308.

Murry, T., & Carrau, R. (2001). *Clinical manual for swallowing and swallowing disorders.* San Diego, CA: Singular Thomson Learning.

Pandolfino, J., Richter, J., Ours, T., Guardino, J., Chapman, J., & Kahrilas, P. (2003). Ambulatory esophageal pH monitoring using a wireless system. *The American Journal of Gastroenterology, 98,* 740–749.

Perlman, A., & Schulze-Delrieu, K. (Eds.). (1997). *Deglutition and its disorders: Anatomy, physiology, clinical diagnosis, and management.* San Diego, CA: Singular Publishing Group.

Potter, P., & Perry, A. (2001). *Fundamentals of nursing* (6th ed.). St. Louis, MO: Mosby.

Robbins, J. (1999). Old swallowing and dysphagia: Thoughts on intervention and prevention. *Nutrition in Clinical Practice, 14*(5), S21–S26.

Rogers, B., Stratton, P., Msall, M., & Andres, M. (1994). Long-term morbidity and management strategies of tracheal aspiration in adults wih severe developmental disabilities. *American Journal on Mental Retardation, 98,* 490–498.

Rosenthal, S., Sheppard, J., & Lotze, M. (Eds.). (1995). *Dysphagia and the child with developmental disabilities: Medical, clinical, and family interventions.* San Diego, CA: Singular Publishing Group.

Sheikh, S., Allen, E., Shell, R., Hruschak, J., Iram, D., Castile, R., et al. (2001). Chronic aspiration without gastroesophageal reflux as a cause of chronic respiratory symptoms in neurologically normal infants. *Chest, 120,* 1190–1195.

Sheppard, J. (1987). Assessment of oral motor behaviors in cerebral palsy. *Seminars in Speech and Language, 8*(1), 57–70.

Sheppard, J. (1994). Clinical evaluation and treatment. In S. R. Rosenthal, J. J. Sheppard, & M. Lotze (Eds.). *Dysphagia and the child with developmental disabilities: Medical, clinical and family interventions* (pp. 37–76). San Diego, CA: Singular Publishing Group.

Sheppard, J. (2002). Swallowing and feeding in older people with lifelong disability. *Advances in Speech-Language Pathology, 4*(2), 119–121.

Sheppard, J., & Hochman, R. (1988). *Screening large residential populations for dysphagia.* Paper presented at the American Academy for Cerebral Palsy and Developmental Medicine, 42nd Annual Meeting, Toronto, Canada.

Sheppard, J., Liou, J., Hochman, R., Laroia, S., & Langlois, D. (1988). Nutritional correlates of dysphagia in individuals institutionalized with mental retardation. *Dysphagia, 3,* 85–89.

Sheppard, J., & Pressman, H. (1988). Dysphagia in infantile cortical hyperostosis (Caffey's disease): A case study. *Developmental Medicine & Child Neurology, 30,* 108–114.

Siktberg, L., & Bantz, D. (1999). Management of children with swallowing disorders. *Journal of Pediatric Health Care, 13,* 223–229.

Smith, D., & Soucy, P. (1996). Complications of long-term jejunostomy in children. *Journal of Pediatric Surgery, 31,* 787–790.

Spremulli, M. (2001). Adherence concerns . . ."Dysphagia: Going down and staying down." *American Journal of Nursing, 101*(3), 13.

Tamura, F., Shishikura, J., Mukai, Y., & Kaneko, Y. (1999). Arterial oxygen saturation in severly disabled people: Effect of oral feeding in the sitting position. *Dysphagia, 14,* 204–211.

Tymchuk, D. (1999). Textural property considerations of food for dysphagia. Proceedings of the fourth annual Ross medical nutrition and device roundtable, Charleston, SC, April 1999. *Nutrition in Clinical Practice, 14*(5), S57–S59.

Woods, E. (1994). The influence of posture and positioning on oral motor development and dysphagia. In S. R. Rosenthal, J. J. Sheppard, & M. Lotze (Eds.), *Dysphagia in the child with developmental disabilities: Medical, clinical, and family interventions* (pp. 153–188). San Diego, CA: Singular Publishing Group.

Zarate, N., Mearin, F., Hidalgo, A., & Malagelada, J. R. (2001). Prospective evaluation of esophageal motor dysfunction in Down syndrome. *American Journal of Gastroenterology, 96,* 1718–1724.

Behavior Management and Mental Health

Sarah H. Ailey, RN, PhD

18

Objectives

At the completion of this chapter, the learner will be able to:

1. Identify the risk for behavioral disorders and/or mental health conditions in persons with intellectual and developmental disabilities (I/DD).
2. Define "diagnostic overshadowing."
3. Discuss theoretical models of mental health care used in the care of persons with I/DD.
4. Critique interdisciplinary methods of assessment, intervention, case management, and evaluation in providing evidence-based behavior and mental health management.

Key Points

- Individuals with I/DD can have all the same mental health problems and disorders as the general population, as well as increased risk of some mental health problems.

- Some syndromes and disorders are associated with increased risk of particular behavioral and mental health disorders.

- Individuals with mental health problems may be overlooked and not receive treatment and/or may be subject to inappropriate medication management.

- Models of mental health care are important in identification and treatment of mental health problems.

- Care of individuals with I/DD and mental health problems may be complex. Ability to assess the interrelationship of physical health, mental health, and behavior problems to the care of persons with I/DD is important.

Key Points *(continued)*

- Planning and implementing care of individuals with I/DD and mental health problems requires the participation of the individuals themselves, family members, and caregivers, and may require the coordination of various professional disciplines.

- Medication management may be part of the treatment of mental health disorders. Regular evaluation is important in order to assess for efficacy, side effects, and interaction with other medications.

- Case management skills are important in planning and implementing care for individuals with I/DD and mental health disorders.

I.   Background

Mental health disorders are often under-recognized and under-treated. This is as true for individuals with I/DD as for the general population. Individuals with I/DD are at increased risk for behavioral disorders and some mental health disorders such as anxiety and depression. Some syndromes and disorders are associated with increased risk of particular behavior and mental health disorders.

A.   Individuals with I/DD have all the mental health problems and disorders of the general population. The prevalence of some disorders may be higher than the general population (Deb, Thomas, & Bright, 2001a; Moss, Emerson, Bouras, & Holland, 1997).

B.   Behavior disorders may or may not be associated with mental health disorders. Estimates of behavior disorder prevalence range to over 60% of individuals with I/DD (Deb, Thomas, & Bright, 2001b).

C.   Poor outcomes such as low levels of social support, social skills deficits, and aggressive behavior and conduct problems are associated with mental health disorders. Mental health disorders may hamper integration into community, residential, and workplace settings.

II.   Interrelationship of I/DD, Physical, and Mental Health Problems

Understanding the interrelationships of physical health, mental health, and behavior problems is important. One of the features of inadequacies in the care of individuals with I/DD is that both physical and mental health symptoms have been attributed to I/DD by health professionals.

A. Attributing mental health disorders to the I/DD has been called "diagnostic overshadowing."

1. Reiss, Levitan, and Szyszko (1982) conducted a classic study on diagnostic overshadowing. When given the same case descriptions, professional psychologists identified psychopathology more often for individuals with I/DD than for individuals with average intelligence. The phenomenon was found for psychologists both with and without experience with individuals with I/DD (Reiss & Szyszko, 1983).

B. Physical disorders may also be attributed to the I/DD, and some physical problems mimic or complicate mental health disorders for individuals with I/DD.

1. Symptoms of sleep disorders include behavior changes, mood swings, depression, and appetite changes. These symptoms may be mistaken as part of the I/DD or as depression, intermittent explosive disorders, or anxiety.

2. Symptoms of hypothyroidism include weight gain, sleep changes, and decreased activity and may mimic depression.

3. Symptoms of hyperthyroidism include nervousness, sleep changes, behavior changes, and fatigue, and might be mistaken for mental health problems.

III. Models of Mental Health Care

Theoretical models of mental health care focus the attention of health professionals and have implications for identification, treatment, and outcomes of mental health disorders.

A. Behavior modification models

1. Important models of care in the treatment of psychopathology in individuals with I/DD (Dosen & Day, 2001).

2. Practices such as analyzing behaviors in relation to settings, antecedents, and consequences, and practices of positive and negative reinforcement to develop desired behavior are well known in the field of I/DD. Many training and habilitation programs for toileting skills, self-help skills, speech skills, obesity, enuresis, and encopresis use behavior modification strategies.

3. Ethical and legal concerns exist with behavior modification strategies including:

   a. Positive and negative reinforcement strategies and punishment strategies (Nezu & Nezu, 1994)

   b. Individuals whose behavior is not problematic may not receive needed treatment for mental health problems.

B. Cognitive models

1. Since the mid-1980s, researchers have established that cognition is involved in mental health disorders in individuals with mild and moderate I/DD. For example, depression is associated with:

a. Negative self-concept (Benson & Ivins, 1992)

b. Frequency of automatic negative thoughts, thoughts of hopelessness, and self-reinforcement (Nezu, Nezu, Rothenberg, DelliCarpini, & Groag, 1995)

c. Social comparison (Dagnan & Sandhu, 1999)

d. Self-hatred (Ailey, 2002)

e. Conversely, the absence of depression in adolescents with I/DD is associated with global self-worth and positive self-image (Zigler, Bennet-Gates, & Hodapp, 1999).

2. In cognitive therapy, emphasis is placed on changing or modifying internal experiences, thoughts, feelings, and attitudes (Clark, Beck, & Alford, 1999). These therapies are increasingly used for individuals with mild and moderate I/DD (Benson & Valenti-Hein, 2001).

3. Cognitive models fail to adequately take account of environmental and interpersonal factors affecting mental health (Hammen, 1999).

C. Ecological and interpersonal models

1. Advances in mental health care over the last quarter century include development of interpersonal and ecological theories and models of mental health care that specifically assess social and environmental conditions as well as cognitive and behavioral variables.

2. Learned helplessness and social skills deficit models have been used to explain mental health problems in individuals with I/DD. Both were originally conceived as behavioral models, reformulated as cognitive models, and today are discussed in the context of interpersonal/ecological models of mental health (Ingram, Miranda, & Segal, 1998; Trower, 1995).

3. Social stigma, isolation, loneliness, and social conflict are important in interpersonal/ecological models of mental health (Dill & Anderson, 1999; Roberts & Monroe, 1999). In the last 20 years, it is established that interpersonal issues are important for individuals with I/DD.

a. Reiss and Benson (1984) indicated that individuals with I/DD have increased expectations of failure and are aware of social stigma.

b. Negative social support and social strain are associated with mental health disorders in individuals with I/DD (Lunsky & Havercamp, 1999; Nezu et al., 1995).

c. Loneliness and life satisfaction are associated with depression in individuals with Down Syndrome (Ailey, 2002).

4. Interpersonal models of mental health care offer improved methods to assess mental health and develop treatments for individuals with I/DD (Ailey & Miller, 2004).

IV. Screening and Referrals

Care of individuals with I/DD may include screening for mental health disorders and identifying and referring individuals for mental health services.

A. Screening

1. Active process to identify and refer individuals who may have previously unrecognized mental health problems.

2. Important in secondary prevention. Most useful if mental health disorders are detected early, so that individuals benefit from the treatment.

3. Health care professionals working in school, employment, residential, and community settings may be interested in screening for mental health disorders as part of providing optimal care to their clients.

4. Screening tools developed for the general population may be used. Tools specifically developed for individuals with I/DD include:

   a. *Psychopathology Instrument for Mentally Retarded Adults* (PIMRA) (Kazdin, Matson, & Senatore, 1983)

   b. *Reiss Screens for Maladaptive Behavior* (RSMB) (Havercamp & Reiss, 1997; Reiss, 1992)

   c. *Reiss Scales for Children's Dual Diagnosis* (Reiss & Valenti-Hein, 1994)

   d. *Strohmer-Prout Behavior Rating Scale* (Strohmer & Prout, 1998)

B. Referrals for mental health care

1. Treatment is generally sought for individuals with I/DD by family or by agency, employment, and housing staff.

2. Staff and family may have problems recognizing when individuals with I/DD need evaluation for mental health disorders.

3. Treatment is more likely to be sought for some mental health disorders than others. For example, Edelstein and Glenwick (2001) used a series of vignettes to assess how direct-care workers identify psychological disorders of adults with I/DD and their need for treatment. Direct care workers were more likely to identify behavioral symptoms of aggressive disorders and psychosis than depression and to identify a need for treatment of aggressive disorders and psychosis than depression.

4. Be aware of signs and symptoms indicating the need for individuals to have mental health referrals, and be able to work with family and staff to identify individuals needing follow-up.

V. Assessment

Once individuals with I/DD have access to mental health services, thorough assessment is critical to appropriate mental health care. Individuals with

I/DD may have physical and mental health issues that require advanced assessment skills. Thorough assessment may necessitate the work of a multidisciplinary team and include a physical examination, a history of current complaints, assessment for presence of particular syndromes or diagnoses, medication history, psychosocial history, family history, and eligibility for programs. As much as possible, information should be obtained from individuals with I/DD themselves.

A. Physical assessment

   1. Multiple physical health problems including seizure disorders, musculoskeletal disorders, cerebral palsy, hypothyroidism, sleep disorders, nutritional problems, and uncommunicated pain may mimic or complicate mental health disorders.

   2. Individuals with I/DD may be difficult to interview, necessitating good physical assessment skills and skill in interviewing caregivers and informants.

B. Assessing the interrelationship of behavior problems and mental health disorders is a complex issue.

   1. Behaviors are a primary reason for psychiatric referral for individuals with I/DD (Moss, 1999). Physical and mental health problems may be manifested by behaviors.

   2. Physicians generally do diagnostic assessment of mental health disorders. However, other health care professionals need to be familiar with the criteria involved. Individuals with mild and moderate I/DD can generally be assessed with standard diagnostic criteria such as the DSM-IV-TR, the principal system for mental health diagnosis in the United States (American Psychiatric Association, 2000).

   3. The high prevalence of behavior disorders in individuals with I/DD may reflect mental health disorders and symptoms that are unique or significantly more common among individuals with I/DD (Einfeld & Aman, 1995). For example, Marston, Perry, and Roy (1997) found that individuals with mild and moderate I/DD could generally be assessed for depression using standard diagnostic criteria such as the DSM or ICD systems, but often had new behavior problems as atypical symptoms, and that individuals with more severe levels of I/DD often have mental health disorder symptoms that are not covered in the standard criteria.

   4. Individuals with mental health disorders whose behaviors are not problematic may not receive adequate mental health treatment.

C. History of current complaints—Might include onset of complaints; changes in sleep patterns; changes in appetite; recent illnesses; recent changes in family, work, and social relationships; and pain and any physical complaints.

D. Presence of particular syndromes—Specific syndromes often have characteristic associated mental health and behavioral problems, and knowledge of the presence of particular syndromes can help guide the assessment.

1. Individuals with Prader-Willi syndrome:

   a. Frequently have obsessive-compulsive disorders, particularly obsessions with food and hoarding food; self-injurious behaviors, including skin picking; depression and anxiety, at times associated with psychosis (Moldavsky, Lev, & Lerman-Sagie, 2001).

   b. May need nutritional management, specific educational approaches, appropriate medication management, and behavioral, cognitive, and environmental interventions (Akefeldt & Gillberg, 1999; Clarke, 1998; State, Dykens, Rosner, Martin, & King, 1999).

2. Individuals with Fragile X syndrome:

   a. Often have attention deficit disorders, obsessive-compulsive behaviors, anxiety disorders, autism disorders, stereotypic behaviors, mood lability, and problems with sensory integration (Baumgardner, Reiss, & Freund, 1995; Hagerman, 1996, 1999).

   b. May need evaluation for behavior and environmental management and specific educational interventions. Consideration can be given to medication management (Hagerman, 1999).

3. Individuals with Down syndrome:

   a. May have obsessive-compulsive behaviors, unrecognized autism spectrum disorders, attention deficit disorders, and depression.

   b. Need appropriate evaluation. If attention deficit problems are present, physical or environmental causes should be ruled out as the cause (McBrien, 1998). Reversible conditions such as depression should be ruled out before a diagnosis of Alzheimer's disease is made (Chicoine, McGuire, & Rubin, 1999). Education and support are important (Rasmussen, Borjesson, Wentz, & Gillberg, 2001). Environmental and psychosocial interventions and medication management may be indicated.

4. Individuals with autism spectrum disorders:

   a. Often have obsessive-compulsive disorders, ritualistic behaviors, poor social skills, and difficulty making decisions.

   b. Interventions include social, psychological, and educational interventions, at times in conjunction with medication management (Hoover, 2001).

5. Individuals with Williams syndrome:

   a. Often have uninhibited behaviors, hypersociability, exaggerated fears, sadness, excitement, somatic complaints, and depression (Einfeld, Tonge, & Florio, 1997; Gosch & Pankau, 1997; Moldavsky et al., 2001).

b. Interventions may include environmental management, psychosocial therapies, and medication management.

6. Individuals with fetal alcohol syndrome:

a. Often have ADHD, impulsivity, depression, panic disorders, and suicidal threats and attempts (Streissguth & O'Malley, 1997).

b. Interventions might include individual and family therapy, environmental and behavioral management, and medication management.

E. Psychosocial history—Social and environment issues are a risk factor for mental health disorders and include:

1. Major life changes such as death of a parent, other family member, or an individual important in one's life; moving; the loss of an important staff member; or other significant change. For example, Hollins & Esterhuyzen (1997) found that 26% of individuals who had lost a parent within 2 years could be characterized as depressed.

2. Social isolation—For example, individuals with I/DD may have limited social contacts. Job and social opportunities may be restricted.

3. Poor self-esteem and stigmatization.

4. History of abuse.

a. Individuals with I/DD are at risk for abuse, including incest, rape and assault, abuse by caregivers and persons in authority, and exploitation (American Academy of Pediatrics, 2001). For example, in a study in the United Kingdom, McCarthy and Thompson (1997) found 61% of women and 25% of men with I/DD have experiences with sexual abuse, while Stromsness (1993), in the U.S., found 79% of women with I/DD likely to have experienced sexual abuse.

b. Aspects of the lives of individuals with I/DD such as different caretakers, the need for help with personal care, being used to obeying and complying, and lack of skills in defending and speaking up for themselves put them at risk for abuse and exploitation (Aylott, 1999).

5. Family history including history of mental health disorders.

6. Eligibility for programs such as Medicaid, special education, vocational rehabilitation, housing services, and respite services.

VI. Planning and Implementation of Care—Medication Management

The combination of medications and psychosocial interventions may be better than each alone in mental health treatment (see Chapter 19).

A. Rationale for psychoactive drugs.

1. A common reason for referral to mental health services for individuals with I/DD is behavior problems, and the diagnoses and clinical symptoms targeted by psychoactive drugs are often behavioral in nature.

2. Psychoactive drugs should be prescribed to treat definite clinical symptoms and diagnoses. However, for individuals with I/DD, psychoactive drugs often are given in the absence of sound clinical rationales and the drugs may not be monitored for efficacy and side effects. Such practice amounts to chemical restraint and is contrary to good clinical practice (Matson et al., 2000).

3. Because of the frequency of behavioral diagnoses, the rationales for drug use by individuals with I/DD may be different than common use by the general population.

B. Key classes of psychoactive medications used with individuals with I/DD

  1. Psychotropic medications

   a. Generally used to treat symptoms of schizophrenia. Include dopamine agonists and atypical drugs (Risperdal and Zyprexa).

   b. In individuals with I/DD, psychotropics are used to treat both psychotic and nonpsychotic disorders such as behavior problems (Friedlander, Lazar, & Klancnik, 2001). For example, in Oklahoma, a statewide survey found that 22% of adults with mental retardation received psychotropic drugs, and the drugs were frequently used to treat behavior disorders (Spreat, Conroy, & Jones, 1997).

   c. Experts suggest that psychotropics may be useful to manage acute behavior problems; there is no sound research supporting long-term use for chronic behavior problems (Matson et al., 2000).

   d. Behavior problems may be reduced, but adaptive behaviors and overall activity may also be reduced (Matson et al., 2000).

   e. Severe and permanent side effects such as tardive dyskinesia are associated with long term use of psychotropics. Individuals with I/DD may be particularly sensitive to developing side effects (Friedlander et al., 2001).

   f. Regular re-evaluation of the appropriateness of psychotropic drug therapy and routine screening for movement disorders for individuals with I/DD is indicated.

  2. Antidepressant medications

   a. Generally used to treat depression and anxiety disorders. Include the selective serotonin reuptake inhibitors (SSRIs), tricyclic antidepressives, and MAOI inhibitors.

   b. May relieve symptoms of depression of persons with I/DD. Methodological problems exist with the research on use of the drugs for individuals with I/DD (Matson et al., 2000).

   c. Used along with other drugs to manage behavior problems for individuals with I/DD (Amaria, Billeisen, & Hagerman, 2002). No methodologically sound research demonstrates efficacy for this purpose.

    d. SSRIs are thought to have fewer side effects than older classes of drugs, but side effects of long term use are not known. Evaluation for side effects and for efficacy is indicated.

  3. Mood stabilization medications

    a. Usually for treatment of symptoms of bipolar disorders. Classic drugs include lithium. Anti-convulsants such as Tegretol, Neurontin, and Depakote shown to have a mood stabilizing effect.

    b. Also used for problem behaviors for individuals with I/DD.

    c. Depakote reported effective in reducing aggressive and self-injurious behavior in individuals with I/DD (Ruedrich, Swales, Fossaceca, Toliver, & Rutkowski, 1999).

    d. Research on mood stabilizers for problem behaviors is limited.

    e. Regular re-evaluation for side effects and efficacy needed.

C. Risks versus benefits should be considered with all medications.

  1. Specific drugs may be beneficial and others inappropriate for specific syndromes (Santosh & Baird, 1999).

    a. Some psychoactive drugs have weight gain as a side effect. May be contra-indicated with Prader-Willi syndrome or Down syndrome.

    b. Individuals with congenital metabolic disorders, children under 2 years of age, and those with severe seizure disorders accompanied by mental retardation need regular evaluation for hepatoxicity if taking Depakote or its derivatives.

  2. Regular evaluation needed for efficacy, side effects, interaction with other drugs, and long-term effects. Part of planning overall care for individuals with I/DD.

D. Adjunct and alternative treatments

  1. In the general population, alternative therapies for mental health disorders such as meditation and exercise are shown to have some benefit.

  2. No research on benefits of alternative therapies for individuals with I/DD.

E. Assess adequacy of medication management and assess for errors. In a study of medication errors for individuals with I/DD living in community residences, 85% of the individuals experienced medication errors in the course of a year (Stupalski & Russell, 1999). Medication errors may be related to the training of unlicensed caregivers giving medications.

VII. Planning and Implementation of Care—Case Management

Care of individuals with I/DD requires coordination with the individual with I/DD, family, various specialists, and community agency personnel. Case management principles are useful in planning and managing the care of individuals with I/DD, as they may have a number of physical and mental health complaints.

A. Case management includes coordination of disciplines including neurologists, endocrinologists, sleep disorder specialists, nutritionists, psychologists, psychiatrists, and nurses with the individual, his or her family, and staff.

B. Includes advocacy, utilization of community resources, training in adaptive social skills, behavioral and cognitive programs, developing objectives, psychiatric services, counseling, and respite services (Coelho, Kelley, Deatsman-Kelley, & Clinton-Eaton-Ingham Community Mental Health Board, 1993).

C. The client in the community should be the focus.

VIII. Planning and Implementation of Care—Evaluation

Evaluating the plan of care is a standard in all settings. Identifying the expected outcomes is important.

A. Overall issues when evaluating care:

1. Mental health problems often negatively impact functioning in society. An expected outcome is to promote maximum functioning of the client. The health professional needs to ask whether the individual's school, work, and/or family functioning improved after implementation of the management plan.

2. Other questions to ask include whether the conceptual model was appropriate for the client; was adequate data collected, were concerns of the individual, family, and staff addressed; and were planning and implementation effective.

3. Answering these questions assists in assessing the total care provided.

B. Evaluation involves describing and measuring the effect of the care on the expected outcomes. For example, an individual might have depressive symptoms of appetite changes, changes in interest levels for usual activities, and sadness along with new behavior problems. One would expect a reduction of symptoms, improved and more adaptive behaviors, and returned interest in usual activities. If the depressive symptoms were intensified by physical health symptoms, one would expect improvement in the physical health symptoms.

C. Feedback from the individuals with I/DD, family, and/or staff is crucial.

IX. Summary

Mental health issues and mental illnesses need to be considered when conducting a health assessment and physical examination. Such conditions may co-exist with I/DDs. Nurses and health professionals need to be knowledgeable about mental health and illness models and available assessment tools.

References

Ailey, S. H. (2002). Evaluating an interpersonal model of depression in adults with Down syndrome. Unpublished doctoral dissertation. Chicago, IL: University of Illinois at Chicago.

Ailey, S., & Miller, A. (2004). Psychosocial theories of depression for individuals with intellectual and development disabilities: A historicist perspective. *Research and Theory for Nursing Practice, 18,* 131–148.

Akefeldt, A., & Gillberg, C. (1999). Behavior and personality characteristics of children and young adults with Prader-Willi syndrome: A controlled study. *Journal of the American Academy of Child and Adolescent Psychiatry, 38,* 761–769.

Amaria, R. N., Billeisen, L. L., & Hagerman, R. (2002). Medication use in Fragile X syndrome. *Mental Health Aspects of Developmental Disabilities, 4,* 143–147.

American Academy of Pediatrics. (2001). Assessment of maltreatment of children with disabilities. *Pediatrics, 108,* 508–512.

American Psychiatric Association. (2000). *Diagnostic and statistical manual of mental disorders* (Rev. ed.). Washington, DC: Author.

Aylott, J. (1999). Preventing rape and sexual assault of people with learning disabilities. *British Journal of Nursing, 8,* 871–874.

Baumgardner, T. L., Reiss, A. L., & Freund, L. S. (1995). Specification of the neurobiological phenotype in males with fragile X syndrome. *Pediatrics, 95,* 744–752.

Benson, B. A., & Ivins, J. (1992). Anger, depression, and self-concept in adults with mental retardation. *Journal of Intellectual Disability Research, 36,* 169–175.

Benson, B. A., & Valenti-Hein, D. (2001). Cognitive and social learning treatment. In A. Dosen & K. Day (Eds.). *Treating mental illness and behavior disorders in children and adults with mental retardation* (pp. 101–188). Northumberland, UK: Northgate & Prudhoe NHS Trust.

Chicoine, B., McGuire, D., & Rubin, S. (1999). Adults with Down syndrome: Specialty clinic perspectives. In M. Janicki & A. J. Dalton (Eds.). *Dementia, aging, and intellectual disabilities: A handbook* (pp. 278–293). New York: Taylor & Francis.

Clark, D. A., Beck, A. T., & Alford, B. A. (1999). *Scientific foundations of cognitive theory and theory of depression.* New York: John Wiley & Sons.

Clarke, D. (1998). Prader-Willi syndrome and psychotic symptoms 2: A preliminary study of prevalence using the Psychopathology Assessment Schedule for Adults with Developmental Disability Checklist. *Journal of Intellectual Disability Research, 42,* 451–454.

Coelho, R. J., Kelley, P. S., Deatsman-Kelley, C., & Clinton-Eaton-Ingham Community Mental Health Board. (1993). An experimental investigation of an innovative community treatment model for persons with a dual diagnosis (I/DD/MI). *Journal of Rehabilitation, 59,* 37–44.

Dagnan, D., & Sandhu, S. (1999). Social comparison, self-esteem, and depression in people with intellectual disability. *Journal of Intellectual Disability Research, 43,* 372–379.

Deb, S., Thomas, M., & Bright, C. (2001a). Mental disorder in adults with intellectual disability. 1: Prevalence of functional psychiatric illness among a community-based population aged between 16 and 64 years. *Journal of Intellectual Disability Research, 45,* 495–505.

Deb, S., Thomas, M., & Bright, C. (2001b). Mental disorder in adults with intellectual disability. 2: The rate of behavior disorders among a community-based population aged between 16 and 64 years. *Journal of Intellectual Disability Research, 45,* 506–514.

Dill, J. C., & Anderson, C. A. (1999). Loneliness, shyness, and depression. The etiology and interrelationships of everyday problems in living. In T. Joiner and J. C. Coyne (Eds.). *The interactional nature of depression* (pp. 93–125). Washington, DC: American Psychological Association.

Dosen, A., & Day, K. (2001). Treatment: An integrative approach. In A. Dosen & K. Day (Eds.). *Treating mental illness and behavior disorders in children and adults with mental retardation* (pp. 519–528). Northumberland, UK: Northgate & Prudhoe NHS Trust.

Edelstein, T. M., & Glenwick, D. S. (2001). Direct-care workers' attributions of psychopathology in adults with mental retardation. *Mental Retardation, 39,* 368–378.

Einfeld, S. L., & Aman, M. (1995). Issues in the taxonomy of psychopathology in mental retardation. *Journal of Autism and Developmental Disorder, 25,* 143–167.

Einfeld, S. L., Tonge, B. J., & Florio, T. (1997). Behavioral and emotional disturbance in individuals with Williams syndrome. *American Journal of Mental Retardation, 102,* 45–53.

Friedlander, R., Lazar, S., & Klancnik, J. (2001). Atypical antipsychotic use in treating adolescents and young adults with developmental disabilities. *Canadian Journal of Psychiatry, 46,* 741–745.

Gosch, A., & Pankau, R. (1997). Personality characteristics and behavior problems in individuals of different ages with Williams syndrome. *Developmental Medicine and Child Neurology, 39,* 527–533.

Hagerman, R. J. (1996). Fragile X syndrome. *Child and Adolescent Psychiatric Clinics of North America, 5,* 895–911.

Hagerman, R. J. (1999). Medical treatment of aggression. *The National Fragile X Foundation.* Retrieved July 7, 2002 from http://www.nfxf.org

Hammen, C. (1999). The emergence of an interpersonal approach to depression. In T. Joiner & J. C. Coyne (Eds.). *The interactional nature of depression* (pp. 21–36). Washington, DC: American Psychological Association.

Havercamp. S. M., & Reiss, S. (1997). *The Reiss Screen for Maladaptive Behavior:* Confirmatory factor analysis. *Behaviour Research and Therapy, 35,* 967–971.

Hollins, S., & Esterhuyzen, A. (1997). Bereavement and grief in adults with learning disabilities. *British Journal of Psychiatry, 170,* 497–501.

Hoover, M. (2001). The role of medication in the management of autistic spectrum disorders. In A. F. Rotatori, T. Wahlberg, & F. Obiakor (Eds.). *Autistic spectrum disorders: Educational and clinical intervention. Advances in special education 14* (pp. 255–267). Oxford, England: Elsevier Science.

Ingram, R. E., Miranda, J., & Segal, Z. V. (1998). *Cognitive vulnerability to depression.* New York: Guilford Press.

Kazdin, A. E., Matson, J. L., & Senatore, V. (1983). Assessment of depression in mentally retarded adults. *American Journal of Psychiatry, 140,* 1040–1043.

Lunsky, Y., & Havercamp, S. M. (1999). Distinguishing low levels of social support and social strain: Implications for dual diagnosis. *American Journal on Mental Retardation, 104,* 200–204.

Marston, G. M., Perry, D. W., & Roy, A. (1997). Manifestations of depression in people with intellectual disability. *Journal of Intellectual Disability Research, 41,* 476–480.

Matson, J. L., Bamburg, J. W., Matville, E. A., Pinkston, J., Bielecki, J., Kuhn, D., et al. (2000). Psychopharmacology and mental retardation: A 10 year review (1990–1999). *Research in Developmental Disabilities, 21,* 263–296.

McBrien, D. (1998). *Attention problems in Down syndrome: Is this ADHD?* Retrieved July 7, 2002 from www.ds-health.com

McCarthy, M., & Thompson, D. (1997). A prevalence study of sexual abuse of adults with intellectual disabilities referred for sex education. *Journal of Applied Research in Intellectual Disabilities, 10,* 105–124.

Moldavsky, M., Lev, D., & Lerman-Sagie, T. (2001). Behavioral phenotypes of genetic syndromes: A reference guide for psychiatrists. *Journal of the American Academy of Child and Adolescent Psychiatry, 40,* 749–761.

Moss, S. (1999). Assessment: Conceptual issues. In N. Bouras (Ed.). *Psychiatric and behavioural disorders in developmental disabilities and mental retardation* (pp. 18–37). New York: Cambridge University Press.

Moss, S., Emerson, E., Bouras, N., & Holland, A. (1997). Mental disorders and problematic behaviours in people with intellectual disability: Future directions for research. *Journal of Intellectual Disability Research, 41,* 440–447.

Nezu, C. M., & Nezu, A. M. (1994). Outpatient psychotherapy for adults with mental retardation and concomitant psychopathology: Research and clinical imperatives. *Journal of Consulting and Clinical Psychology, 62,* 34–42.

Nezu, C. M., Nezu, A. M., Rothenberg, J. L., DelliCarpini, L., & Groag, I. (1995). Depression in adults with mild mental retardation: Are cognitive variables involved? *Cognitive Therapy and Research, 19,* 227–239.

Rasmussen, R. P., Borjesson, O., Wentz, E., & Gillberg, C. (2001). Autistic disorders in Down syndrome. *Developmental Medicine & Child Neurology, 43,* 750–754.

Reiss, S. (1992). Assessment of a man with dual diagnosis. *Mental Retardation, 30,* 1–6.

Reiss, S., & Benson, B. A. (1984). Awareness of negative social conditions among mentally retarded, emotionally disturbed outpatients. *American Journal of Psychiatry, 141,* 88–90.

Reiss, S., Levitan, G. W., & Szyszko, J. (1982). Emotional disturbance and mental retardation: Diagnostic overshadowing. *American Journal of Mental Deficiency, 86,* 567–574.

Reiss, S., & Szyszko, J. (1983). Diagnostic overshadowing and professional experience with mentally retarded persons. *American Journal of Mental Deficiency, 87,* 396–402.

Reiss, S., & Valenti-Hein, D. (1994). Development of a psychopathology rating scale for children with mental retardation. *Journal of Consulting & Clinical Psychology, 62,* 28–33.

Roberts, J. E., & Monroe, S. M. (1999). Vulnerable self-esteem and social problems in depression: Toward an interpersonal model of self-esteem regulation. In T. Joiner & J. C. Coyne (Eds.). *The interactional nature of depression* (pp. 149–187). Washington, DC: American Psychological Association.

Ruedrich, S., Swales, T. P., Fossaceca, C., Toliver, J., & Rutkowski, A. (1999). Effect of divalproex sodium on aggression and self-injurious behavior in adults with intellectual disability: A retrospective review. *Journal of Intellectual Disability Research, 43,* 105–111.

Santosh, P. J., & Baird, G. (1999). Psychopharmacotherapy in children and adults with intellectual disabilities. *Lancet, 354*(9174), 233–242.

Spreat, S., Conroy, J. W., & Jones, J. C. (1997). Use of psychotropic medication in Oklahoma: A statewide survey. *American Journal of Mental Retardation, 102,* 80–85.

State, M. W., Dykens, E. M., Rosner, B., Martin, A., & King, B. H. (1999). Obsessive-compulsive symptoms in Prader-Willi and "Prader-Willi-like" patients. *Journal of the American Academy of Child and Adolescent Psychiatry, 38,* 329–334.

Streissguth, A. P., & O'Malley, K. D. (1997). Fetal alcohol syndrome/fetal alcohol effects. *Treatment Today, 9*(3). Retrieved July 7, 2002 from http://depts.washington.edu/fadu/Tr.today.97.html

Strohmer, D. C., & Prout, H. T. (1998). *Strohmer-Prout behavior rating scale.* Schenectady, NY: Genium.

Stromsness, M. (1993). Sexually abused women with mental retardation: Hidden victims, absent resources. *Women and Therapy, 14,* 139–152.

Stupalski, K. A., & Russell, G. E. (1999). Reported medication errors in community residences for individuals with mental retardation: A quality review. *Mental Retardation, 37,* 139–146.

Trower, P. (1995). Adult social skills: State of the art and future directions. In W. O'Donohue & L. Krasner (Eds.). *Handbook of psychological skills training* (pp. 54–80). Needham Heights, MA: Allyn & Bacon.

Zigler, E., Bennett-Gates, D., & Hodapp, R. M. (1999). Assessing personality traits of individuals with mental retardation. In E. Zigler & D. Bennett-Gates (Eds.). *Personality development in individuals with mental retardation* (pp. 206–225). New York: Cambridge University Press.

Psychopharmaceutical Management of Comorbid Psychiatric Diagnoses

Roy Q. Sanders, MD and Leslie Rubin, MD, FAAMR

19

Objectives

At the completion of this chapter, the learner will be able to:

1. List common psychiatric diagnoses that lead to problem behavioral symptoms in people with intellectual and developmental disabilities (I/DD).

2. Recognize medication treatment options commonly prescribed for comorbid diagnoses and problem behavior symptoms.

3. Discuss medication options related to particular symptoms and/or diagnoses.

4. Discuss side effects and other "risk" issues related to medication choices.

Key Points

- People with I/DD often suffer from other medical and psychiatric diagnoses that many times have behavioral manifestations that require intervention.

- Nurses and other professionals play a critical role in helping to recognize the need for intervention and in the implementation of appropriate treatment strategies.

- Appropriate diagnosis and reduction of symptoms leads to significant improvement in quality of life for people with I/DD, their families, and other caregivers.

I.   Introduction

People with I/DD experience medical and psychiatric diagnoses and behavior problems at a greater rate than the general population. These diagnoses and behavior problems lead to significant impairment for people with I/DD, restricting their ability to be fully included and productive members of the community.

A.   Common comorbid psychiatric diagnoses and behavioral problems

1.   Disorders of concentration and attention

2.   Anxiety disorders

3.   Affective disorders including bipolar disorder

4.   Obsessive-compulsive disorder

5.   Perseverations and preoccupations

6.   Tourette's disorder

7.   Self-injurious behavior

8.   Aggression

9.   Psychotic disorders

II.   Disorders of Concentration and Attention

Children with I/DD are more likely than children without I/DD to have problems with concentration, attention, and activity regulation (O'Neal, Talga, & Preston, 2002; Schatzberg & Nemeroff, 2004; Stahl, 2000; Varcarolis, 2003).

A.   The mainstay of therapy for problems with concentration and attention is stimulant medication. Although stimulants are very effective medications, there have been problems with their use because of the relatively short half-life of each of these preparations. Even at their longest, the medications rarely last greater than 8 hours and often patients can experience a sort of rebound hyperactivity once the medication has "worn off."

1.   Methylphenidate (Ritalin) is one of the oldest of the stimulant medications used in the treatment of attention and concentration problems.

a.   In general, methylphenidate is well tolerated and works well to increase concentration and attention and to decrease hyperactivity. It works about 80% of the time to reduce up to 80% of the symptoms a person is experiencing.

b.   Side effects include decreased appetite, decreased or disturbed sleep, and sometimes headaches and gastrointestinal pains. At times motor or vocal tics emerge. There can also be problems with mood instability and irritability. In overdose, you can see psychotic symptoms or symptoms of delirium.

    c. Problems can also arise with methylphenidate because of the short half-life of the standard formulation. Theoretically dosing can occur every 4 hours, but clinical experience leads to dosing as frequently as every 150 minutes. Other forms of the medication have longer duration of action including, but not limited to, Ritalin LA, Metadate CD, and Concerta.

2. Mixed amphetamine salts have also been available in the treatment of attention and concentration for many years. They are currently available in generic form and under the trade name of Adderall and AdderallXR.

    a. These medications are very effective in decreasing the symptoms of poor attention, poor concentration, and hyperactivity. Their effectiveness is similar to methylphenidate and they are very widely used.

    b. Side effects are also similar to those listed above with methylphenidate, but in clinical experience they are slightly more likely to create some mood lability and irritability than the other stimulant medications.

3. Dextroamphetamine has also been used for years in the treatment of problems with attention, concentration, and the regulation of activity level. It is sold under the trade name of Dexedrine or Dexedrine Spanules.

    a. Dextroamphetamine is effective in reduction of symptoms at a level consistent with the treatments listed above.

    b. Side effects are similar to those listed above.

B. Other medication used in the treatment of problems with attention, concentration, and regulation of activity level.

1. Atomoxitine (Strattera) is a noradrenergic reuptake inhibitor that appears to have relatively good effectiveness in decreasing levels of hyperactivity and in helping with increasing attention, concentration, and organization. It has been approved for use in children as young as 6 years old weighing above 40 pounds. It generally has lasting effects throughout the day and into the evening. Problems have included changes in appetite, nausea, and some sleep problems.

2. Centrally acting alpha adrenergic agonists such as clonidine and guanfacine have also been very useful in decreasing levels of hyperactivity and in increasing attention and concentration. They are not necessarily as effective as stimulant medications but they are effective in a group of very-aroused patients. Side effects are limited to problems with drowsiness and with hypotension.

3. Venflaxamine (Effexor) is a mixed serotonin and noradrenergic reuptake inhibitor that has been used in the treatment of difficulties related to concentration, attention, and regulation of activity level with some limited success. Recently, venflaxamine has come under increasing scrutiny because of issues related to possible increased suicidal ideation and suicidal behaviors in children

and adolescents taking serotonin reuptake inhibitors. Other problems have included increased irritability and possible increases in blood pressure.

4. Buproprion (Wellbutrin) is an antidepressant medication that is sometimes used in the treatment of problems with attention and concentration. Buproprion can be reasonably effective in the reduction of symptoms but must be used with caution in children or adolescents with history of seizures, head injury, or bulimia.

5. Tricyclic antidepressants have also been used successfully in the treatment of problems with attention, concentration, and regulation of activity levels. The tricyclics used in children most often include imipramine and nortrityline. They generally have good effectiveness over 24 hours but they can have troublesome side effects that include a widening of the QRS as measured on EKG. Also they can lead to drowsiness, weight gain, dry mouth, and constipation. It is also generally important to check serum levels of these medications while a child is being treated.

III. Anxiety Disorders

Anxiety disorders as a group are very common in children in general and, as with other psychiatric concerns, are more likely to affect children and adults with I/DD. These problems seem particularly acute and problematic in individuals diagnosed with any of the pervasive developmental disorders (PDD), but can also be the overwhelming symptom in other disorders such as Prader-Willi syndrome (O'Neal, Talga, & Preston, 2002; Rush & Frances, 2000; Schatzberg & Nemeroff, 2004; Stahl, 2000; Varcarolis, 2003).

A. Since their introduction in the last several years, the serotonin reuptake inhibitors have been the first choice in the treatment of anxiety. They include fluoxetine (Prozac), sertraline (Zoloft), paroxitine (Paxil), citalopram (Celexa), escitalopram (Lexapro), and fluvoxamine (Luvox). These medications taken as a whole have been very effective in reducing anxiety and also in decreasing anxiety-related symptoms associated with perseveration and preoccupation. In general they should be used starting at low doses for most patients, but especially with those diagnosed with PDD. The medications should be gradually titrated to desired effect. Care should be given to look for the emergence of any agitation or irritability, and these medications have been known to induce mania in predisposed patients. Also, added care should be given to observe for any signs or symptoms associated with increased suicidal ideation or suicidal behaviors.

B. Buspirone (Buspar) is an anxiolytic that can have some success in the treatment of anxiety. Although not always successful in relieving anxiety, it is a medication with very few side effects and is well tolerated. Generally, problems arise from needing to dose up to three times a day and it has a relatively slower onset of action, sometimes taking up to 3 weeks to achieve clinically significant effect.

C. Venflaxamine (Effexor) is a combination serotonin reuptake inhibitor and noradrenergic reuptake inhibitor that has been clinically effective in decreasing anxiety symptoms. It has generally been well tolerated but there have been problems with sleep disturbance and even drowsiness on the medication. There have also been problems with elevations in blood pressure.

D. Benzodiazepines as a class are excellent anti-anxiety medications. They can be very effective in the treatment of anxiety-related problems in persons with I/DD. These medications include, but are not necessarily limited to, diazepam, alprazolam, lorazepam, chlordiazepoxide, clonazepam, chlorazepate, oxazepam, flurazepam, and temazepam. Problems that can arise in these medications most often relate to somulence, difficulty with short-term memory, development of tolerance requiring increasingly higher doses, and also with the half-life and active metabolites of some of the medications in this class leading to unwanted prolonged effects.

E. Tricyclic antidepressants such as imipramine and nortriptyline can also be effective anxiolytics. However, they may take up to 4 weeks to work effectively once an adequate serum level has been obtained. As when using these medications in the treatment of other symptoms, care must be given to monitor the EKG to insure a QTc that is within acceptable clinical parameters. Also as stated above, problems with high anticholinergic side effects can lead to problems like dry mouth, constipation, and drowsiness.

F. There are times when antihistamines such as hydroxyzine or diphenhydramine are prescribed to relieve anxiety. Although these medications may be effective in the short run, sedating a patient and calming the "crisis," they are generally not good medications for long-term use in the treatment of ongoing anxiety symptoms.

IV. Affective Disorders Including Bipolar Disorder

Although rates are hard to find and there have not been definitive studies done looking at the comorbidity of affective/mood disorders in persons with I/DD, from clinical practice it is clear that these problems are common and probably occur at a higher rate than the general population (O'Neal, Talga, & Preston, 2002; Rush & Frances, 2000; Schatzberg & Nemeroff, 2004; Stahl, 2000; Varcarolis, 2003).

A. Major depression

1. Several antidepressant medications are used to treat depression.

a. The generally accepted first line of treatment for depression is the choice of a selective serotonin reuptake inhibitor. These medications, which were listed above, include fluoxetine (Prozac), sertraline (Zoloft), citralopram (Celexa), escitralopram (Lexapro), fluvoxamine (Luvox), and paroxetine (Paxil). All of these medications generally have the same level of effectiveness in the treatment of depression, and choices are often made based upon side-effect profiles or the past response to a particular medication by the patient or a close relative of the patient. These are generally safe and effective medications, although their use in children has not been studied.

    i.   Side effects in this class of medication are generally related to gastrointestinal problems, sometimes problems with sleep, and all generally tend to create problems with sexual function (in adults) that are usually related to decreased orgasm, but there can also be decreased desire.

    ii.   These medications can also cause problems with increased irritability and at times they can induce mania in individuals with that predisposition. Care should be given, especially when giving to individuals with a strong family history of bipolar disorder. Individuals with PDD also can be very susceptible to side effects of irritability and mood instability. These medications should be used at low doses and with appropriate caution.

b.   Buproprione (Wellbutrin) is effective in the treatment of depression and in general has been well tolerated. It has advantages over the other antidepressants used in adults in that it is generally accepted that it has fewer sexual side effects. This medication has also appeared to be less likely to create difficulties with inducing mania in individuals that may be vulnerable.

    i.   Buproprion must be used in caution with individuals who have a history of head injury or those with seizure disorder or history of bulimia. These individuals may be at higher risk for seizure on this medication. Newer formulations of buproprion have lengthened the half-life of the medication and this has led to less risk of seizure in individuals. It still should not be given to individuals with the risk factors noted above.

c.   Venflaxamine (Effexor) is a combination selective serotonin reuptake inhibitor and noradrenergic reuptake inhibitor. It has been effective in the treatment of depression and is generally well tolerated. There have been problems as noted above with increased blood pressure and there have also been complaints related to sexual function.

d.   Tricyclic antidepressants have long been, and in some circles continue to be, the gold standard for the treatment of depression. These medications, although they do have quite a few side effects in general, have been well tolerated and are effective in relieving symptoms. These medications include imipramine, nortriptyline, amitriptyline, and clomipramine. They all work in varying degrees on the same neurotransmitter systems that have been mentioned above, but each to a different degree and with a different level of specificity for a particular neurotransmitter. This difference in neurotransmitter effect and the side-effect profiles of each allows a clinician to attempt a good match for treatment with these medications.

    i.   All of these medications generally have high anticholinergic profiles. Side effects are usually problems with sleepiness, weight gain, dry mouth, constipation, and so on.

    ii.   Each of these medications generally causes an increase in the time interval associated with the QRS complex as measured with an EKG. This can lead to dangerous arrhythmias during the course of treatment.

    iii.   Because of each of the side effect difficulties listed above, these medications can be fatal in overdose. This is generally not seen with the other medications that have been listed above for the treatment of depression. Given that by its very nature depression can have as a core symptom morbid preoccupation and suicidality, these medications must be given cautiously and monitored closely.

  e. Other medications have been used effectively as adjuncts to those listed above when treating depression. So-called mood stabilizers such as lithium or valproic acid or other anticonvulsants have been used to try to decrease symptoms in a marginally responsive or nonresponsive patient. Other medications that have been used with some effectiveness include stimulants and even thyroid hormone supplementation.

    i.   Adolescent girls and women with I/DD who have achieved menarche sometimes respond well to adjuncts of oral or depo contraceptive medications for depressive symptoms.

  2. Although medications have been very effective in relieving the symptoms of depression, it should be noted that electroconvulsive therapy is also a very effective somatic treatment. There are side effects associated with short-term memory problems and the risk associated with anesthesia, but overall the patients respond well and quickly to this somatic treatment. Many centers have even moved to offering this treatment in a day hospital setting with no overnight stays.

B. Bipolar disorder

  1. Bipolar disorder is seen in individuals with I/DD and, although it is a discussion not within the scope of this chapter, it can often present in an atypical fashion. Determining core symptoms of grandiosity, racing thoughts, or flight of ideas with increased goal-oriented pursuits may be difficult to discern, and features related to irritability and hypersexuality may be difficult to tease from behaviors typical for the particular individual. Medications used to treat bipolar disorder are generally called mood stabilizers, but there are mood stabilizers in several different classes of medications.

a. Lithium has long been the treatment standard in the psychopharmaco-logic treatment of bipolar disorder. It is an exceptionally effective mood stabilizer and is generally well tolerated. It does, however, have several side effects and has a very narrow therapeutic window, making it potentially dangerous in overdose.

   i. Side effects include weight gain, diarrhea, acne, and, less commonly, problems with renal function, possible hypothyroidism, and cardiac rhythm problems.

   ii. Blood levels need to be monitored carefully and care has to be taken in patients who are on medications or participate in activities that would potentially increase the drug's serum level.

b. Divalproex (Depakote) is also a very effective mood stabilizing medication. It is generally used as an anticonvulsant, but it does currently have approval from the FDA for use as a treatment of acute mania. Most patients tolerate divalproex (Depakote) with few problems but there can be side effects. It can lead to some gastrointestinal problems and there can be increased appetite with weight gain. Additionally, in women there has been a correlation between divalproex (Depakote) use and polycystic ovaries. There have also been problems with liver function and bone marrow changes, usually with a decrease in megakaryocytes and subsequently platelets. In very rare cases critical pancreatitis has been a problem. Blood levels need to be monitored while the patient is on divalproex (Depakote) in addition to laboratory investigation of other systems that might be affected.

c. Other anticonvulsants used to treat bipolar disorder include but are not limited to, Neurontin, Lamictil, Tegretol, Trileptal, and Topomax. These medications have been generally helpful in treating some of the symptoms of bipolar disorder. They have been generally well tolerated, some more than others. They have varying side effects and require different levels of monitoring, but all are currently part of the armentareum used for treatment.

d. Some of the new so-called "atypical" antipsychotic medications are also being used in the treatment of bipolar disorder, especially to treat the acute manic phase. These include Zyprexa, Geodon, Abilify, Risperdal, and Seroquel. These medications also have been well tolerated by patients, but there are some side effects. Although they do not have the risk of tardive dyskensia associated with them that the so-called "typical" antipsychotics possess, there is still a risk of this potentially irreversible movement disorder. Also, each carries a risk of acute extra-pyramidal side effects including acute dystonias, parkinsonism, and akathesia. All have generally been associated with increased appetite and weight gain and possible increase in baseline glucose levels and lipid levels.

V.   Obsessive-Compulsive Disorder (OCD)

Obsessive-compulsive disorder usually responds well to an appropriate medication regimen. In addition to medication treatment, cognitive and behavioral therapies are important. Symptoms of preoccupations and perseveration are not OCD. The rigidity sometimes seen in I/DD individuals, especially those with PDD, and their preoccupations with particular behaviors or items are not OCD. These symptoms tend to have a somewhat different response to medications and require different interventions than classic OCD symptoms (O'Neal, Talga, & Preston, 2002; Rush & Frances, 2000; Schatzberg & Nemeroff, 2004; Stahl, 2000; Varcarolis, 2003).

A. Psychopharmacologic treatment for OCD revolves around the use of medications that affect the serotonergic functions in the brain.

1. Any of the selective serotonergic reuptake inhibitors can be very useful in the treatment of OCD. As noted above, these medications are well tolerated and possess few side effects. Dosages used to treat OCD are sometimes greater than those used for the treatment of depression and other anxiety disorders.

a. These medications include the ones listed under Anxiety Disorders, fluoxetine (Prozac), paroxetine (Paxil), sertraline (Zoloft), fluvoxamine (Luvox), citalopram (Celexa), and escitalopram (Lexapro). As noted above, care should be taken in prescribing these medications related to recent concerns about increased suicidal ideations and/or suicidal behavior in children and adolescents taking these medications.

B. Clomipramine (Anafranil) is a tricyclic antidepressant medication that has a primary serotonergic action in the brain that has been used for many years in the treatment of obsessive-compulsive disorder symptoms.

1. Side effects with clomipramine (Anafranil) include the usual side effects associated with tricyclic antidepressants. These are anticholinergic side effects that include increased appetite and weight gain, dry mouth, and constipation. There are also the same concerns associated with a widening in the QRS complex, as seen on an EKG. Such a widening in the QRS complex, as noted above, can lead to problematic arrhythmias. This medication is also extremely toxic in overdose and can lead to death because of the anticholinergic and cardiac side effects associated with it.

2. Routinely, clomipramine (Anafranil) serum levels should be evaluated periodically. Baseline EKG with routine follow-up EKG should be part of the post-prescription care given with this medication.

C. Other medications are used to treat symptoms associated with OCD. These include other medications that help relieve anxiety. These medications are in the benzodiazepine class and others, in addition to clomipramine, that are in the tricyclic antidepressant class. There are at times severe OCD symptoms that seem to be helped by the addition of antipsychotic medications, in particular the newer atypical antipsychotic medications that have been discussed above.

VI. Perseverations and Preoccupations

Perseveration and preoccupation symptoms are often seen in people with I/DD, in particular, people with PDD. Many times, this group of symptoms can be misdiagnosed as OCD. It can be difficult to differentiate these symptoms from OCD. However, individuals with these symptoms rarely show classic symptoms of OCD, for example, counting, checking, and hand washing (O'Neal, Talga, & Preston, 2002; Rush & Frances, 2000; Schatzberg & Nemeroff, 2004; Stahl, 2000; Varcarolis, 2003).

A. Perseverations and preoccupations generally respond well to medications. Tics are not generally completely alleviated by medications, but with medication in conjunction with behavioral therapy patients can see a significant reduction in these troublesome symptoms. Medications helpful with these symptoms include the selective serotonin reuptake inhibitors and alpha adrenergic agonists. At times, the use of atypical antipsychotics, in particular, Risperdal, can be helpful. Additionally, anxiolytic medications such as benzodiazepines and tricyclic antidepressants may also alleviate the drive associated with pursuing particular perseverations or preoccupations.

VII. Tourette's Disorder

Tourette's disorder is a collection of symptoms associated with chronic vocal and motor tics. Sometimes these tics can be very complex. In addition to the chronic vocal and motor tics, comorbid issues associated with emotional lability and attention/concentration problems can also be present. OCD is also likely to be comorbid in individuals and in families of individuals with Tourette's. Both Tourette's disorder and OCD can be the result of a post-strep infection autoimmune syndrome (O'Neal, Talga, & Preston, 2002; Schatzberg & Nemeroff, 2004; Stahl, 2000; Varcarolis, 2003).

A. Medications that have been used to treat Tourette's disorder include medications that inhibit tic production and also those that decrease anxiety. Of the medications that inhibit tic symptoms, whether vocal or motor, the most effective group of medications is the antipsychotic group. These seem to be helpful because they block dopamine activity in the subcortical structures of the brain that are associated with movement. They are generally quite effective in reducing tics, both vocal and motor, but do have substantial side effects, as have been noted above.

1. A frequently used antipsychotic medication in the treatment of Tourette's is Risperdal. Just as in the treatment of other disorders with antipsychotic medications, care must be taken to monitor for both short-term acute side effects that include extrapyramidal symptoms of parkinsonism, akathisia, and acute dystonias as well as longer-term side effects such as tardive dyskinesia. Additionally, with the chronic use of Risperdal as well as most of the older so-called "typical" antipsychotics, prolactin levels are increased and this can lead to difficulties associated with possible gynecomastia in males, particularly adolescents, and possible lactation and decreased menstruation in females. These atypical antipsychotics, as noted above, are also possibly linked to increased glucose levels in individuals taking the medication and possible increased lipid levels. Other atypical antipsychotics that have been used in the treatment of Tourette's disorder include Geodon, Seroquel, and Zyprexa. The newer atypical antipsychotic Abilify would probably also be useful in decreasing tics in these patients.

2. Older so-called typical antipsychotics such as Pimozide and Haloperidol have also been shown to be very effective in the treatment of Tourette's disorder. These medications decrease disruption secondary to tics, both vocal and motor. Both Haloperidol and Pimozide have substantial side effects. These side effects occur at a somewhat higher rate than the typical antipsychotic group. Neither Haloperidol nor Pimozide have been shown to increase glucose levels or increase lipid levels, but they have been associated with permanent, long-term side effects such as tardive dyskinesia, and at a much higher rate than the atypical antipsychotics. These two older antipsychotics are also much more likely to have problems associated with acute extrapyramidal side effects. At times, adjunctive anticholinergic medications are needed to decrease some of the worrisome acute side effects of movement associated with the older antipsychotics. Such medicines as Cogentin, Vistoril, Artane, and Benadryl have been used.

3. Other medications have also been used with relative success in decreasing tics in patients with Tourette's disorder. They also may have some adjunctive effect in decreasing some of the anxiety associated with Tourette's disorder and in helping with some of the comorbid symptomatology associated with decreased attention and concentration. The medications most often used in this particular category are the alpha adrenergic agonists that are centrally acting. These include Quanfacine and Clonidine. Both of these are essentially antihypertensives, and acting centrally seem to have some effect on the decrease in tic production. Also, by decreasing the overall arousal level, they seem to have a mild anxiolytic effect and seem to increase concentration and attention. Side effects associated with these medications include sleepiness and/or feelings of being tired, both associated with a somnolent effect of the

medications and their ability to decrease blood pressure. Care has to be given to monitor blood pressure to ensure that blood pressure levels do not drop too precipitously. Usually, patients need to be slowly titrated onto these medications and then subsequently slowly titrated off.

4. Other medications that have been useful in decreasing anxiety levels have also been helpful in controlling symptoms associated with Tourette's disorder. These include the anxiolytics that have been noted above, including but not limited to, benzodiazepines, selective serotonin reuptake inhibitors, tricyclic antidepressants, and other more atypical anxiolytics, including BuSpar.

VIII. Self-Injurious Behavior

Self-injurious behavior is a very common problem associated with individuals with I/DD. It seems to be correlated to a degree with more severe I/DD, but certainly can be seen in individuals with I/DD at all levels of cognition. This particular problem can be dangerous to the individual and is significantly distressing to people who live and work with the patient engaged in these behaviors. The behaviors can be as mild as someone slapping their arms or legs relatively lightly to individuals who frequently bang their head either with their fist or against other objects or people. They may actually attempt to damage themselves by gouging at eyes or biting away tissue. Considerable effort has gone into coming up with strategies to decrease self-injurious behavior and, for the most part, behavioral interventions remain the most reliable treatment. However, often these behavioral treatments are quite effectively assisted with the use of appropriate medication. This is especially true if the self-injurious behavior has some other underlying cause beyond some as yet not understood idiopathic difficulty. For example, if the self-injurious behavior is being driven by anxiety, the use of anxiolytics is appropriate. If it has been driven by psychotic symptomatology, then treatment of the psychosis is appropriate. If it is caused by some specific pain or some pain syndrome, then treatment of the pain is appropriate in alleviating the symptoms, and so on (O'Neal, Talga, & Preston, 2002; Schatzberg & Nemeroff, 2004; Stahl, 2000; Varcarolis, 2003).

A. Generally, if no apparent or hypothesized underlying driving factor can be discerned for the self-injurious behavior, use of any and all of the medications that have been listed above have been at times useful in treatment. Antipsychotics, especially atypical antipsychotics, are probably used more often at this point to decrease self-injurious behavior, but also selective serotonin reuptake inhibitors, tricyclic antidepressants, and anxiolytics have been used. Anticonvulsants have also been used in attempts to decrease these troublesome behaviors.

B. There has been considerable attention paid to the potential use of opiate antagonists in the treatment of these symptoms, and some clinicians have reported success with such treatments. Our experience has been that these symptoms are not often affected by the use of these particular medications, which include Naloxone and Naltrexone. The theory behind using such medications has been that the patients engaging in self-injurious behavior perhaps do not fully appreciate the extent of the pain that they are causing and if their natural opiate response is somehow blocked that they will then experience the pain more significantly and subsequently move to extinguish the behavior.

IX. Aggression

Aggression directed toward others in people with I/DD is probably one of the most incapacitating symptoms that clinicians face in the treatment and care of this population. Probably more than any other problem, this behavior symptom alienates and isolates people from participation in the broader society. It also leads to significant morbidity and stress within the family system itself and also hinders the individual with I/DD from being able to participate fully in life and realize their full potential (O'Neal, Talga, & Preston, 2002; Schatzberg & Nemeroff, 2004; Stahl, 2000; Varcarolis, 2003).

A. The gold standard for treating aggressive behavior in individuals with I/DD remains intensive behavioral interventions through applied behavioral analysis. This being said, however, as with self-injurious behavior, aggression is sometimes curbed by the addition of appropriate psychopharmacologic medication. As stated above, with self-injurious behavior, care needs to be given to teasing out any specific or presumed underlying etiologies for the aggression, and these causes need to be treated. This is important with regard to appropriate psychiatric diagnoses associated with aggression, as well as appropriate physical diagnoses associated with the aggression.

1. Medications that are most often used for the treatment of aggression in people with I/DD include antipsychotic medications, selective serotonin reuptake inhibitor medications, tricyclic antidepressant medications, at times stimulant medications, and various other pharmacologic treatments, including blood pressure medications that specifically interact with the adrenergic and noradrenergic systems. Benzodiazepine medications used as both tranquilizers and anxiolytics are also sometimes helpful in decreasing aggression.

2. Antihypertensive medications are sometimes used in the treatment of aggression. These medications include both alpha adrenergic medications and beta adrenergic medications. These include, but are not limited to, medications such as Propanolol, Pinodol, Prazosin, Clonidine, and Quanafacine. It is unclear how these medications may be helpful, but it appears that there is perhaps

some sort of inhibition of the autonomic nervous system so that the ability to become anxious or to become rageful is partially blocked by decreasing the overall autonomic tone in individuals taking these medications. This leads to a decreased likelihood of developing serious rages and/or tantrums. These medications are not as helpful in decreasing some of the out-of-the-blue impulsive aggressive acts that individuals with I/DD may perpetrate from time to time, but do seem to be helpful in decreasing episodes of rage and tantruming as noted above.

X. Psychotic Disorders

Psychotic disorders are difficult to diagnose in people with I/DD, especially people with I/DD who are lower-functioning. However, this being said, individuals with I/DD do suffer from psychotic disorders at a higher rate than individuals in the general population based on clinical experience (O'Neal, Talga, & Preston, 2002; Rush & Frances, 2000; Schatzberg & Nemeroff, 2004; Stahl, 2000; Varcarolis, 2003).

A. Any psychotic medications, both the newer atypical antipsychotic medications and the older typical antipsychotic medications, are the mainstays for treatment of psychosis in any individual, including those with I/DD. The medications that are used in the treatment of psychotic disorders are those that have been mentioned above, including but not limited to Risperdal, Zyprexa, Geodone, Seroquel, Abilify, and the older, more typical antipsychotic medications that include Haldol, Thorazine, Prolixin, Mellaril, Loxitane, and many others. All of these medications, as has been noted above, have substantial side effects associated with them, not the least of which is the possibility of permanent movement difficulty associated with syndromes of tardive dyskinesia.

B. In addition to these antipsychotic medications in the treatment of psychosis in people with I/DD, benzodiazepines can also sometimes be helpful in treating agitation and irritability that exist alongside the psychotic symptomatology in people with I/DD. The use of benzodiazepines such as Ativan, Klonopin, Valium, and so on, can be very helpful in decreasing the morbidity associated with psychotic symptoms. Issues related to dependence and abuse are less of a concern in the population of persons with I/DD, but because these medications can sometimes impair short-term memory, use of them needs to be carefully monitored to make sure that the patient is still able to interact and to learn in a way that enhances their potential.

XI. Summary

The treatment of comorbid psychiatric diagnoses in persons with I/DD is complex. The primary care provider prescribing medications needs to be knowledgeable of current and new psycho-pharmaceutical drugs, including their side effects and interactions with other drugs. Frequent monitoring is necessary.

References

O'Neal, J. H., Talga, M. C., & Preston, J. D. (2002). *Handbook of clinical psycho-pharmacology for therapists* (3rd ed.). Boston: Cambridge University Press.

Rush, A. J., & Frances, A. (Eds.). (2000). Expert consensus guideline series: Treatment of psychiatric and behavioral problems in mental retardation. *American Journal of Mental Retardation, 105,* 159–228.

Schatzberg, A. F., & Nemeroff, C. B. (2004). *The American Psychiatric Publishing textbook of psychopharmacology* (3rd ed.). New York: American Psychiatric Press.

Stahl, S. M. (2000). *Essential psychopharmacology: Neuroscientific basis and practical applications* (2nd ed.). Boston: Cambridge University Press.

Varcarolis, E. M. (2003). *Manual of psychiatric nursing care plans: Diagnoses, clinical tools, and psychopharmacology* (2nd ed.). Philadelphia: W. B. Saunders.

Case Identification and Case Management

Barbara Hanley, BSN, MSW, MPH, PhD

20

Objectives

At the completion of this chapter, the learner will be able to:

1. Identify persons with intellectual and developmental disabilities (I/DD) and those at-risk for I/DD in multiple service settings.
2. Understand how the challenges of individuals with I/DD affect the quality of services provided.
3. Describe the elements of consistent case management for children, adolescents, and adults with I/DD.
4. Discuss case management as a continuing care concept.

Key Points

- Case identification includes a knowledge and skill base that addresses a variety of I/DD that chronically affect life span issues and care services.
- Case management is a life-long activity needed to coordinate care services for a family who has a member identified with an I/DD.

I.   Identification of Individuals at Risk for or Presenting with an I/DD

Nursing and other health professionals serve persons with I/DD in numerous settings. Many of these children, adolescents, and adults may not have been recognized as members of this vulnerable population. Nurses and health professionals need knowledge and skills for early and late case identification as well as case management.

A. Services provided in multiple settings by nurses and health professionals present opportunities to identify previously unnoticed I/DD in childhood, adolescence, and adulthood.

1. Some multiple settings where nursing and health professionals practice include health care centers, mental health centers, criminal justice environments, and geriatric care clinics/long term care facilities.

2. Nurses and health professionals in preschool and school settings, for example, are often the first to be presented with a child who is struggling with academics. Vision, hearing, speech, motor, and/or sensory difficulties may present at this time (see Chapters 9 and 10).

3. Some challenges may have been overlooked earlier in the individual's life or evaluated as being a weakness that would self-correct with maturation and growth.

B. A child who is identified as being at risk for an I/DD needs a comprehensive evaluation.

1. Neonates at increased risk include:

a. CNS abnormalities

b. <32 weeks prematurity

c. <3rd percentile gestational age

d. Dysmorphic features

e. Abnormal chromosomes

f. Ventilation >2 weeks

g. Hypoglycemia

h. Congenital infection

i. Hyperbilirubinemia

j. Associated medical problems (e.g., cardiac) (Batshaw, 2002; Liptak, 1995; Shevell et al., 2003)

2. Sociocultural factors affect development and interact with the biological factors.

3. Child-rearing conditions that support and enrich development can compensate for biologic deficits, except in children with catastrophic conditions.

C. Early treatment can significantly influence the course of diseases associated with I/DD such as:

1. Hearing loss

2. Strabismus

3. Galactosemia

4. Lead intoxication

5. Hypothyroidism

6. PKU

7. Maple syrup urine disease

8. Recurrent otitis media

9. Malnutrition (Batshaw, 2002; Liptak, 1995)

II. Connecting Challenges and Services

A. Obtaining a formal diagnosis depends often on the nurses' and health professionals' observational and diagnostic skills. The ability to assess the degree of a presenting developmental limitation(s) and interpret the significance will impact on the quality of life, health care, and supports needed.

1. The behaviors associated with specific I/DDs are of paramount importance as well.

2. Features of communication patterns, behavioral presentations, and ritualistic routines may initiate the further exploration for autism spectrum disorders (ASD); the knowledge of the early pregnancy history with drug/alcohol use may be related to identify fetal alcohol syndrome (FAS), fetal alcohol effects (FAE), or other outcomes related to chemical abuse.

3. Early identification by the nurse and health professional includes, for infants and toddlers, an ability to identify:

   a. Dysmorphic features

   b. Physical presentations such as hand formations

   c. Bone ages

   d. Subtle as well as overt seizure activity

4. Later identification includes analyzing factors associated with attention deficit hyperactivity disorder (ADHD), attention deficit disorder (ADD), deafness, blindness, orthopedic problems, and learning disabilities (LD).

5. Much later identifications may include co-existing/multiple disabilities such as mental illness and I/DD.

B. Nurses and health professionals participate in multidisciplinary assessments and interdisciplinary conferences that result in family-centered approaches to sharing diagnosis and planning for care management.

1. A team-based approach to planning can begin the response for individualized services.

2.   The team includes the individual with I/DD and his or her family as possible.

C.   Some barriers that interfere with quality of care services include:

    1.   Low-cognition clients

        a.   May not be able to present symptoms and/or history

        b.   May not be able to tolerate waiting room stay

        c.   May be fearful of the physical examination and/or strangers

        d.   May physically confront examiner

        e.   May need family member or friend to assist

    2.   Physically impaired clients

        a.   May be compromised in getting into a required position

        b.   Communication/speech difficulties

        c.   Appearance may misrepresent intellectual abilities

    3.   Attitudes and beliefs of the health care professional

        a.   lack of training to deal with individual who has special difficulties

        b.   Negative biases regarding individuals with I/DD

        c.   Personal discomfort or uneasiness with an individual with I/DD

        d.   Belief that the individual with I/DD will need more demands in time and effort (Doostan & Wilkes, 1999; Lewis, Lewis, Leake, King, & Lindemann, 2002)

III.   Elements in Case Management

A.   Case management is often described as the process that coordinates and integrates the care of the client and his or her family in the community, and which is driven by the client's goals and not the system's goals. Four unique activities as performed by the case manager are:

    1.   Forming a relationship

    2.   Planning for services

    3.   Linking clients with services

    4.   Advocating for service improvements (Anthony, Cohen, Farkas, & Cohen, 2000; Barley, 1989; Hromco, Lyons, & Nikkel, 1997)

B.   "Case management must be seen as a uniquely human response to the client's specific service needs and overall goals. For persons with long-term psychiatric (and I/DD), case management brings to life the human dimension of the human service system(s)" (Anthony et al., 2000, p. 415).

    1.   Strategies and techniques of case management are as varied as the different types of models available to this practice for this population. Some elements identified as paramount in any model are as follows:

  a. Mutuality in decision making between the client, the client's family as available, and the case manager, but person-centered when possible.

  b. The primary responsibility is identification: client, service network, or case management system.

C. The term case management is often referred to as care coordination.

 1. Care coordination occurs when a specified care plan is implemented by a variety of service providers and programs in an organized fashion (American Academy of Pediatrics Committee on Children with Disabilities, 1999).

 2. Care coordination centers on the client's need for:

  a. Treatments

  b. Prevention activities

  c. Promoting developmental activities

  d. Rehabilitation

  e. Prevention of secondary complications

 3. Care coordination reduces the factors contributing to maintaining risk or impairment.

  a. Poor environments

  b. Cultural issues

  c. Eligibility for care services

  d. Accessibility to care services

 4. Care coordination can reduce inpatient care for people with I/DD.

  a. As a group, people with I/DD have increased requirements for health care services.

  b. People with I/DD have increased utilization of inpatient services.

  c. Community-based supports decrease mental health hospitalizations for the I/DD population (Walsh, Kastner, & Criscione, 1997).

D. A model of case coordination was developed in 1901 by Mary Richmond (Weil & Karls, 1985). Other models have been developed over the years for different types of service delivery systems as well as service delivery systems for the I/DD population.

 1. Fifteen service provision roles of case managers have been identified:

  a. *Problem solver*—"Acts on behalf of clients to assist them to function as independently as possible" (Grisham, White, & Miller, 1983, p. 6).

  b. *Advocate*—Represents clients and helps them speak for themselves.

  c. *Diagnostician or assessor*—Analyzes client's situation, needs, and system arrangements that will facilitate or impede service delivery; recommends services and initial plans for care.

  d. *Planner*—Designs case plans, treatment, service integration, and agency collaboration to meet the needs of clients and the service network.

e.   *Community or service organizer*—Develops arrangements to facilitate interagency cooperation and coordination and/or plans for needed services with agencies and citizens.

f.   *Employee and system boundary spanner*—Occupies a specific position to provide service coordination; must move beyond the agency to develop coordination and collaboration with agency members of the service network.

g.   *Service monitor and system modifier*—Keeps track of what goes well and what does not in case management and in the interagency collaboration process. Studies effects on a particular client and on the overall target population and service network. Identification of problems is key to correcting them.

h.   *Recordkeeper*—Documents what happens to clients and to case service coordination, agency interaction, and interagency coordination efforts.

i.   *Evaluator*—Analyzes effectiveness of services for individual clients, for the caseload, and for the service network.

j.   *Consultant*—Analyzes organizational or client problems and develops strategies to solve them.

k.   *Colleague and collaborator*—Develops productive working relationships within the service agency and service network to help accomplish task.

l.   *Service coordinator*—Sees that things work, that client needs and provided services mesh, and that monitoring, feedback, and evaluation take place.

m.   *Counselor or therapist*—Provides support, mental health interventions, and consultation to assist clients in decision making and planning.

n.   *Expeditor*—Secures cooperation, carries out tasks, and analyzes results.

o.   *Cost-container*—Assesses available funds of client, balances needs and funds, and serves as a service negotiator (Leahy, Chan, Shaw, & Lui, 1997; Rapp, 1998; Weil & Karls, 1985).

2.   Thirteen basic tasks of case managers have been identified:

a.   Complete the initial interviews with the client and his or her family to assess the client's eligibility for services.

b.   Gather relevant and useful data from the client, family, other agencies, and so on to formulate a psychosocial assessment of the client and his or her family.

c.   Assemble and guide group discussions and decision-making sessions among relevant professionals and program representative, the client and his or her family, and significant others to formulate goals and design an integrated and comprehensive intervention plan.

d.   Monitor adherence to the plan.

e.   Provide "follow-along" to the client and his or her family to speed identification of unexpected problems in service delivery and to serve as a general troubleshooter on behalf of the client.

f.   Provide counseling and information to help the client and his or her family in situations of crisis and conflict with service providers.

g.   Provide ongoing emotional support to the client and his or her family so they can cope better with problems and utilize professionals and complex services.

h.   Complete the necessary paperwork to maintain documentation of client progress and adherence to the plan by all concerned.

i.   Act as a liaison between the client and his or her family and all relevant professionals, program, and informal resources involved in the overall intervention plan to help the client make his or her preferences known and secure the services needed.

j.   Act as a liaison between programs, providing services to the client to ensure the smooth flow of information and minimize conflict between the subsystems.

k.   Establish and maintain credibility and good public relations with significant formal and informal resource systems to mobilize resources for current and future clients.

l.   Perform effectively and as a "good bureaucrat" within the organization to be in a position to develop and modify policies and procedures affecting clients and the effectiveness of the service delivery system.

m. Secure and maintain the respect and support of those in positions of authority so their influence can be enlisted on behalf of the client and used, when necessary, to encourage other individuals and agencies to participate in the coordination effort (Freedman & Boyer, 2000; Weil & Karls, 1985).

E. Case management/care coordination is complex due to the variety of types of I/DD as well as the increased availability of technology and the recent developments in managed care (Ronder, Kastner, Parker, & Walsh, 1999).

1. Whether case management is practiced by a parent, family member, nurse, or health professional, the avoidance of fragmentation and duplication is essential in order to promote family-based care.

2. The coordination of care is the ideal, resulting in quality community concern, cooperation, and service (American Academy of Pediatrics Committee on Children with Disabilities, 1998).

IV. Case Management as Continuing Care

A. It is an established fact that this population and their families have needs that extend further than the practice of any one discipline or profession.

1. The role of a particular case manager may be short term or span a long period in the lives of families.

2. Even if the individual changes, the care management will extend over the lives of the individuals, especially for:

   a. Periods of transition such as birth to early intervention

   b. School age to middle school

   c. Adolescence to adulthood

   d. Other social and financial changes

3. At different times and in different settings, case management leadership may be the responsibility of the families' public health nurse, other health professionals, a teacher, a grandfather, and so on, depending on the priorities, relationship developments, and skills needed at the time.

B. A case management assessment does not lead to treatment but to the coordination/referral of treatment/services.

   1. Evidence is needed for setting and prioritizing goals.

   2. An ongoing plan for service provision includes assessment of priorities (e.g., getting housing and food precedes enrollment in a social interaction group).

C. There is a special seriousness regarding infants born with specific problems that interfere with development.

   1. The case manager needs to establish supportive relationships with the parents that enhance environments for prevention and intervention related to the effects of risk factors and/or disabling conditions.

   2. Few families are ready for the changes that result from having a child with an I/DD.

   3. The case manager needs to understand the interrelatedness of the biopsychosocial factors that impinge on the goal of helping families adjust to life with a child who has an I/DD (e.g., Down syndrome, cerebral palsy, neurofibromatosis).

D. It is essential that there are mutually agreed upon coping strategies to meet the individual and joint needs of family members.

   1. Learning that takes place in the early childhood years has life-long implications.

   2. Active support from the case manager assists in educating the primary caretakers regarding public laws and rights and the Individualized Family Support Plan, Individualized Education Plan, and Individualized Health (or Habilitation) Plan as appropriate.

E. Other principles that guide case management practice relate to monitoring and coordination.

   1. Monitoring on an ongoing basis to assure the accessibility and continued appropriateness of the identified service.

2. Trouble-shooting, negotiating, and renegotiating are often needed activities in the implementation of the care/service plan.

3. Coordinating professional roles and collaborating can prevent and/or reduce conflicts that can arise in the service delivery system (e.g., two services are only available at the same time on the same day).

4. Expanding of linkages may be needed to other services related to the case management program.

5. Guiding, supporting, and supervising of case managers to enhance their services. Administrators should be knowledgeable regarding guiding principles of case management practice.

F. Continuity of care over the lifespan is identified as assisting with the quality of life available for an individual with an I/DD.

1. The case manager can be called upon to assist with a crisis situation for the client.

2. The case manager must be aware of the five stages that identify a crisis situation and those emotional and behavioral responses that can be associated with each.

3. Crises often emerge as the result of chronic stressful situations. There is usually a precipitating event. The other components or stages are:

    a. A hazardous condition—one or more stressful events prior to the crisis event

    b. A vulnerable state—the subjective reaction to the hazardous condition

    c. An experience of disequilibrium

    d. Coping without success and seeking help

    e. Re-integration—developing new strategies for problem solving (Dixon & Sands, 1983)

    f. It is not unusual that the case manager, who has such an influential and powerful role/relationship with the client and his or her family, is the one called upon to lead the client/family to develop new coping skills and achieve resolution of the issues.

V. Summary

Case management has become important and at times essential, as the health care and service system begins to appreciate the need for lifespan care when an individual has a diagnosis of I/DD. The role of the case manager may be undertaken by a nurse or other health care professional, and it is important that those health care professionals working with individuals with I/DD understand and are able to fulfill this role.

References

American Academy of Pediatrics, Committee on Children with Disabilities. (1998). Managed care and children with special health care needs: A subject review. *Pediatrics, 102,* 657–660.

American Academy of Pediatrics, Committee on Children with Disabilities. (1999). Care coordination: Integrating health and related systems of care for children with special health care needs. *Pediatrics, 104,* 978–981.

Anthony, W. A., Cohen, M., Farkas, M., & Cohen, B. F. (2000). Clinical care update: The chronically mentally ill case management—more than a response to a dysfunctional system. *Community Mental Health Journal, 36,* 99–106.

Bailey, Jr., Donald, B. (1989). Case management in early intervention. *Journal of Early Intervention, 13*(2),120–134.

Batshaw, M. L. (Ed.). (2002). *Children with disabilities* (5th ed.). Baltimore: Paul H. Brookes.

Dixon, S. L., & Sands, R. G. (1983). Identity and the experience of crises. *Social casework: The Journal of Contemporary Social Work, 64,* 223–230.

Doostan, D., & Wilkes, M. (1999). Best practice: Treating the developmentally disabled. *Western Journal of Medicine, 171,* 92–96.

Freedman, R. I., & Boyer, N. C. (2000). The power to choose: Supports for families caring for individuals with developmental disabilities. *Health & Social Work, 25,* 59–68.

Grisham, M., White, M., & Miller, L. S. (1983). Case management as a problem-solving strategy. *Pride Institute Journal of Long-Term Home Health Care, 2*(4), 21–28.

Hanley, B. (1989). *Case management/care coordination for children with special health care needs: Individualized curriculum workbook.* MCH Project #MCJ0092, Columbus, OH: Ohio State University.

Hromco, J. G., Lyons, J. S., & Nikkel, R. E. (1997). Styles of case management: The philosophy and practice of case managers. *Community Mental Health Journal, 33,* 415–428.

Leahy, M., Chan, F., Shaw, L., & Lui, J. (1997). Preparation of rehabilitation counselors for case management practice in health care settings. *Journal of Rehabilitation, 63,* 53–59.

Lewis, M. A., Lewis, C., Leake, B., King, B. H., & Lindemann, R. (2002). The quality of health care for adults with developmental disabilities. *Public Health Reports, 117,* 174–184.

Liptak, G. (1995). The role of the pediatrician in caring for children with developmental disabilities: An overview. *Pediatric Annals, 24,* 233–237.

Mary, N. L. (1998). Social work and the support model of services for people with developmental disabilities. *Journal of Social Work Education, 34*(2), 50–56.

Rapp, C. A. (1998). The active ingredients of effective case management: A research synthesis. *Community Mental Health Journal, 34,* 363–380.

Ronder, R. W., Kastner, T., Parker, S. J., & Walsh, K. (1999). Serving people with developmental disabilities in Medicaid managed care. *Managed Care Quarterly, 7*(2), 23–30.

Shevell, M., Ashwal, S., Donley, D., Flint, J., Gingold, M., & Hirtz, D. (2003). Practice parameter: Evaluation of the child with global developmental delay: Report of the Quality Standards Subcommittee of the American Academy of Neurology and the Practice Committee of the Child Neurology Society. *Neurology, 60,* 367–380.

Walsh, K. K., Kastner, T., & Criscione, T. (1997). Characteristics of hospitalizations for people with developmental disabilities: Utilization, costs, and impact of care coordination. *American Journal of Mental Retardation, 10,* 505–520.

Weil, M., & Karls, T. (1985). *Case management in human service practice: A systematic approach to mobilizing resources for clients.* San Francisco: Jossey-Bass.

Infection, Infectious Disease, and Infection Control

21

Felissa R. Lashley, RN, PhD, FACMG, FAAN

Objectives

At the completion of this chapter, the learner will be able to:

1. Identify factors that influence infectivity or the ability of the microorganism to cause disease.
2. Discuss general categories of microbial agents of infectious diseases.
3. Describe the transmission of infectious disease agents.
4. Discuss specific infectious diseases and their impact on persons with intellectual and developmental disabilities (I/DD).
5. Identify interdisciplinary interventions to prevent spread of infectious diseases, including specific precautions for persons with I/DD.

Key Points

*   There are a variety of factors that influence the development and transmission of infectious disease.
*   Infectious diseases greatly affect morbidity and mortality in all age groups.
*   It is crucial that nurses and other health care professionals know the outcomes of exposure to infectious agents.
*   Pulmonary tuberculosis and viral hepatitis A through C are specific infectious diseases that should be understood by nurses and other health care professionals.
*   The transmission of infectious disease can be prevented or interrupted if several steps are followed.
*   It is important for nurses and other health care professionals to understand isolation precautions.

I.   Introduction

A. Infectious diseases take a considerable toll both on morbidity and mortality. Worldwide, in 2002, of approximately 53 million deaths, about one-third were due to infectious diseases, especially respiratory diseases such as tuberculosis and pneumonia; gastroenteritis, such as diarrheal illnesses; malaria; and human immunodeficiency virus infection causing acquired immune deficiency syndrome.

B. Infectious diseases have become important again in the U.S. for many reasons including re-emergence of various pathogens, identification of new pathogens and new infectious diseases, declining rates of immunization in some areas, antimicrobial resistance, social and behavioral factors, demographic changes, health care advances and invasive techniques, weather events and climate changes, and lack of attention to, and funding of, some public health and preventative measures (Lashley, 2004; Smolinski, Hamburg, & Lederberg, 2003).

II.   Infection Development

For infection to develop, three components are required—a disease-causing agent, usually a microorganism; a susceptible host, which may be human, animal, or plant; and an environment that allows interaction of the host and agent so that transmission is facilitated. Each is discussed below. A source of disease-causing microorganism may be a sick person or animal, an asymptomatic carrier (human or animal), or an inanimate reservoir. A vector may facilitate transfer of the organism from a source or reservoir to a new host.

A. Factors influencing infectivity or the ability of microorganism to cause disease

1. Ability to reach host

2. Virulence factors such as adhesiveness and toxin production

3. Number of organisms needed to cause disease

4. Ability to survive such as by forming spores

5. Ability to replicate in host cells

6. Ability to protect self and overcome host defenses

7. Invasiveness

8. Ease of transmission

9. Antimicrobial resistance

10. Ability to infect new hosts (e.g., jump from animals to humans)

B. Factors influencing host susceptibility

1. Age—infants, children, and the elderly are more susceptible to infections

2. Nutritional status—malnutrition, dehydration, and various vitamin deficiencies can result in immune compromise and greater susceptibility to infection

   3. Immunization status

   4. Presence of other infections or disease states

   5. Immune status and compromise—may be from underlying disease such as cancer, from therapy such as with corticosteroids, or from immunosuppressive therapy due to medical advances such as transplantation

   6. Genetic make-up and innate characteristics of host

   7. Quality, type, and strength of the host response to antimicrobial agents

   8. Type and number of resident microorganisms

   9. Integrity of skin and other barriers

   10. Whether or not other access to body areas occurs, such as through medical devices allowing a portal of entry and providing access for microorganisms to areas they would not ordinarily be able to reach

C. Environmental factors

   1. Cleanliness

   2. Sanitation

   3. Crowding factors

   4. Air exchange and volume

   5. Adequate, appropriately trained staff in a facility for appropriate care and supervision

III. Microbial Agents

A. General categories of microbial agents of infectious diseases and examples of diseases they may cause are:

   1. Bacteria—*Mycobacterium tuberculosis*, tuberculosis; *Campylobacter jejuni*, enteritis

   2. Viruses—Sin Nombre hantavirus, hantavirus pulmonary syndrome; human herpesvirus 7, roseola

   3. Fungi—*Candida albicans*, candidiasis; *Cryptococcal neoformans*, meningitis, and pulmonary disease

   4. Parasites, including protozoa, helminths, and others—*Cryptosporidium parvum*, gastrointestinal illness, especially diarrhea; *Plasmodium vivax*, malaria

   5. Prions—Are believed to be infectious proteins that have an abnormal shape compared to the normal version; cause Creutzfeldt-Jakob disease (Lashley & Durham, 2002)

B. Microbial agents may be divided into categories based on pathogenesis.

   1. Pathogens are microorganisms that can cause disease.

2. Nonpathogens are agents that rarely cause clinical disease in a normal host, and are usually benign. When they cause disease under certain circumstances, such as in an immunocompromised person, they may be known as opportunists.

3. Other agents that are part of the usual body microbial flora are capable of causing disease when they are moved to a different body location, such as when bowel flora may enter the abdominal cavity and cause peritonitis (Goldman & Ausiello, 2004).

IV. Transmission of Infectious Disease Agents

An organism may be transmitted by a single or multiple routes.

A. Transmission by contact

1. Direct or person-to-person including touching, sexual contact, transplacental and perinatal, through contact with blood or body fluids, fecal-oral, or respiratory droplets

2. Direct or animal-to-person including touching

3. Indirect from a reservoir or source via inanimate objects (fomites)

B. Vehicle transmission

1. So-called because various substances are taken into (serve as vehicles into) the body such as foods, water, and air.

2. Foodborne contamination may occur at any stage of the food-handling process including planting, growing, harvesting, processing, transporting, storing, preparing, and handling. Most often occurs in food preparation, often through exposure to contaminated hands of the food handler.

3. Waterborne contamination may occur via ingestion of contaminated drinking water, usually contaminated by sewage, or may occur during recreational activities.

4. Airborne as very small droplets or aerosols or dust particles.

C. Vector-borne transmission

1. Transmission is usually via arthropods, particularly insects that transmit microbes from a source to a vertebrate host. Examples are mosquitoes, which transmit the West Nile virus resulting in West Nile fever, or the deer tick, which transmits *Borrelia burdorferi* resulting in Lyme disease.

V. Possible Outcomes of Exposure to a Microorganism

A. Outcomes after exposure to a microorganism may be

1. No infection

2. Infection that is asymptomatic or subclinical

3.   Infection that is clinically apparent

B.   Persons who contact an infectious disease may develop long- or short-term immunity, no immunity, or may become carriers. An example of a carrier state is in the case of typhoid fever caused by *Salmonella enteritidis* serotype Typhi in which some individuals, such as the infamous Typhoid Mary, become harborers of the organism without having any overt signs of infection, but who may transmit disease organisms to others. One type of carrier is the individual who becomes colonized with an infectious agent. In this case, again the infectious agent is present in the body flora and causes no symptoms in the carrier but can spread the organism to others. People can become colonized with *Staphylococcus* in the nose or on the skin, where the organism has established a niche and may replicate (Goldman & Ausiello, 2004).

VI.   Specific Infectious Diseases

While persons with I/DD may acquire any of the infectious diseases that anyone may come in contact with, several diseases may be seen more often in persons who attend day care or live in group homes, institutions such as nursing homes, or other congregate living facilities. These may include diarrheal diseases; conjunctivitis; scabies; fungal diseases such as athletes foot; respiratory diseases such as influenza, pneumonia, and tuberculosis; as well as viral hepatitis. In any of these, the nurse's and other health care professionals trained and ongoing assessments are vital to appropriate interventions, treatment, and prevention.

Discussed below are tuberculosis and viral hepatitis A, B, and C. Other infectious diseases are discussed elsewhere in this book. Information about other infectious diseases can be found through the Centers for Disease Control and Prevention (CDC) Web site at http://www.cdc.gov, using the search engine for specific information.

A.   Pulmonary tuberculosis (TB)

1.   Etiology—Usually due to *Mycobacterium tuberculosis,* which are rod-shaped nonspore-forming bacilli also known as tubercle bacilli. Must distinguish between infection with *M. tuberculosis* and those who have tuberculosis. Persons may be exposed to *M. tuberculosis* and may or may not develop infection. If they do develop infection, they may or may not go on to develop active tuberculosis in the shorter term or at a future time. Thus, not all exposed to *M. tuberculosis* develop infection, and not all who develop infection develop tuberculosis. Of those who develop infection, 90% do not develop active disease. Of the other 10%, 5% are estimated to develop tuberculosis in under 2 years, and the others will do so sometime in their life. Those who are infected, often called latent TB infection, may experience later re-activation of disease, especially if their immune system is compromised.

2. Epidemiology—In the U.S. about 10 to 15 million persons are estimated to be infected with *M. tuberculosis,* with about 20,000 new cases per year. Worldwide, about one-third of the world's population is latently infected and 8 to 10 million new active cases arise each year. There was a period of higher incidence and prevalence from 1985–1993 in the U.S.

3. Persons at higher risk for exposure to or infection with *M. tuberculosis* include residents and employees of high-risk congregate settings; health care workers with high-risk clients; close contacts of persons with TB; persons born in countries with a high TB incidence or prevalence; high-risk racial or ethnic minority populations defined locally as having an increased prevalence of TB; persons who inject illicit drugs; and infants, children, and adolescents exposed to adults in high risk categories. Persons who are at higher risk to develop actual TB disease once they are infected with *M. tuberculosis* include persons with HIV infection, persons who were infected with *M. tuberculosis* in the past 2 years, persons who have certain medical conditions such as diabetes mellitus, silicosis, immunosuppressive therapy, end stage renal disease, low body weight, intestinal bypass or gastrectomy, cancer of head and neck, certain hematologic diseases, and persons who inject illicit drugs or abuse other substances such as crack cocaine.

4. Transmission and spread—Usually spread from person-to-person through the air after a person with TB coughs, sneezes, sings, or speaks and thus releases aerosolized droplet nuclei with *Mycobacterium tuberculosis* into the air. These droplet nuclei are usually 1–5 microns and can remain suspended in the air for hours. Rarely spread by ingestion of unpasteurized contaminated milk or other fluids or foods or by direct inoculation. Places where air does not circulate well and contained spaces facilitate transmission if a person with active TB is present.

5. Incubation period—Infection may occur 6 to 8 weeks after exposure.

6. Signs and symptoms—For pulmonary TB, clinical presentation is generally insidious with gradual development of vague symptoms, but other onsets may occur such as with flu-like symptoms to start. Common symptoms include fatigue; malaise; anorexia; weight loss; cough, which usually becomes productive and may become bloody; low grade fever, often occuring in the afternoon, which may be intermittent; sweating and/or chills at night; and chest tightness. A tuberculin test may be done as part of diagnosis.

7. Treatment—For active TB without HIV infection or knowledge that the organism is multidrug-resistant, therapy is usually begun with isoniazid, rifampin, pyrazinamide, and ethambutol for 2 months. At that time, a sputum smear and culture are done and, if negative, either isoniazid with rifampin or isoniazid with rifpentine are given to complete a total treatment regimen of 6 months. Other detailed regimens are available for various age groups, characteristics of the disease, microorganism characteristics, and dis-

ease state of the infected person in various combinations. For those with TB infection who are considered at high risk for development of TB disease, a course of preventive pharmacotherapy is often prescribed, often called treatment of latent tuberculosis infection.

8. Prevention—Prevention is multipronged and includes that high-risk persons with TB infection complete preventative therapy or treatment of latent TB infection regimens. Targeted tuberculin testing with PPD is used as part of TB control to detect latent infection in those who are at high risk of developing TB disease. If coughing, the infected person should wear a mask around others, and use one themselves especially with visitors or if being transported. For active TB cases in institutions, a three-tiered system of administrative measures should be instituted, such as recognition and immediate isolation of possible active cases, educational programs, and staff tuberculin skin testing; environmental programs such as effective isolation with negative pressure rooms and the appropriate decontamination or HEPA filtration; and personal respiratory protection and the use of the appropriate airborne isolation procedures for care staff with the appropriate education to use them (Centers for Disease Control and Prevention (CDC), 2000, 2001, 2003; Lashley & Durham, 2002).

B. Acute viral hepatitis

May be caused by at least five distinct viruses: hepatitis A, B, C, D, and E. Others such as the hepatitis G virus and others caused by non-A–E viruses have been implicated in acute hepatitis. Hepatitis B and, to a lesser extent, hepatitis A infection prevalence were associated with duration of residence in a study of hepatitis in a developmental center (Woodruff & Vazquez, 2002). Hepatitis A through C are most important, and are considered below.

1. Hepatitis A

    a. Etiology—Small RNA virus, the hepatitis A virus (HAV) is a picornavirus.

    b. Epidemiology—Has decreased to all-time lows in the U.S., higher in western and southwestern U.S. Highest incidence is in children under 5 years; 5–14 years. There are about 25,000 reported cases in the U.S. each year, but it is believed the actual incidence is about 260,000 cases.

    c. Transmission and spread—Highly contagious. Largely spread through fecal-oral route by direct contact with an infected person or a contaminated object; through ingestion of contaminated food or water, especially when there are poor sanitary conditions; and exposure to contaminated blood or blood products.

    d. Persons at greatest risk—Children, parents, and workers in day care settings; men who have sex with men; persons in institutions; and travelers to developing countries.

    e. Incubation period—15 to 45 days, typically 25–30 days.

f. Signs and symptoms—Nausea, diarrhea, fatigue, abdominal pain, fever, loss of appetite, and possibly myalgia. Jaundice (occurs in about 70% of adults but is less frequent in children), dark colored urine, or light colored stools may follow. Abdominal tenderness and hepatomegaly may be seen. Lasts several weeks, and in about 10% relapse occurs. In children, it is common not to see jaundice and they may be asymptomatic. This is believed to contribute to transmission in multichildren settings.

g. Treatment—Not specific. May use post-exposure prophylaxis with immune globulin for close contacts. Standard isolation precautions are recommended unless client is incontinent or in diapers or is not capable of complying with regimen, in which case contact precautions are recommended.

h. Prevention—Vaccine available and recommended for children 2 years and older in states or areas with high rates of hepatitis A (CDC, 2004a; Fiore, 2004; Goldman & Ausiello, 2004; National Digestive Disease Information Clearinghouse, 2003b).

2. Hepatitis B

a. Etiology—The hepatitis B virus is a DNA virus of the hepadnavirus family.

b. Epidemiology—Endemic in parts of Asia and sub-Saharan Africa. Hepatitis B is the second most common cause of acute hepatitis in the U.S., where there currently are about 75,000 cases per year. There has been a marked decrease in cases in the U.S. since the 1980s, largely attributed to the availability of hepatitis B vaccine for prevention. In the U.S., the highest rate of infection is in those 20–49 years of age.

c. Transmission and spread—Largely spread through parenteral route, exposure to infected blood or blood products (now relatively rare in blood transfusions in developed countries), through sexual contact with an infected person, or vertically from an infected mother to her infant.

d. Persons at greatest risk—Include men who have sex with men, injecting drug users, persons with multiple sex partners, persons with another sexually transmitted disease, infants born to HBV-infected mothers, health care and public safety workers, household contacts of chronically infected persons, hemodialysis patients, and those who work in congregate settings.

e. Incubation period—30–150 days, commonly 75 days.

f. Signs and symptoms—Range from subclinical disease to liver failure. Acute disease may present as a flu-like illness with fever, fatigue, loss of appetite, nausea, vomiting, joint pain, and abdominal pain. Jaundice, dark urine, itchy skin, and light, clay colored stools may develop later. Up to 50% may show no or very mild symptoms. Most infections are self-limited, but in about 5% viremia is persistent. Outcomes include development of a chronic state that can progress to cirrhosis or, in some cases, primary liver cancer. Chronic hepatitis B infection is a common cause of cirrhosis and liver cancer. Some persons develop a chronic carrier state and usually do not show symptoms but are potentially infectious.

g. Treatment—Acute disease is not usually treated unless very severe. Lamivudine is recommended in such cases. Treatment for those who are HBeAg positive (have replicative disease) and chronic hepatitis B are generally treated with interferon-alpha, peginterferon, lamivudine, and/or adefovir alone or in combination therapy. Those who are infected should avoid drinking alcohol. Standard isolation precautions are recommended unless client is incontinent or in diapers or is not capable of complying with regimen, in which case contact precautions are recommended.

h. Prevention—Vaccination against HBV is recommended routinely for newborns and children and for adults at high risk, such as health care workers. Postexposure prohylaxis with hepatitis B immune globulin is recommended followed by vaccination, but in some cases HBV vaccination alone is recommended. Infants born to hepatitis B-infected mothers should receive hepatitis B vaccine within 12 hours after birth. Other prevention includes not sharing personal care items such as razors, nail clippers, or toothbrushes, which may become contaminated with blood; not having unprotected sex; not injecting drugs or sharing drug needles or equipment; and for health care workers, being vaccinated against hepatitis B and following standard precautions using barrier nursing and other applicable methods and appropriately handling needles and other sharps. Pregnant women should be screened for hepatitis B infection (CDC, 2004b; Ganem & Prince, 2004; Goldman & Ausiello, 2004; National Digestive Disease Information Clearinghouse, 2003b).

3. Hepatitis C

a. Etiology—The hepatitis C virus (HCV) is a single-stranded RNA virus in the flavivirus family with various genotypes and subtypes that vary in distribution. Clinical course and treatment response may vary according to the genotype and subtypes present.

b. Epidemiology—Worldwide more than 1 million cases are reported each year. The worldwide prevalence is about 170 million persons. The National Digestive Disease Information Clearinghouse (2003b) indicates that hepatitis C causes about 10,000 deaths annually in the U.S., and accounts for up to 50% of cirrhosis end stage liver disease and liver cancer in the U.S. Most cases in the U.S. occur in those over 25 years of age.

c. Transmission and spread—Largely spread through the parenteral route, exposure to infected blood or blood products (now relatively rare in blood transfusions in developed countries), through sexual contact with an infected person, and vertically from an infected mother to her infant. In about 10% of cases, no source of infection is determined and they are referred to as sporadic.

d. Persons at greatest risk—Include men who have sex with men, injecting drug users, persons with multiple sex partners, persons with another sexually transmitted disease, infants born to HCV-infected mothers (not common), health care and public safety workers, household contacts of chronically infected persons, hemodialysis patients, and those who work in congregate settings. Screening of blood and blood products has reduced the number of cases from transfusion.

e. Incubation period—15–120 days, mean of 50 days.

f. Signs and symptoms—About 60% to 70% may show no symptoms. In others, clinical signs in the acute phase may be fatigue, abdominal tenderness, nausea, poor appetite, and muscle and joint pain. Jaundice may appear later, but anti-HCV may not be detected in the serum until later. A high proportion of persons with acute HCV develop chronic disease, and may also develop extrahepatic manifestations. Chronic disease may involve extrahepatic manifestations.

g. Treatment—In acute hepatitis C, treatment is recommended only if disease does not resolve within 2 to 3 months. In chronic hepatitis C, the recommended regimen is a combination of peginterferon and ribavirin. Therapy is adjusted to genotype of organism and viremia. Standard isolation precautions are recommended.

h. Prevention—No vaccine is currently available. Other prevention includes reducing risk of exposure to HCV; avoiding body piercing and tattooing; not sharing personal care items such as razors, nail clippers, or toothbrushes, which may become contaminated with blood; not having unprotected sex; not injecting drugs or sharing drug needles or equipment; and for health care workers, following standard precautions using barrier nursing and other applicable methods and appropriately handling needles and other sharps (Booth, O'Grady, & Neuberger, 2001; CDC, 2004c; Chou, Clark, & Helfand, 2004; Goldman & Ausiello, 2004; Lashley & Durham, 2002; National Digestive Disease Information Clearinghouse, 2003a, 2003b).

VII. Intervention in Transmission and Development of Infectious Diseases

A. Can be in regard to the microbial agent's transmission, the host, the environment, and/or their interaction. The extent of responsibility for any interventions depends on the job function of the individual nurse and any other health care professional. However if, for example, the nurse observes that a facility kitchen is not clean and trash is not appropriately contained, the nurse should know the steps to take in the organization and follow through to assure compliance.

1. Reduce transmission of the microbial agent

    a. Crowding is known to increase risk for infectious disease transmission, especially airborne or via contact. Limit program participants to the number allowed by state or local laws, and which are appropriate for the level of staffing.

    b. Effective and appropriate handwashing (see IX below) is the single most important way to decrease microorganism transmission between persons or between a person and an object or animal host.

    c. Appropriate use of standard precautions, and other isolation precautions as appropriate.

    d. Using antimicrobial agents appropriately only when needed and assuring adherence with the prescribed regimen to minimize opportunity for the development of antimicrobial-resistant organisms.

2. Modifying environment

    a. Maintain a safe, clean environment following any state, local, or accreditation guidelines using appropriate cleaning agents.

    b. Be sure there are adequate bathroom facilities that are kept clean with appropriate hand cleaning agents and disposable towels available.

    c. All equipment must be in adequate supply, accessible, and in good working order.

    d. Assure adequate fresh air ventilation and indoor air volume.

    e. Be sure room temperatures are in appropriate ranges.

    f. Be sure all spills are cleaned immediately with the appropriate precautions and cleaners.

    g. Ensure that there are not too many program participants for the capacity of the facility.

    h. Ensure adequate numbers of well-educated and trained personnel for the facility.

    i. Be aware that bringing pets into a facility has certain benefits but may be sources for microbial agents, and use appropriate screening, handwashing, and cleanliness techniques.

3. Maximizing host defenses

    a. Provide food that is clean and nutritious.

    b. Observe clients for any signs of impaired nutrition or hydration, and take appropriate action if needed.

    c. Assure that appropriate immunizations and screenings such as tuberculin skin testing are in place for clients and staff.

d. Perform ongoing assessment for any signs or symptoms needing medical attention.

e. Be sure appropriate regular medical and health care is rendered.

f. Follow through with any medications or treatments to appropriate completion, thus minimizing risk for antimicrobial resistance as well as maintaining client's health.

g. Provide additional assistance and appropriate teaching to clients with I/DD in terms of personal hygiene such as not sharing toiletries, health practices such as are appropriate during menstrual cycle and covering mouth when coughing, appropriate responses, and so on (Cohen & Tartasky, 1997; Lashley & Durham, 2002; Roth & Clausen, 1994).

VIII. Patient Isolation Precautions

A. Patient isolation precautions are generally discussed in terms of:

1. Standard precautions

2. Contact precautions

3. Droplet precautions

4. Airborne precautions

B. Standard precautions are used in all care settings routinely for all patients, and replace universal and body substance precautions. In addition, patient care units are usually mainly concerned with contact, droplet, and airborne transmission, although care must be taken to prevent transmission of microorganisms through such common vehicle means as medications, devices, and equipment as well as food and water, as discussed earlier as modes of transmission. All other transmission-based precautions include (are in addition to) standard precautions. Additional isolation precautions are based on a patient's known or suspected infection, what is known about the microorganism causing it, and its route of transmission. In most hospitals in the U.S. vector-borne transmission is not relevant, but there may be vector control issues in other settings that require pest control. In addition, contact between residents or program participants and vectors such as mosquitoes, fleas, or ticks may occur not only within a building but during recreational and other outside activities. Detailed preventive protocols for food-borne, water-borne, recreational water-borne, tick-borne, mosquito-borne, and rodent-borne transmission of infection may be found in Lashley and Durham (2002).

C. Standard precautions

1. Are used for all patient care regardless of diagnosis or infection status. Applies to blood, body fluids, excretions, and secretions regardless of whether they contain visible blood, mucous membranes, and nonintact skin. Presumes that

any person being treated is a potential source of infection. Protect patients from microbes on hands of staff. Precautions for handling needles and disposable sharps may be found through the OSHA Web site at http://www.osha.gov/SLTC/bloodbornepathogens/index.html.

    a. Wear gloves when touching blood, body fluids, secretions, excretions, mucus membranes, nonintact skin, and contaminated items. These provide a protective barrier.

    b. Change gloves after patient contact.

    c. Wash hands before putting on gloves and after gloves are removed.

    d. Wear mask, eye protection, and gown during procedures likely to generate splashes or spray of blood, body fluids, secretions, or excretions.

    e. Handle contaminated patient-care equipment and linen in a manner that prevents the transfer of microorganisms to people or equipment.

    f. Use care when handling sharps and use a mouthpiece or other ventilation device as an alternative to mouth-to-mouth resuscitation when practical.

    g. If the person has a known infection, place the patient in a private room, when feasible, as they may contaminate the environment, especially if they practice poor hygiene, have altered mental status, or are infants/children. If not available, cohort patients infected with the same microorganism after consulting with an infection control expert.

D. Contact precautions—Consist of standard precautions plus contact precautions (indirect and direct). Direct contact transmission includes activities with direct personal contact between a susceptible host and an infected person. Indirect contact involves contact between a susceptible host and a contaminated, usually inanimate, object such as contaminated needles, instruments, or dressing, or contaminated hands that were not properly washed or gloves not changed between patients. An example of use is with acute diarrhea in an incontinent patient.

    1. Use gloves when entering the room. Gloves should cover wrist of gown. Change gloves after contact with infective material. Remove gloves before leaving the room. Wash hands after glove removal. Do not then touch infective material or surface.

    2. Use isolation impenetrable gown when entering the room if contact with patient is anticipated or if the patient has diarrhea, colostomy, or wound drainage that is not covered by a dressing. Remove gown prior to leaving room.

    3. Limit the movement or transport of the patient from the room. Know precautions for transport. Let receivers know of precautions.

    4. Ensure that patient-care items, bedside equipment, and frequently touched surfaces receive daily cleaning.

5. Dedicate use of noncritical patient-care equipment to a single patient, or a cohort of patients with the same pathogen. If not feasible, adequate disinfection between patients is necessary. Dedicated thermometer and B/P apparatus preferred.

E. Airborne precautions—Consist of standard contact precautions plus specifics for airborne precautions. Airborne precautions apply to particles 5μm or smaller in size or dust particles with a microbe such as with TB. Microbes transmitted via this route can be from a host nearby or a distance away. An example is TB.

1. Place the patient in a private room that has monitored negative air pressure in comparison to surrounding air, at least six air changes per hour.

2. Room doors are to be kept closed except for entry and exit.

3. Air is appropriately filtered before it is discharged from the room.

4. Use NIOSH-approved respiratory protection when entering the room, such as N-95 respirator. Limit movement and transport of the patient. Use a mask and other appropriate barriers on the patient if they need to be moved.

F. Droplet precautions—Consist of both standard and contact precautions plus droplet precautions. Droplets are larger than airborne transmission and are usually generated via sneezing or coughing as well as certain procedures. Droplets from source person are transmitted to another person's mouth, conjunctiva, or nasal mucosa. Different from airborne precautions because droplets do not remain suspended in the air. An example of use is with pertussis.

1. Place the patient in a private room that has negative air pressure, at least six air changes per hour.

2. Air is appropriately filtered before it is discharged from the room.

3. Use respiratory protection when entering the room.

4. Limit movement and transport of the patient. Use a mask on the patient if they need to be moved.

5. Use eye protection/shielding.

IX. Handwashing

A. The most important protection against transmission of microbes and disease.

B. Should be used before gloving and after removing gloves.

C. Should occur after touching blood, body fluids, tissues, secretions, excretions, or any contaminated items; between patients; and after procedures on some patients to prevent cross-contamination of different body sites.

D. Wash with soap and water at least 15 seconds when hands are visibly soiled. Follow institutional procedures.

E. Can use alcohol-based rubs to decontaminate hands if not soiled.

F. Fingernails should be short, clean, and free from polish.

G. Artificial nails should be avoided.

H. Rings should not be worn.

I. Watches and bracelets should be removed.

J. For alcohol-based rubs, apply to palm of one hand and rub hand together, covering all surfaces of hands and fingers until hands are dry.

K. Detailed information on handwashing may be found in CDC (2002).

L. Outside the patient-care arena, use handwashing after using the bathroom, after touching any potentially contaminated objects or surfaces such as diapers or contaminated linens, or touching any animals, and before eating or feeding anyone else.

X. Gloves and Glove Use in Infection Control

A. Wear gloves when anticipating contact with patient's blood, body fluids, and tissue.

B. Are not a substitute for appropriate hygiene.

C. Do not need to be sterile unless procedure requires it.

D. Should be appropriate for hand size.

E. Material may be latex, vinyl, or surgical, but thin. May need to consider latex allergies and not use latex gloves.

F. Must be long enough to reach above the wrist (4–6 inches from wrist along arm) and overlap cuff of gown.

G. Change gloves between procedures with the same patient after contact with material or tissue that may contain a high number of microbes.

H. Remove gloves immediately after use and before caring for another patient.

I. Wash hands before and after gloves are removed.

J. Use care in removing gloves if soiled so as not to contaminate hands or environment.

K. Single use gloves should *not* be washed or reused.

L. Glove selection is task-appropriate.

XI. Preventing Infectious Diseases Among the Intellectually or Developmentally Disabled

The same basic principles of infectious disease prevention are operational for those with I/DD as for those without. However, for reasons detailed above, particular emphasis should be put in various areas.

A. Physical capability limitations, either by a congenital anomaly associated with a genetic or nongenetic condition or by limitations due to some type of impairment from other causes such as lack of mobility; incontinence; or susceptibility to illness due to a particular I/DD, such as in the case of disorders that result in impairment of airway clearance due to muscular weakness or poor pulmonary reserve due to chest wall or spinal deformities may result in increased susceptibility to and mortality from respiratory infections.

B. Feeding problems may lead to aspiration and pneumonia, and poor neuromuscular function may lead to ineffective cough, which can result in lung problems.

C. Cognitive conditions or limitations that relate to judgment, ability to understand instructions, impaired decision making, patterns of behavior such as lack of assertiveness, and ability to be manipulated or persuaded can all contribute to the acquisition or transmission of infectious agents. An example would be vulnerability to sexual contact with someone who may transmit a sexually transmitted disease.

D. Clients who have impaired bowel or bladder function or control may be sources of or at risk for acquiring microorganisms spread by the fecal-oral route. This might also be true of a person who does not understand the need to wash hands after toileting or before eating, or who does not remember to do so without reminders.

E. Particular health risks and susceptibilities may also be associated with a particular condition such as cystic fibrosis and susceptibility to *Burkholderia cepacia*, or immunodeficiencies that are from genetic conditions.

F. Those who have I/DD may also have difficulty in obtaining appropriate, ongoing health care provided by knowledgeable and caring providers. (Lashley, in press; Roth & Clausen, 1994; Toder, 2000).

XII. Summary

Nurses and other health care professionals have consistently been educated on infectious diseases and their care and prevention. Today there are many emerging infections, as well as known infections, that threaten the public. It is vital that health care professionals caring for persons with I/DD know and practice this information because persons with I/DD may be more vulnerable to these infectious diseases.

References

Booth, J. C. L., O'Grady, J., & Neuberger, J. on behalf of the Royal College of Physicians of London and the British Society of Gastroenterology. (2001). Clinical guidelines on the management of hepatitis C. *Gut, 49*(Suppl 1), i1–i21.

Centers for Disease Control and Prevention (CDC). (2003). American Thoracic Society, CDC, and Infectious Disease Society of America. Treatment of tuberculosis. *Morbidity and Mortality Weekly Report, 52*(RR-11), 1–77.

Centers for Disease Control and Prevention (CDC). (2001). *Core curriculum on tuberculosis. Division of TB Elimination.* Retrieved June 6, 2004 from http://www.cdc.gov/nchstp/tb/pubs/corecurr/default.htm

Centers for Disease Control and Prevention (CDC). (2002). Guidelines for hand hygiene in healthcare settings. *Morbidity and Mortality Weekly Report, 51*(RR-16), 1–44.

Centers for Disease Control and Prevention (CDC). (2000). Targeted tuberculin testing and treatment of latent tuberculosis infection. *Morbidity and Mortality Weekly Report, 49* (RR-6), 1–54.

Centers for Disease Control and Prevention (CDC). (2004a). *Viral hepatitis A. Fact Sheet.*

Centers for Disease Control and Prevention (CDC). (2004b). *Viral hepatitis B. Fact Sheet.*

Centers for Disease Control and Prevention (CDC). (2004c). *Viral hepatitis C. Fact Sheet.*

Chou R., Clark, E., & Helfand, M. (2004). Screening for hepatitis C virus infection: A review of the evidence for the U.S. Preventive Services Task Force. *Annals of Internal Medicine, 140,* 465–479.

Cohen, F. L., & Tartasky, D. (1997). Microbial resistance to drug therapy: A review. *American Journal of Infection Control, 25,* 51–64.

Fiore, A. E. (2004). Hepatitis A transmitted by food. *Clinical Infectious Diseases, 38,* 705–715.

Ganem, D., & Prince, A. M. (2004). Mechanisms of disease: Hepatitis B virus infection—natural history and clinical consequences. *New England Journal of Medicine, 350,* 1118–1129.

Goldman, L., & Ausiello, D. (Eds.). (2004). *Cecil textbook of medicine* (22nd ed.). Philadelphia: WB Saunders.

Lashley, F. R. (2004). Emerging infectious diseases: Vulnerabilities, contributing factors, and approaches. *Expert Review of Anti-infective Therapy, 2,* 299–316.

Lashley, F. R. (in press). *Clinical genetics in nursing practice* (3rd ed.). New York: Springer.

Lashley, F. R., & Durham, J. D. (Eds.). (2002). *Emerging infectious diseases: Trends and issues.* New York: Springer.

National Digestive Disease Information Clearinghouse, National Institute of Diabetes, Digestive & Kidney Diseases. (2003a). *Chronic hepatitis C: Current disease management.* NIH publication No. 03-4230.

National Digestive Disease Information Clearinghouse, National Institute of Diabetes, Digestive & Kidney Diseases. (2003b). *Viral hepatitis: A through E and beyond.* NIH publication No. 03-4762.

Roth, S., & Clausen, P. W. (1994). The role of the nurse in infection control. In S. P. Roth & J. S. Morse (Eds.). *A life span approach to nursing care for individuals with developmental disabilities* (pp. 305–349). Baltimore: Paul H. Brookes.

Smolinski M. S., Hamburg M. A., & Lederberg J. (Eds.). (2003). *Microbial threats to health: Emergence, detection, and response.* Washington, DC: Institute of Medicine, National Academy Press.

Toder, D. S. (2000). Respiratory problems in the adolescent with developmental delay. *Adolescent Medicine, 11,* 617–631.

Woodruff, B. A., & Vazquez, E. (2002). Prevalence of hepatitis virus infections in an institution for persons with developmental disabilities. *American Journal of Mental Retardation, 107,* 278–292.

Quality of Life and Outcomes Management

22

Robert L. Schalock, PhD

Objectives

At the completion of this chapter, the learner will be able to:

1. Identify the three uses of the concept of quality of life.

2. Understand the multidimensional nature (that is, core domains and indicators) of the quality-of-life construct.

3. Understand the importance of using multiple methods (that is, methodological pluralism) in the assessment of one's quality of life.

4. Use quality enhancement techniques related to (a) providing personalized supports in each quality-of-life domain, and (b) implementing caregiver guidelines to enhance individual quality-of-life domains.

5. Measure quality-of-life-related outcomes and manage for results.

Key Points

- There is currently an increased concern for the social and psychological dynamics of perceived well-being, including factors related to social support, social integration, interpersonal trust, internal control, autonomy/independence, self-confidence, aspirations/expectations, and values having to do with family, job, and life in general.

- Disability and change associated with impairments are conditions that affect people's ability to make self-determined choices and live life to the fullest. For individuals with intellectual and developmental disabilities (I/DD), living an ordinary life requires support beyond that normally needed by others at a similar age and stage of life. Such support may include a variety of forms such as specialized training, guidance, structured opportunities, or specially designed environmental or social arrangements. Providing these forms of

Key Points *(continued)*

support has been a major function of education, health, and human service programs. In this process, the concept of quality of life has become increasingly central in developing programmatic policies and practices as well as evaluating the impact that programs have on the lifestyles of their users.

• Individuals with I/DD often experience problems concerning participation in society, which means that such persons and their families are in danger of being excluded from many situations and opportunities that normally are available to others. The concept of quality of life is beginning to impact social policy and serve as the conceptual basis for developing environments that allow access to people, places, and resources for all persons.

I. Historical Context and Current Use

A. Over the past two decades, the concept of quality of life has increasingly been applied to persons with I/DD (Brown & Brown, 2003; Felce, 2000; Goode, 1994; Keith, 2001; Schalock & Bonham, 2003; Schalock, Bonham, & Marchand, 2000).

B. Historically, the interest in quality of life has come from four sources (Schalock & Verdugo, 2002):

1. A shift in focus away from the belief that scientific, medical, and technological advances alone would result in improved life, towards an understanding that personal, family, community, and societal well-being emerge from complex combinations of these advances plus values, perceptions, and environmental conditions

2. The next logical step from the normalization movement that stressed community-based services to measuring the outcomes from the individual's life in the community

3. The rise of consumer empowerment and patients' rights movements and their emphasis on person-centered planning, personal outcomes, and self-determination

4. The emergence of sociological changes that introduced the subjective or perceptual aspects of quality of life and the individual and personal characteristics involved

C. Currently, the quality-of-life concept is being used as a:

1. *Sensitizing notion* that gives us a sense of reference and guidance from the individual's perspective, focusing on the person and the individual's environment

2. *Unifying theme* that is providing a framework for conceptualizing, measuring, and applying the quality of life construct

3. *Social construct* that is being used as an overriding principle to enhance an individual's well-being and to collaborate for programmatic, community, and societal change

II. Quality-of-Life Domains

A. The term *quality-of-life domains* refers to the set of factors composing personal well-being.

B. A recent analysis (Schalock, 2004a) of the literature on individual-referenced quality-of-life domains found considerable agreement regarding these domains. The 16 published articles analyzed yielded a total of 125 indicators. The vast majority (74.4%) of these indicators related to eight core quality-of-life domains: interpersonal relations, social inclusion, personal development, physical well-being, self-determination, material well-being, emotional well-being, and rights. The number of times each of these domains was listed in the 16 published articles is summarized in Table 22.1, along with a listing of the other individual-referenced quality-of-life domains.

C. Core quality-of-life indicators are quality-of-life domain-specific perceptions, behaviors, or conditions that give an indication of the person's well-being. These indicators, which are listed in Table 22.2, are currently being operationalized and used in quality-of-life measurement and application.

III. Methodological Pluralism or Using Multiple Methods in the Study of Quality of Life

A. There is a need to incorporate the systems perspective (Bronfenbrenner, 1979) into the conceptualization, measurement, and application of the concept of quality of life because people live in a number of systems (micro, meso, macro) that influence the development of their values, beliefs, and attitudes. The major parameters of this methodological pluralism approach applied to quality-of-life measurement are summarized in Table 22.3.

B. An analysis of the international quality-of-life literature (Schalock & Verdugo, 2002) indicates clearly four quite different uses for quality indicators (sometimes referred to as performance measures): personal reactions, research, program evaluation, and decision making.

1. Two important points regarding quality indicators:

    a. As one employs quality indicators for the purposes of program evaluation and decision making, the use of objective quality-of-life measures is essential.

Table 22.1 Quality Indicators: Content Analysis of Individual-Referenced Domains	
DOMAIN	**NUMBER OF TIMES REFERENCED (IN 16 REFERENCES)**
Interpersonal Relations	15
Social Inclusion	14
Personal Development	13
Physical Well-Being	13
Self-Determination	12
Material Well-Being	12
Emotional Well-Being	8
Rights	6
Environment (home/residence/living situation)	6
Family	5
Recreation and Leisure	5
Safety/Security	4
Satisfaction	3
Dignity and Respect	2
Spiritual	2
Neighborhood	2
Services and Supports	1
Practical Being	1
Civic Responsibility	1

Based on individual-referenced domains published by: Andrews & Withey (1976), Bonham et al. (2004), Campbell (1981), Cummins (1997), Felce & Perry (1996), Ferdinand & Smith (2000), Flanagan (1982), Gardner & Nudler (1997), Gettings & Bradley (1997), Hughes, Hwang, Kim, Eisenman, & Killian (1995), Karon & Bernard (2002), Lehman, Postrado, & Rachuba (1993), Parmenter (2001), Renwick, Brown, & Raphael (2000), Schalock (1996), Schalock & Keith (1993), The World Health Organization Quality of Life Group (1995).

b. One should keep in mind the following criteria for selecting particular indicators (Karon & Bernard, 2002):

   i.   Indicator has strategic importance for maximizing well-being.

   ii. Indicator measurement is expected to show variation and/or potential for improvement.

   iii. Indicator is useful for improving outcomes.

   iv. Indicator can be affected by actions taken by the provider organization and staff.

   v.   Indicator measure is meaningful and interpretable.

   vi. Data collection is feasible with reasonable efforts.

Table 22.2   Core Indicators and Descriptors per Core Quality-of-Life Domain

QOL Core Domain	Indicators and Descriptors
Emotional Well-Being	Contentment (satisfaction, moods, enjoyment)
	Self-Concept (identity, self-worth, self-esteem)
	Lack of Stress (predictability and control)
Interpersonal Relations	Interactions (social networks, social contacts)
	Relationships (family, friends, peers)
	Supports (emotional, physical, financial, feedback)
Material Well-Being	Financial Status (income, benefits)
	Employment (work status, work environment)
	Housing (type of residence, ownership)
Personal Development	Education (achievements, status)
	Personal Competence (cognitive, social, practical)
	Performance (success, achievement, productivity)
Physical Well-Being	Health (functioning, symptoms, fitness, nutrition)
	Activities of Daily Living (self-care skills, mobility)
	Leisure (recreation, hobbies)
Self-Determination	Autonomy/Personal Control (independence)
	Goals and Personal Values (desires, expectations)
	Choices (opportunities, options, preferences)
Social Inclusion	Community Integration and Participation
	Community Roles (contributor, volunteer)
	Social Supports (support network, services)
Rights	Human (respect, dignity, equality)
	Legal (citizenship, access, due process)

vii.   Costs of data collection are justified by the expected improvements in service and outcomes.

viii. Indicator is sensitive to cultural and linguistic differences.

ix.   Indicator is applicable across populations and programs.

x.   Indicator is based on sound theory or concepts as determined by consensus in the I/DD field.

C.   Four guidelines for the use of methodological pluralism in quality of life research:

1.   Satisfaction is a trait-like entity that correlates little with objective indicators, is not predicted by personal characteristics such as adaptive behavior levels,

Table 22.3 Methodological Pluralism Applied to Quality-of-Life Measurement		
Systems Level	**Measurement Focus**	**Measurement Strategies**
Microsystem	Subjective nature of QOL ("Personal appraisal")	Satisfaction survey Happiness measures
Mesosystem	Objective nature of QOL ("Functional assessment")	Rating scales (level of functioning) Participant observation Questionnaires (external events and circumstances) Engagement in everyday activities Self-determination and personal control Role status (education, employment, living)
Macrosystem	External conditions ("Social indicators")	Standard of living Employment rates Literacy rates Mortality rates Life expectancy

is not predicted by environmental characteristics, and produces scores around the expected 70–75% mark (Cummins, 1998).

2. One needs to be careful considering empirical results related to quality of life to distinguish whether the assessment methods measure subjective well-being or objective life circumstances and experiences.

3. If one wants to determine whether people with I/DD are as satisfied with life as other population subgroups, then assess subjective well-being and compare.

4. If one wants to evaluate environmental design or service programs in a sensitive way, one should use objective indicators of personal experience and circumstances (Schalock & Felce, 2004).

IV. Quality Enhancement Techniques

A. Personalized supports—The supports paradigm is widely recognized as an effective way to enhance one's quality of life (Schalock, 2004b). Supports are defined as resources and strategies that aim to promote the development, education, interests, and personal well-being of a person and that enhance individual functioning. Services are one type of support provided by professionals and agencies (Luckasson et al., 2002). Support functions aggregated by quality-of-life core domains are presented in Table 22.4.

Table 22.4   Support Functions Aggregated by Quality-of-Life Core Domain

QUALITY-OF-LIFE DOMAIN	SUPPORT FUNCTIONS
Emotional Well-Being	Emotional support, support groups, counseling, mental health or substance abuse counseling, treatment
Interpersonal Relations	Friendships, development of networking skills, socializing, promotion of peer support groups, communication aids
Material Well-Being	Income support, assistance with money management, access to financial assistance, adjustment of work benefits, job creation
Personal Development	Compensatory strategies (e.g., memory aids), problem-solving strategies, adaptive behavior, self-management, transportation training strategies
Physical Well-Being	Provision of home health care, therapy-related activities, medical intervention, transfer and mobility, emergency procedures
Self-Determination	Incorporating personal preferences into daily activities, instructing in decision making, making choices and taking initiatives, developing self-advocacy skills, social inclusion, identifying supports in the environment
Rights	Protection and legal assistance, advocating for person

B. Caregiver guidelines—A person's quality of life cannot be separated from the care provided or the people (for example, family members and nurses) providing the care. Thus, it is important to consider a number of quality-of-life-related techniques that families can use to enhance the recipient's subjective well-being and quality of life. Guidelines for these techniques, aggregated by core quality-of-life domains, are presented in Table 22.5.

V.   Outcomes Management

A. Outcomes management needs to be based on a program-evaluation model and measurement methods that clearly delineate organization and individual-referenced outcomes that reflect performance and value standards, and that meet the dual requirements of increased accountability and continuous program improvement. Key aspects of such a model are presented in Table 22.6 (Schalock & Bonham, 2003).

B. Outcomes management also requires a program-logic model that helps program managers see the relationship among inputs (for example, resources), program processes, program outputs, and short- and long-term outcomes, along with the key roles played by formative feedback and contextual variables in managing for results (Schalock, 2001).

Table 22.5 Quality-of-Life-Related Caregiver Guidelines	
QUALITY-OF-LIFE DOMAIN	**CAREGIVER GUIDELINES**
Emotional Well-Being	Freedom from fear, harm, injury, neglect, or hurt
	Opportunity to act on or pursue personal beliefs
	Positive feedback about capabilities
	Freedom from worry involving aspects of family, friends, where to live, financial situation
Interpersonal Relations	Involvement and relationships with family members
	Involvement and relations with friends and acquaintances
	Involvement and relationships with those providing organized activities such as church and recreation
Material Well-Being	Money with which to buy things and do activities
	Availability and use of furniture, pictures, radio, and similar preferred items
Personal Development	Opportunities for developing new skills
	Opportunities to engage in arts, crafts, and other personal enhancing activities
Physical Well-Being	Allowing person to eat, dress, bathe, walk, and care for self
	Receipt of appropriate health care
	Nutritional well-being
	Proper medication dosages
	Opportunities for physical activity and exercise
Self-Determination	Freedom to make choices or decisions about daily activities
	Freedom to make choices or decisions about preferred food and clothing
	Opportunities to express personal opinions and values
	Opportunities to achieve personal goals
Social Inclusion	Being liked and accepted by cohabitants and having cohabitants involved with person's activities
	Being liked and accepted by caregiver(s); having caregiver(s) involved in activities and conversations
	Receiving help and support from cohabitants or caregivers
Rights	Respect for person's privacy
	Opportunities to give input regarding rules or schedules
	Opportunities to own things
	Opportunities to receive legal aid or advocacy assistance
	Protection from negative or potentially harmful events or situations

Table 22.6 Key Aspects of Program Evaluation Model

ASPECT	OUTCOMES	PREFERRED MEASUREMENT METHODS
Organization Performance ("program process")	Health and safety, financial stability, staff development, and organization efficiency	Performance assessment measures that include performance planning and reporting, licensure requirements, staff certification, performance indicators (such as critical performance indicators or report cards), and financial accountability measures (such as financial audit)
Organization Value ("organization outcomes")	Access to services, consumer satisfaction, staff competencies, family/consumer supports, wrap-around services, and community support	Consumer appraisal measures that include consumer satisfaction surveys, measures reflecting fidelity to service delivery model, benchmarks, and standards of excellence
Individual Performance ("program outputs")	Physical and mental health, functional status (activities of daily living and instrumental activities of daily living), financial well-being, residential status, and educational development	Functional assessment measures that include rating scales, observation, objective behavioral measures, and status indicators (such as education, living, and employment)
Individual Value ("individual outcomes")	Self-determination, social inclusion, social relationships, friendships, rights and personal dignity, and personal development	Personal appraisal methods that include quality of life evaluations, personal interviews, surveys, or focus groups

C. Outcomes management also requires a mechanism to manage for results that includes feedback to the consumer and service provider(s), a quality improvement process, and performance standards (Dewa, Horgan, Russell, & Keates, 2001).

VI. Summary Statements

A. The last two decades have seen considerable progress in understanding the significant role that the concept of quality of life has played in the lives of individuals with I/DD and the systems that interact with those lives. Indeed, the concept has extended beyond the person and has now influenced an entire service delivery system because of its power as a sensitizing notion, unifying theme, and social construct.

B. At its core, the concept of quality of life gives us a sense of reference and guidance from the individual's perspective, an overriding principle to enhance an individual's well-being and collaborate for change, and a common language and systematic framework to guide our current and future endeavors (Schalock et al., 2002).

C. It is important to point out that the concept of quality of life is still emerging in the field of I/DD, and that currently there is still considerable debate about its application and impact. There are at least three contextual issues around which this debate is occurring: economic rationalism and the allocation of resources to people with I/DD; the disability reform movement, including the rapid emergence of the self-advocacy movement; and which outcomes best provide evidence that services and supports provided to people with I/DD have indeed enhanced personal well-being (Rapley, 2000; Reinders, 2002).

VII. Questions to Consider

A. What examples have you seen lately regarding the three uses of the quality-of-life concept: sensitizing notion, unifying theme, and social construct?

B. Although the eight core domains are universal, their relative value differs across people, the life span, and cultures. Rank order (#1 = most important) these eight core domains (see Table 22.2) for yourself and one or more clients with whom you are working (their ranking should be based on *their* input). How do these ranks differ and what does that difference say about the concept of quality of life?

C. For each core domain (see Table 22.2) give an example of a subjective indicator and an objective indicator. Subjective indicators are frequently expressed as the person's level of satisfaction; objective indicators are personal experiences and circumstances. What do these different examples suggest in regard to the measurement of one's quality of life?

D. Develop an individualized supports plan for two of your clients, focusing on appropriate supports for each of the eight core quality-of-life domains (see Table 22.4). What do the differences in these two support plans suggest about using personalized supports to enhance a life of quality?

E. Discuss the concept of "caregiver supports" (see Table 22.5) with one or more of the families with whom you are working. How do they respond to the concept of caregiver supports and the guidelines presented in Table 22.5? What do they need to implement them?

F. What outcomes (see Table 22.6) might you measure or evaluate given your current position and clientele? How would you measure them and what strategies would you employ to use the resulting information to enhance the individual's personal well-being, or focus the organization with whom you are working to increase their efforts at measuring outcomes and managing for results?

G. Summarize the five key ideas you have gained from reading this chapter. How do these ideas reflect changes in what you thought previously about the concept of quality-of-life?

VIII. Summary

Each individual has a right to have and experience their optimum quality of life. In this chapter, methods for assessing, implementing, intervening, and evaluating quality of life in persons with I/DD have been explored.

References

Andrews, F. M., & Withey, S. B. (1976). *Social indicators of well-being.* New York: Plenum Press.

Bonham, G. S., Basehart, S., Schalock, R. L., Marchand, C. G., Kirchner, N., & Rumenap, J. M. (2004). Consumer based quality of life assessment: The Maryland Ask Me! Project. *Mental Retardation, 42,* 338–355.

Bronfenbrenner, U. (1979). *The ecology of human development.* Cambridge, MA: Harvard University Press.

Brown, I., & Brown, R. I. (2003). *Quality of life and disability: An approach for community practitioners.* London: Jessica Kingsley.

Campbell, A. (1981). *The sense of well-being in America: Recent patterns and trends.* New York: McGraw-Hill.

Cummins, R. A. (1997). Assessing quality of life. In R. I. Brown (Ed.). *Assessing quality of life for people with disabilities: Models, research, and practice* (pp. 116–150). London: Stanley Thornes.

Cummins, R. A. (1998). The second approximation to an international standard for life satisfaction. *Social Indicators Research, 43,* 307–334.

Dewa, C. S., Horgan, S., Russell M., & Keates, J. (2001). What? Another form? The process of measuring and comparing service utilization in a community mental health program model. *Evaluation and Program Planning, 24,* 239–247.

Felce, D. (2000). Engagement in activity as an indicator of quality of life in British research. In K. D. Keith & R. L. Schalock (Eds.). *Cross-cultural perspectives on quality of life* (pp. 173–190). Washington, DC: American Association on Mental Retardation.

Felce, D., & Perry, J. (1996). Assessment of quality of life. In R. L. Schalock (Ed.), *Quality of life: Volume I: Conceptualization and measurement* (pp. 63–73). Washington, DC: American Association on Mental Retardation.

Ferdinand, R., & Smith, M. A. (2000). *2000 Nebraska developmental disabilities provider profiles.* Lincoln, NE: The ARC of Nebraska.

Flanagan, J. C. (1982). Measurement of quality of life: Current state of the art. *Archives of Physical Medicine and Rehabilitation, 63,* 56–59.

Gardner, J. F., & Nudler, S. (1997). Beyond compliance to responsiveness: Accreditation reconsidered. In R. L. Schalock (Ed.). *Quality of life: Vol. II: Application to persons with disabilities* (pp. 135–148). Washington, DC: American Association on Mental Retardation.

Gettings, R. M., & Bradley, V. J. (1997). *Core indicators project.* Alexandria, VA: National Association of State Directors of Developmental Disabilities Services.

Goode, D. A. (Ed.). (1994). *Quality of life for persons with disabilities: International perspectives and issues.* Boston: Brookline Books.

Hughes, C., Hwang, B., Kim, J., Eisenman, L. T., & Killian, D. J. (1995). Quality of life in applied research: A review and analysis of empirical measures. *American Journal on Mental Retardation, 99,* 623–641.

Karon, S. L., & Bernard, S. (2002). *Development of operational definitions of quality indicators for Medicaid services to people with developmental disabilities.* Submitted to Centers for Medicare and Medicaid Services, January 1, 2002.

Keith, K. D. (2001). International quality of life: Current conceptual, measurement, and implementation issues. *International Review of Research in Mental Retardation, 24*, 49–74.

Lehman, A., Postrado, I., & Rachuba, L. (1993). Convergent validation of quality-of-life assessments for persons with severe mental illness. *Quality of Life Research, 2*, 327–333.

Luckasson, R., Borthwick-Duffy, S., Buntinx, W. H. E., Coulter, D. L., Craig, E. M., Reeve, A., et al. (2002). *Mental retardation: Definition, classification, and systems of supports* (10th ed.). Washington, DC: American Association on Mental Retardation.

Parmenter, T. (2001). The contribution of science in facilitating the inclusion of people with intellectual disability into the community. *Journal of Intellectual Disability Research, 45*, 183–193.

Rapley, M. (2000). The social construction of quality of life: The interpersonal production of well-being revisited. In K. D. Keith & R. L. Schalock (Eds.), *Cross-cultural perspectives on quality of life* (pp. 155–172). Washington, DC: American Association on Mental Retardation.

Reinders, J. S. (2002). The good life for citizens with intellectual disability. *Journal of Intellectual Disability Research, 46*(1), 1–5.

Renwick, R., Brown, I., & Raphael, D. (2000). Person-centered quality of life: Contributions from Canada to an international understanding. In K. D. Keith & R. L. Schalock (Eds.), *Cross-cultural perspectives on quality of life* (pp. 5–22). Washington, DC: American Association on Mental Retardation.

Schalock, R. L. (2001). *Outcome-based evaluation* (2nd ed.). New York: Kluwer Academic/Plenum.

Schalock, R. L. (1996). Reconsidering the conceptualization and measurement of quality of life. In R. L. Schalock (Ed.). *Quality of life: Vol. I: Conceptualization and measurement* (pp. 123–139). Washington, DC: American Association on Mental Retardation.

Schalock, R. L. (2004a). The concept of quality of life: What we know and do not know. *Journal of Intellectual Disability Research, 48*, 203–216.

Schalock, R. L. (2004b). The emerging disability paradigm and its challenges to the field. *Journal of Disability Policy Studies, 14*, 204–215.

Schalock, R. L., & Bonham, G. S. (2003). Measuring outcomes and managing for results. *Evaluation and Program Planning, 26*, 229–235.

Schalock, R. L., Bonham, G. S., & Marchand, C. B. (2000). Consumer based quality of life assessment: A path model of perceived satisfaction. *Evaluation and Program Planning, 23*(1), 77–88.

Schalock, R. L., Brown, I., Brown, R., Cummins, R. A., Felce, D., Matikka, L., et al. (2002). Conceptualization, measurement, and application of quality of life for persons with intellectual disabilities: Results of an international panel of experts. *Mental Retardation, 40*, 457–470.

Schalock, R. L., & Felce, D. (2004). Quality of life and subjective well-being: Conceptual and measurement issues. In E. Emerson, T. Thompson, T. Parmenter, & C. Hatton (Eds.), *International handbook of methods for research and evaluation in intellectual disabilities*. New York: Wiley.

Schalock, R. L., & Keith, K. D. (1993). *Quality of life questionnaire*. Worthington, OH: IDS.

Schalock, R. L., & Verdugo, M. (2002). *Handbook on quality of life for human service practitioners*. Washington, DC: American Association on Mental Retardation.

The World Health Organization Quality of Life Group. (1995). The World Health Organization Quality of Life Assessment (WHOQOL): Position paper from the World Health Organization. *Social Science Medicine, 41*, 1403–1409.

Oral Health

Steven Corbin, MPH, DDS and Sanford J. Fenton, DDS, MDS

23

Objectives

At the completion of this chapter, the learner will be able to:

1. Identify the crucial role that oral health plays in the overall health of individuals with intellectual and developmental disabilities (I/DD).
2. Discuss the historical role that oral health for persons with I/DD has played in the health policy, health professional training, health programs, and health care financing areas.
3. Identify the most prevalent oral diseases that affect persons with I/DD across the life stages.
4. Describe appropriate oral care (planning, delivery, management) for persons with I/DD.
5. Describe specific clinical factors that present for persons with I/DD and how they should be managed relative to maintaining oral health.
6. Identify the critical roles that nurses and other health care professionals should play in promoting oral health among the population with I/DD.
7. Describe current oral health educational, care, and coordination resources that exist for persons with I/DD.

Key Points

- Oral diseases and conditions can dramatically compromise the health and functioning of persons with I/DD and significantly reduce their quality of life.
- Persons with I/DD need assessment, education, prevention strategies, and oral health treatment services throughout their lifespan, regardless of the particular setting in which they reside.

Key Points *(continued)*

- The health sector has done an inadequate job to date in meeting the oral health needs of people with I/DD.

- Nurses and other healthcare professionals can play critical roles in educating caretakers and family members about oral health needs and concerns, delivering clinical oral health services, recognizing the need for referral, and coordinating overall oral care services for persons with I/DD.

I. The Importance of Oral Health

A healthy mouth plays a basic and fundamentally essential role in maintaining human health. The teeth are responsible for chewing and proper speech, and aid in appearance and an improved self-image. Nursing professionals and other direct care professionals must be able to distinguish a healthy mouth from an unhealthy mouth in order to ensure that assigned patients, including those individuals with I/DD, do not unduly experience oral pain, bleeding, or infection without appropriate professional intervention (U.S. Department of Health and Human Services (DHHS), 2000a, 2001).

A. Traditional views were that oral diseases and conditions were an inevitable part of aging and that they were of little consequence beyond avoidance of pain and maintaining a "bright smile."

B. Dental caries declined dramatically in the general population during the 1960s and later due largely to expansion of fluoride use through various modalities, both systemic and topical.

C. Gingivitis and periodontal infections (periodontitis) are highly prevalent and responsible for most tooth loss among adults.

D. New science indicates that oral infections relate to other systemic issues, including heart disease, diabetic exacerbation, and possibly preterm birth.

E. Oral health relates to general functioning (oral, general physiologic, occupational, social) and quality of life.

II. Oral Diseases/Conditions and Implications

A. Dental caries

1. Affects people of all ages with or without I/DD.

2. Major factor responsible is dental plaque, a sticky film that accumulates on the teeth and can particularly be felt in the morning before brushing.

3. Bacteria in plaque thrive on sugary foods (i.e., candy, cake, soft drinks), converting sugar into acid. Acid beaks down the enamel and a cavity eventually results. The longer plaque is present on teeth, the more damage it will cause.

B. Factors that contribute to an individual's susceptibility to dental caries:

1. Physical disabilities—Some people may lack the manual dexterity to perform daily tooth brushing and flossing skills necessary for removing plaque from all tooth surfaces.

2. Cognitive deficiencies—Some people may not have the mental capacity to understand the importance of proper oral health care. Even individuals with average to above-average intelligence may have a low dental I.Q., making them unaware of the routine procedures necessary to prevent dental disease.

3. Malocclusion—Teeth that are crooked or misaligned make plaque removal a difficult task.

4. Oral defects—Teeth located in cleft lip and palate defects or teeth with unusual shapes, pits, or grooves may also complicate the removal of plaque.

5. Decreased self-cleansing ability—Diminished or thick salivary flow resulting from radiation treatment or drug therapy can interfere with the normal bathing of the teeth by saliva. Poor oral muscle control also reduces the individual's oral self-cleansing ability. This self-cleansing process buffers acids in the mouth and reduces the risk of decay.

C. Periodontal disease

1. Periodontal disease (gum disease) in its various forms or severities affect people of all ages.

2. Most common cause of tooth loss after age 35 years.

3. Plaque is also the major cause of periodontal disease. If plaque is left on the teeth for long periods of time (1–3 days) it crystallizes and becomes hard, forming "tartar" or calculus.

4. Bacteria in plaque and calculus are responsible for irritating and destroying the structures that support the teeth (e.g., gingival, periodontal ligament, and bone). If these deposits are not removed, eventual tooth loss will result.

D. Factors contributing to periodontal disease include:

1. Soft diets that do not stimulate the structures supporting the teeth and may cause eventual deterioration of the gingival, periodontal ligaments, and bone due to their disuse.

2. Metabolic disturbances (e.g., diabetes or leukemia) impair an individual's resistance to infection and healing. Bleeding and tender gums often result.

3. Nutritional deficiencies associated with diet or metabolic disturbances resulting in depletion of vitamins A and/or C may aggravate a periodontal condition. Gingiva may appear deep red in color and may bleed easily.

4. Malocclusions, oral habits (grinding of teeth, chewing on objects) and oral defects (e.g., cleft palate) may make plaque removal more difficult because of a change in the contour of the mouth and structure of the teeth. Mouth breathing causes drying and irritation of the gingival tissue. Grinding of the teeth (bruxism) is an oral habit that places excessive force on the periodontal ligaments holding the teeth in their bony sockets. This pressure may eventually cause the ligaments to deteriorate.

III. Treatment Planning and Coordination

Most people require regular dental care (1–2 times/year) for preventing and managing oral diseases. Persons with disabilities, including I/DD, may require more frequent dental visits because of underlying risk factors. Nursing and other health care professionals should be able to recognize the need for dental care and advise someone who will be able to arrange for necessary treatment of the patient's dental problems. The following detectable conditions require treatment by a dental professional:

A. Periodontal disease—Observable signs include: (1) foul mouth odor; (2) swollen gums; (3) gums that bleed when brushed; (4) teeth that become loose or spread apart; (5) gums that recede down the roots of the teeth; (6) gums that pull away from the teeth; and (7) painful gums. The treatment necessary is a professional cleaning and gingival therapy. The dentist may also recommend other oral hygiene aids such as a specialized brush or may prescribe rinses and/or antibiotics.

B. Dental caries—Observable signs include: (1) grey, brown, or black spots on the teeth; (2) cavities in the teeth; and (3) pain when eating sweets or other foods. These teeth should be treated by the dentist before they become nonrestorable.

C. Abscesses—Observable signs include: (1) swelling of the face, neck, or under the tongue; (2) a throbbing or constant pain; and (3) an area of draining pus in the mouth, under the chin, or on the face. An abscess should be treated immediately as it may spread infection to the brain or neck and thus become life threatening.

D. Fractured teeth, malocclusion, and missing teeth—Fractured teeth should be examined immediately and restored to avoid future problems such as abscesses. Malocclusion or irregular alignment of the teeth: (1) makes the teeth more susceptible to decay and periodontal disease due to difficulty in cleaning; (2) makes chewing and speaking more difficult; and (3) adversely affects facial appearance. Malocclusion may be seen as drifting teeth, loss of teeth, crowding, or excessive overbite. Missing teeth should be replaced by a partial denture, fixed bridge, or complete denture whenever practical. This will aid eating and speaking, will help keep the remaining teeth in proper alignment, and will help avoid jaw discomfort.

E. Oral tissue changes—Observable signs include: (1) white patches on the gingival, lips, cheeks, or tongue; (2) lumps in the mouth or on the neck; (3) numbness, bleeding, dryness, or burning of the mouth without any apparent reason; (4) a red sore on the lips or inside the mouth that does not heal within a 2–3 week period; and (5) a sudden difficulty in speaking or swallowing. These changes should be noted and a dentist contacted as soon as possible for evaluation of the condition.

IV. Oral Diseases/Conditions Prevalence among the Population of Persons with I/DD and Surveillance Mechanisms—Epidemiology

A. Oral epidemiology surveillance systems for persons with I/DD—virtually non-existent except for Special Olympics International (Corbin, 2001; Siperstein, Norins, Corbin, & Shriver, 2003).

　　1. Epidemiology/surveillance

　　　　a. National Health and Nutrition Examination Survey (noninstitutionalized) core and supplement

　　　　b. National Health Interview Survey (self-report)

　　　　c. State oral health surveys

　　　　d. Special surveys (e.g., The Henry J. Kaiser Family Foundation, 2003)

V. History and Current Status: Oral Care Programs, Dental Care Providers, Curricula, and Resources

A. Current access to care and adequacy of services

　　1. Utilization rates among the population of persons with I/DD (41% for non-elderly adult disabled versus nearly 70% for nonelderly adult population)

　　2. Government (federal, state, local) programs, initiatives, and regulations (Medicaid, EPSDT, SCHIP, Special Medical Funds, Medicare, direct delivery, *Healthy People 2010*, nursing home regulations, Maternal Child Health Bureau, etc.)

　　　　a. Only 14% of Medicaid eligible children receive any dental care each year (DHHS, 2000b)

　　　　b. Medicare has virtually no dental care coverage other than oral conditions related directly to a Medicare covered services (e.g., surgical case management)

　　　　c. Nursing home regulations (federal): initial examination and treatment requirements

　　　　d. Spend down provisions under Medicaid

　　3. Volunteer programs (university, professional, other; e.g., Special Olympics Special Smiles, National Foundation of Dentistry for the Handicapped)

　　4. Individual and institutional community providers (community health centers, dental schools, university developmental disability centers, hospital dental clinics, dental residency programs)

5. Private dental insurance—Scope of coverage is over 100 million Americans dentally uninsured (DHHS, 2000b).

6. Private dental insurance status relates directly to employment status, and 95% of persons with I/DD are unemployed.

   a. Indemnity plans

   b. HMOs

   c. PPOs

   d. Medical savings accounts and cafeteria plans

   e. Direct reimbursement plans

B. Dental care providers

1. Type and numbers—Approximately 154,000 active dentists in U.S. (DHHS, 2000b) and 120,000 licensed dental hygienists (personal communication, Stanley Peck, E.D., American Dental Hygienists Association, March 2004).

2. Training—80% of dentists are general practitioners.

3. Pediatric dentists carry the burden of providing most care to children with I/DD and actually provide much adult care also.

4. Location—Preoccupation with institutional settings for care even though most persons with I/DD can be seen in outpatient settings.

5. Few dental schools offer adequate training and experience in I/DD and treating such persons.

   a. Dental students report little confidence in treating this population (U.S. Public Health Service, 2002; Wolff, Waldman, Milan, & Perlman, 2004)

6. Very little continuing professional education offered in the treatment of persons with I/DD.

7. Dental hygienists

   a. In most cases, work under direct supervision of dentists.

   b. Emerging dental practice acts in some states are permitting dental hygienists to work under general supervision of dentists in institutions with people with special care needs, including I/DD.

C. Coordination of care with other professionals (physicians, pharmacists, vocational therapists, psychologists, social workers, teachers, etc.)

D. Academic standards for providers

1. Post-graduate degrees

2. Certificates—general practice residencies

VI. Preventive and Educational Services

Bacterial plaque and inadequate diet affect the teeth and their supporting structures, making them highly susceptible to dental disease. In order to prevent or minimize periodontal disease and dental caries, a daily oral hygiene program must be followed to remove plaque from the teeth and gums. This routine includes tooth brushing, flossing, and fluoride. Diet and eating habits are also important to oral health. Each individual should have a personalized oral hygiene program suited to his or her needs.

A. Infection control—Before the oral hygiene prevention program begins, infection control precautions must be considered (Centers for Disease Control and Prevention (CDC), 2003).

    1. Whenever possible, patients should be encouraged to perform dental hygiene tasks.

    2. For patients who depend on the nurse, direct care support professional, or family member for oral care, blood from bleeding gums, saliva, and oral tissues will be contacted. Splashing of oral fluids often occurs during brushing and flossing. To protect staff and patients, infection control recommendations given by the CDC must be followed to prevent the spread of hepatitis B, AIDS, herpes, and other infectious diseases.

    3. Recommended precautions when providing daily oral care for the patients:

        a. Gloves must always be worn when touching blood, saliva, mucous membranes, blood-soiled items, body fluids or secretions, as well as surfaces contaminated with them. Wash hands before gloving. Use new gloves for each patient. Hands must always be washed with soap following removal of gloves since the gloves may have been perforated during use, thus allowing bacteria or viruses beneath the glove to multiply. Also, thoroughly wash hands after touching objects contaminated with blood or saliva.

        b. Masks and protective eyewear or chin-length plastic face shields must be worn when the splashing of blood or other body fluids is likely.

        c. Scrubs, laboratory coats, reusable gowns, or disposable gowns must be worn when clothing may be soiled with blood or other body fluids.

        d. Surfaces contaminated with blood or saliva should be wiped with an absorbent towel and then disinfected with a chemical germicide.

        e. Waste materials such as paper tissues contaminated with blood or other body fluids should be placed in sealed, sturdy, impervious bags to prevent leakage of contained materials. Dispose of these bags according to local regulations.

B. Tooth brushing—Tooth brushing is very important to remove plaque and food debris from the teeth and gums. Brushing after each meal and snack is ideal but not always possible or practical. Therefore, it may be necessary to thoroughly brush the teeth once per day, preferably in the evening. The patient's daily schedule may determine the time for additional brushing. When the patient has eaten and brushing is not possible, the mouth should be rinsed with water to remove food particles.

1. Disclosing agents (liquid or tablet) may be used (chewed or swished and spit out, not swallowed) to stain plaque prior to brushing to increase its visibility, but should not be swallowed. The liquid solution may be placed on the teeth with a cotton-tipped applicator.

2. Toothpaste

   a. An American Dental Association (ADA)-approved fluoride toothpaste (pea-sized amount for children) should be used. Rinsing and expectoration should follow.

   b. For patients who cannot expectorate or have difficulty expectorating, Nasadent (nonfoaming toothpaste) may be used. It does not contain fluoride, but can be swallowed without concern.

   c. A tartar (calculus) control toothpaste may be necessary for individuals who produce excessive tartar (e.g., people with cerebral palsy, people taking certain kinds of medications).

   d. In some cases, a dentist may recommend a desensitizing toothpaste for persons with sensitive teeth. A patient should receive a dental examination before using this toothpaste since dental problems requiring treatment may be causing the sensitivity.

   e. If for some reason a patient cannot tolerate any toothpaste, a small amount may be rubbed over the teeth, if possible, after brushing.

3. Toothbrush selection and modification—An appropriate toothbrush should have the following characteristics:

   a. Soft, end-rounded, or polished bristles, which are less likely to injure the gums

   b. Size and shape that allows access to every tooth (e.g., child-sized brushes for small mouths)

   c. Level plane of bristles

   d. Toothbrushes can be adapted to meet the needs of each patient. For individuals with impaired motor coordination with hand, arm, or shoulder problems or with limited dexterity, the following toothbrush modifications may be helpful:

      i. Attach the brush to the patient's hand with a wide rubber band.

      ii. Enlarge the handle with a rubber ball, sponge, or bicycle hand grip.

      iii. Lengthen the handle with a ruler, tongue depressor, or a piece of wood or plastic.

      iv. Bend the handle after running it under hot water (do not place the head of the brush in hot water) or purchase a brush with a bent handle.

   e. An electric toothbrush may also be helpful for some patients. The use of a suction toothbrush may be necessary for patients with excessive salivary secretions.

    f. A toothbrush should be changed every three to four months or sooner if worn or frayed. If a patient has the flu, a cold, or the like, his or her toothbrush should be replaced during and after the illness since toothbrushes may perpetuate the infectious disease. After use, the brush should be rinsed and stored where it can air dry.

4. Proper brushing technique

    a. Place the head of the toothbrush on the teeth with the bristles at a 45-degree angle to the gum line. Plaque is usually thickest near the gum line.

    b. In the angled position, move the brush with a short (half-a-tooth wide) back-and-forth stroke several times; scrub the teeth gently in this manner using firm pressure but not mashing bristles against the teeth since their tips do the cleaning.

    c. Brush the teeth in a specific sequence so that the inner (tongue side) and outer (cheek side), and chewing surfaces of each tooth will be cleaned. For example, start with the outer surfaces of the left upper molar (back) teeth. The mouth may be partially closed to aid in reaching the back teeth.

    d. To adequately clean the teeth, they should be brushed three to five minutes at each session. Always brush the top of the tongue to freshen the breath and remove bacteria. After brushing thoroughly rinse the mouth with water. As previously mentioned, patients who cannot rinse and expectorate can use Nasadent or no toothpaste at all. If a suction toothbrush or another form of suction is available, toothpaste and a water rinse may be used with these patients.

5. Positioning—When the nursing or other health care professional must brush the patient's teeth, positioning of the patient is very important for easy and effective cleaning. A number of modifications to normal patient positioning are available depending on the particular circumstances of the patient.

    a. A physician or dentist may need to be consulted in certain cases since some positions are not safe for some patients. For example, a patient with cerebral palsy or one with breathing problems should not have the head tilted back as the airway may be blocked. When positioning a patient, always be alert to possible problems and be ready to quickly reposition him or her if difficulties occur. Experiment with different positions to find one best suited for the caretaker and the patient.

    b. For uncooperative patients, more than one person and/or restraints may be needed to help control movements. Restraint may be a valid treatment modality for noncompliant developmentally disabled patients because significant oral disease can lead to serious systemic problems like aspiration pneumonia. However, restraint must be justified and absolutely necessary. Use the least restrictive method that does not cause physical injury to the patient or caretaker and involves the least possible discomfort (Fenton et al., 1987). For example, one may hold the head gently with his or her hands while someone else holds the arms and legs in place and the third person brushes and flosses the teeth. If the patient's combative behavior continues through several attempts over a day or two, a consultation with a dentist should be scheduled to develop an appropriate modified plan for providing safe and effective oral hygiene for the patient (Fenton et al., 1987; Fenton & Horbelt, 2001).

6. Flossing—Flossing removes plaque from between the teeth and under the gum line where toothbrush bristles cannot easily reach. Since dental caries and periodontal disease often begin in these areas, flossing must be performed at least once each day in conjunction with tooth brushing. Flossing may be difficult at first, but it can be mastered with a few days of practice. Many patients will not be able to floss and the caretaker must accomplish this for them.

   a. Either waxed and unwaxed dental floss can clean effectively, but waxed floss will make flossing easier for persons with tight contacts between the teeth. Flavored floss may help with patient compliance.

   b. Use about 18 inches of floss wrapped around one end of your middle fingers with the majority of the floss on one finger. Hold the floss tightly between the thumb and index finger on each hand. Leave about one inch of floss between these fingers with which to floss. As the floss becomes soiled or frayed, unwind clean floss from one finger about two turns and take up the used floss on the other finger.

   c. Gently slide the floss between the teeth; a gentle sawing motion should be used so that the floss does not snap down into the gums and damage them.

   d. After the floss is between the teeth, curve it around one of the teeth in a C-shape. Slide the floss gently under the gum line until some resistance is felt; do not go down very far as the gums may be cut or injured. While holding the floss tightly against the tooth, scrape the side of the tooth by sliding the floss up and down. Now put the floss between the same two teeth and floss the side of the tooth adjacent to the one just flossed.

   e. Always floss in a specific sequence so that no teeth will be missed. Floss the backs of the last teeth and also around teeth with no adjacent tooth on one or both sides. Often plaque accumulates to a greater extent in these areas.

   f. Rinse mouth.

   g. Patient positioning for flossing the teeth is the same as described for tooth brushing.

   h. If the patient or caretaker has limited finger dexterity, a floss holder may be used.

7. Fluoride—Fluoride administration should be an integral part of any oral hygiene program.

   a. Systemic fluoride is necessary for children while the teeth are developing so that the fluoride will be incorporated into the enamel and make it harder. The source for this fluoride is fluoridated drinking water and some foods. If this route is inadequate, the dentist may recommend supplemental fluoride tablets or liquid.

   b. Topical fluoride application to the teeth provides fluoride's benefits to both children and adults. Fluoride toothpaste should be used daily if tolerated by the patient. In addition, some patients should rinse daily with a nonprescription fluoride mouth rinse. A dentist may recommend this rinse for patients with moderate dental caries, dry mouth, or sensitive teeth. Only persons with the ability to expectorate should use this rinse; it should not be swallowed. For patients with moderate to severe caries, dry mouth, or exposed tooth roots or dentin, a dentist may prescribe a daily home-care fluoride gel.

8. Twice daily chlorhexidine rinse swished or applied may be prescribed by the dentist for those patients demonstrating severe gingivitis or periodontal disease.

9. Nutritional considerations—Foods containing sugar play an important role in the dental caries process. The bacteria found in plaque convert sugar to an acid. Each time a food containing sugar is consumed, 20 minutes of acid production occurs. The greater the frequency of sugar exposures, the greater the risk for developing cavities. Sweets, therefore, should be provided with meals rather than as between-meal snacks and the teeth should be brushed following eating.

   a. Nutritional counseling aimed at both dietary personnel and clinical psychologists is essential. Dietary staff responsible for meal planning and preparation must be familiar with semisoft diets that are low in sugar. Semisoft foods are often highly processed, containing hidden sugars and additives, and are low in nutritional value.

   b. Staff psychologists must be educated to offer alternative behavior modification reinforcers that are low in sugar and high in nutrients when trying to promote desired behaviors in persons with I/DD.

VII. Referral Services and Immediacy

A. If a person with I/DD presents with urgent or emergency oral health care needs including pain, infection, or trauma, a dentist or oral surgeon must be consulted. The hospital's emergency department or medical affairs office usually maintains a list of dental professionals who are members of the hospital medical staff and have clinical privileges.

B. Other possible resources for locating dentists who are willing to treat persons with I/DD in their dental practices include local or state dental professional societies, colleges/schools of dentistry, Special Olympics community or state director, state dental director, or medical director at a community facility for persons with I/DD.

VIII. Educating Personal Care Providers

A. The provision of acceptable daily oral hygiene for persons with I/DD is absolutely necessary to optimize oral health. Periodic preventive and treatment interventions by dental health professionals are no substitute for daily plaque removal and a healthy diet.

B. Training personal care providers is best accomplished by a formal dental health education program (Fenton & Horbelt, 2002):

1. Phase One

a. Pre-test—Evaluates the level of dental knowledge of each trainee.

b. Formal dental health education presentation—Provides the trainees with information regarding the etiology of dental diseases, preventive techniques, and appropriate modifications.

c. Demonstration of personal oral hygiene ability—Provides the instructor with information about the trainee's level of motivation, dexterity, and knowledge. Trainees are given the opportunity to practice oral hygiene skills until they can demonstrate competency.

d. Trainees are encouraged to practice these new skills prior to the second training session.

2. Phase Two

a. Evaluation of personal oral hygiene competency by the dental instructor for each trainee. Discovered deficiencies are addressed by the instructor.

b. Demonstration of adaptive preventive dentistry techniques

i. Modification of patient positioning to ensure good visibility and behavior control if necessary

ii. Adaptive toothbrush design and brushing technique

iii. Modification of flossing technique

3. Phase Three

a. Evaluation of trainee oral hygiene competency—Each trainee must demonstrate that he/she can provide effective and safe plaque removal on a selected person with I/DD.

b. Demonstration of fluoride gel application by dental instructor.

c. Post-test—Each trainee must demonstrate didactic dental health education competence before being allowed to provide oral hygiene services without monitoring.

4. Phase Four

    a. Graduates of the dental health education program establish similar training programs for other staff

IX. Administrative Management, Supervision, and Evaluation of Oral Care Services for Institutionalized Persons with I/DD

A. State facilities frequently have difficulty in securing adequate in-house professional dental services, and administrators must often seek dental services support from outside sources.

B. A comprehensive dental program is composed of four major components:

1. In-service training of facility personnel, emphasizing a daily oral hygiene regimen for each facility resident.

2. Nutritional dental counseling service educates in-house dietary staff and psychologists.

3. Dental treatment service provides comprehensive dental care for each facility resident, either in-house or off site.

4. Continuing evaluation of the dental health education and monthly reports on the overall level of daily oral hygiene for each residential unit is essential. Any detected oral hygiene deficiency is immediately addressed and corrected (Fenton, DeBiase, & Portugal, 1982).

X. Outreach Oral Health Care for Noninstitutionalized Persons with I/DD

Access to comprehensive dental services in their local communities by individuals with I/DD remains a major problem. A lack of private dental practitioners with the necessary clinical training coupled with an inadequate level of reimbursement are significant barriers to universal access to care.

A. Several professional resources are available for persons with I/DD, their parents or legal guardians, and other health care professionals including nurses to locate dental professionals willing and competent to provide comprehensive services.

1. Contact the local or state dental society to solicit the names of dental practitioners in your community who provide comprehensive dental services for persons with I/DD.

2. If the patient lives near a university that has a University Center for Excellence in Developmental Disabilities Education, Research, and Service (UCEDD) on campus, contact them for the name of a dental practitioner that treats patients with I/DD in their dental office.

3. The following Web site for the Association of University Centers on Disabilities (AUCD) provides a directory of all of the UCEDDs (www.aucd.org/directory/directory.cfm).

4. If you have exhausted all available resources and still cannot find a dentist willing to treat the patient, contact the director of your state's Developmental Disabilities Planning Council and director of your state's Protection & Advocacy Agency for advice and direction on the following Web site: www.acf.dhhs.gov/programs/add/state.htm (Fenton, DeBiase, & Portugal, 1982).

XI. Modification in Education, Care, and Referral Routines for Persons with I/DD

A. Medical assessment—A patient's health history should always be thoroughly examined before beginning an oral hygiene program. Some patients require prophylactic antibiotics prior to any dental treatment that may cause bleeding. The patients who require antibiotic coverage include those who have had rheumatic fever; who have certain types of congenital heart disease; who have had prosthetic heart valves, or a prosthetic joint replacement; who have had a spleen removed; or those experiencing uncontrolled diabetes or receiving chemotherapy.

B. Many patients require some type of medication. Some drugs may manifest side effects in the oral cavity. A dry mouth is a common problem for persons who take sedatives, barbiturates, antihistamines, diuretics, and drugs used for muscle control (Perlman, Friedman, & Tesini, 1991). Radiation therapy to the head and neck will also reduce salivary flow. Saliva has protective effects that lubricate the oral cavity, help clean the teeth, and neutralize the acid produced by the bacteria in plaque. Decreased salivary flow promotes dental caries. These patients will benefit from daily fluoride rinses or artificial saliva. Sucking on candy to keep the mouth moist should be avoided as this will aggravate the caries problem.

C. Excessive tooth decay may result from taking drugs with a syrup base for long periods of time. In this case, care should be taken to clean the teeth after medication is given.

D. Gingival hyperplasia, an abnormal overgrowth of the gums, is often observed in patients taking phenytoin (Dilantin) to control seizures (Tesini & Fenton, 1994). This hyperplasia is an exaggerated response to plaque and other gingival irritants in combination with the drug therapy. To reduce the possibility or severity of the hyperplasia and resultant periodontal disease, the patient must have optimal oral hygiene care. Gingival hyperplasia has also been associated, in some instances, with mephenytoin, sodium valproate, phenobarbital, primidone, cyclosporine A, and nifedipine.

XII. Tobacco Habits

Any type of tobacco habit may lead to oral lesions and/or oral cancer. Excessive smoking of cigarettes, cigars, or pipes also contributes to periodontal disease. Smokeless tobacco or snuff has many harmful effects including oral cancer, cancer of the throat or esophagus, high blood pressure, periodontal disease, and dental caries from the sugar content of tobacco. The tobacco or snuff pouch area in the mouth becomes white and wrinkled-looking over time. Regular dental examinations will diagnose any signs of cancer. However, all tobacco habits should be stopped to prevent future problems.

XIII. Appliance Care

An oral hygiene program is also necessary for patients with complete dentures. The dentures should be rinsed with water after eating to remove food particles from under the dentures. At least once a day, all surfaces of the dentures should be gently brushed with a denture brush and a denture-cleaning paste. A regular soft toothbrush may also be used. Occasionally, a denture-cleaning solution can be used, but it is not necessary on a daily basis.

A. Dentures and partial dentures must be removed for 6–8 hours each night. Remove them and place in a container of cool water. Before reinserting the denture, gently brush the gums, tongue, and palate with a soft toothbrush.

XIV. Specific Patient Care Considerations

A. Mental retardation—Patients with mental retardation might experience motor difficulties such as gagging easily or poor tongue control.

   1. Planning an oral hygiene program for this patient requires patience. Progressing slowly and rehearsing each technique with the patient until he or she masters it is a must. Praise the patients continually and reinforce desirable behavior with small material rewards such as stars or stickers.

   2. Modifying the toothbrush for those patients who are unable to grasp and manipulate small objects as described earlier (see VIb: Toothbrush Selection and Modification) may be necessary. A floss holder can assist the nurse in moving the floss between the teeth.

B. Cerebral palsy—Patients with cerebral palsy often exhibit inadequate control of the muscles of the body (including the mouth), encouraging the collection of food debris and plaque.

   1. Excessive drooling due to poor muscle tone in the lips and the frequency of mouth breathing make this patient highly susceptible to calculus formation and inflammation of the gums.

   2. Enlarged and extended toothbrush handles can assist individuals with cerebral palsy in directing or coordinating their movements.

   3. Supportive mouth opening devices (e.g., Specialized Care Company) are often required to maintain the mouth in an open position during oral hygiene care.

4. Dietary considerations are also necessary as these patients are likely to be consuming more highly processed foods that are high in sucrose. This factor makes the individual with cerebral palsy more susceptible to tooth decay.

C. Seizure disorder—Oral hygiene is the major component of dental care for the patient with a seizure disorder managed with Dilantin.

1. If an individual taking Dilantin does not practice meticulous plaque removal, gums will become enlarged, pale, and fibrous in texture. This overgrowth of the gums may be reversible if proper dental care is provided.

D. Sensory impairments—When one loses the sense of sight, the senses of touch, taste, smell, and hearing become very acute. These senses should be utilized to their fullest capacity during the dental health education experience of the patient with vision impairment, ideally using demonstrations.

E. Physical abuse and neglect—The nurse or other health care professional should evaluate thoroughly all oral or perioral injuries in patients (adults and children) with I/DD because physical and sexual abuse is observed in greater frequency in children with I/DD than the general population (Perlman et al., 1991).

1. A complete history and clinical examination should enable the health care professional to distinguish oral injuries that were self-inflicted from those that were the result of abuse (Fenton, Bouquot, & Unkel, 2000; Tesini & Fenton, 1994).

2. Neglect is defined as an intentional denial of adequate food, clothing, shelter, supervision, or medical and dental care. Dental neglect should be suspected if oral infection with associated rampant tooth decay, causing chronic pain, difficulty eating, and delayed growth and development are observed, particularly in the absence of financial or transportation impediments (Jessee, 1995).

XV. Summary

One of the major health disparities for persons with I/DD is appropriate and comprehensive oral health care that is accessible. It is vital that nurses and health care professionals know and inform persons with I/DD and their family members about appropriate oral health education and preventive practices.

References

Centers for Disease Control and Prevention (CDC). (2003). Guidelines for infection control in dental health-care settings—2003. *MMWR, 52*(RR17), 1–76.

Corbin, S. B. (2001). *Prompting the health of persons with mental retardation: A critical journey barely begun.* Washington, DC: Special Olympics.

Fenton, S. J., Bouquot, J. E., & Unkel, J. H. (2000). Orofacial considerations for pediatric, adult, and elderly victims of abuse. *Emergency Medical Clinics of North America, 18,* 601–617.

Fenton, S. J., DeBiase C., & Portugal B. V. (1982). A strategy for implementing a dental health education program for state facilities with limited resources. *Rehabilitation Literature*, 43, 290–293.

Fenton, S. J. and the ADH Ad Hoc Committee. (1987). ADH Ad Hoc Committee Report: The use of restraints in the delivery of dental care for the handicapped: Legal, ethical and medical considerations. *Special Care Dentistry*, 7, 253–256.

Fenton, S. J., & Horbelt, C. V. (2001). The A, B, C's for successful dental treatment. *Exceptional Parent*, 31(9), 133–135.

Fenton, S. J., & Horbelt, C. V. (2002). Vigilance—involvement—persistence: The keys to ensure access to dental care. *Exceptional Parent*, 32(10), 109–112.

Jessee, S. A. (1995). Orofacial manifestations of child abuse and neglect. *American Family Physician*, 52, 1829–1834.

Perlman, S., Friedman, C., & Tesini, D. (1991). *Prevention and treatment considerations for people with special needs*. Skillman, NJ: Johnson & Johnson.

Siperstein, G., Norins, J., Corbin, S., & Shriver, T. (2003). *Multinational study of attitudes toward individuals with intellectual disabilities*. Washington, DC: Special Olympics.

Tesini, D. A, & Fenton, S. J. (1994). Oral health needs of persons with physical and mental disabilities. *Dental Clinics of North America*, 38, 483–498.

The Henry J. Kaiser Family Foundation. (2003). *Understanding the health-care needs and experiences of people with disabilities. Findings from a 2003 survey*. Menlo Park, CA: Author.

U.S. Department of Health and Human Services. (2000a) *Healthy people 2010*. (2nd ed.). Washington, DC: U.S. Government Printing Office.

U.S. Department of Health and Human Services. (2001b). *Healthy people 2010. Disability and secondary conditions. Vision for the decade: Proceedings and recommendations of a symposium, Atlanta, Georgia*. Atlanta, GA: U.S. Department of Health and Human Services, Centers for Disease Control and Prevention.

U.S. Department of Health and Human Services. (2000b). *Oral health in America: A report of the Surgeon General*. Rockville, MD: U.S. Department of Health and Human Services, National Institute of Dental and Craniofacial Research, National Institutes of Health.

U.S. Public Health Service. (2002). *Closing the gap: A national blueprint to improve the health of persons with mental retardation*. Rockville, MD: U.S. Department of Health and Human Services.

Wolff, A., Waldman, B., Milan, M., & Perlman, S. (2004). Dental students' experiences with and attitudes toward people with mental retardation. *Journal of the American Dental Association*, 135, 353–357.

Family Perspectives

V

Family Issues Across the Lifespan

24

Sandra A. Faux, RN, PhD

Objectives

At the completion of this chapter, the learner will be able to:

1. Describe three family theories that contribute to family adaptation to intellectual and developmental disabilities (I/DD).
2. Delineate family, parental, and sibling issues specific to family life cycle stages across the lifespan.
3. Discuss how positive health care professional relationships can be formed with families of children with I/DD.
4. Describe five family management styles.
5. Develop health care professional interventions with families across the lifespan.

Key Points

- The family impact of an I/DD is seen across the family lifespan with certain issues at the forefront dependent upon family development cycle and developmental stage of the family member with an I/DD.

- Family perceptions of the illness and its meaning for the family include both individual and collective family definitions.

- Family stress and change affect all family systems and members.

- The majority of families having a family member with an I/DD are adaptable, flexible, and able to change.

- Health care professionals must respect and collaborate with families to achieve positive child and family outcomes.

I.   Theories of Family Functioning and Adaptation to Chronic Disability

Family adaptation to an I/DD is an ongoing, evolving process. As the family member with the I/DD ages and faces new life challenges, the family and its responses must also evolve and develop new ways of dealing with the associated challenges. To understand the issues that families confront, family and family adaptation need to be defined as well as the underlying family theories that guide interventions with families.

A. Definitions of family (include "self-identification, dynamic interaction through some bond, and functioning to reach mutual goals" (Clawson, 1998, p. 53))

1. Blood or legal definitions as determined by each state; important in adulthood related to issues of competence and consent.

2. Two or more persons who define themselves as family based on emotional closeness, commitment, mutual decision making, and shared goals who live together or in close geographic proximity (Clawson, 1998).

B. Family adaptation to I/DD

1. Adaptation is an ongoing process in which families and/or family members cope, change, and adjust to the challenge of having a family member with an I/DD.

2. Families may adapt or fail to adapt and subsequently experience positive or negative outcomes for the family or individual family members.

3. Basic assumptions about I/DD and the family

a. Diagnosis and progress of an I/DD is a stressful event for the family.

b. The family member's condition has bidirectional effects on both the family and family member.

c. Families have the capacity to adapt and develop styles of managing the I/DD.

d. Illness and/or limitations in a family member require the family system to adapt.

e. The family member's I/DD can result in both positive and negative outcomes (Clawson, 1998).

C. Family theories

1. Stress and systems theory—I/DD is the stressor event that interacts with the family definition of the I/DD and the family's coping abilities and resources. This process results in a positive or negative family outcome. Factors impacting outcome include:

a. Family definition of seriousness of change

b. Family vulnerability to stress

c. Family adaptability

d. Family integration

e. Frequency and severity of events related to the I/DD

f. Family resources

2. Social ecology theory—The family is defined as a "system nested within a number of other societal systems" (Seligman & Darling, 1997, p. 15). In order to change family behavior, one has to change the environments in which they exist.

   a. Microsystem—The pattern of activities and interpersonal relations experienced by various family members within the context of the family.

   b. Mesosystem—The settings within which the family actively participates, including:

      i. Medical and health care workers

      ii. Extended family

      iii. Friends/neighbors

      iv. Work/recreation associates

      v. Early intervention programs

      vi. Other parents

      vii. Local community

   c. Exosystem—Settings in which the family is not actively involved but which may affect the family

      i. Mass media, which may affect attitudes about persons with I/DD

      ii. Health care

      iii. Social welfare (e.g., SSI)

      iv. Education

   d. Macrosystem—Values inherent in society and social situations

      i. Ethnic, cultural, religious, and socioeconomic values impact how families define an I/DD, interact with service delivery systems, and access available resources.

      ii. Economic and political

3. Family life cycle—Developmental theory based on life stage of the children in the family. Each stage has tasks the family needs to accomplish. This theory has been adapted to include the stress experienced by families of someone with an I/DD.

   a. Childbearing—Getting an accurate diagnosis, making emotional adjustments, informing other family members

   b. School-age—Clarifying personal views regarding mainstreaming versus segregated placements, dealing with reactions of child's peer group, arranging for child care and extracurricular activities

    c. Adolescence—Coping with the chronicity of the child's I/DD, dealing with issues of sexuality, coping with peer isolation and rejection, planning for the child's vocational future

    d. Launching—Adjusting to the family's continuing responsibility, deciding upon appropriate residential placement, dealing with the lack of socialization opportunities

    e. Postparental—Re-establishing relationships with spouse; if child has been successfully launched, interacting with disabled member's residential service providers; planning for the future (Seligman & Darling, 1997, p. 14).

II. Childbearing Stage—Initial Diagnosis

The initial diagnosis is a time of stress for parents and other family members. The diagnosis may occur prenatally (e.g., genetic testing, sonogram), at birth, or during the first two years of life. Parental and family responses are similar regardless of timing. Crucial for the family and child is how they cope with the diagnosis, accept the child, and deal effectively with the changes in family life engendered by the presence of a child with I/DD in the family.

A. Initial diagnosis—Families experience a series of responses to the stress of the initial diagnosis. These responses have been understood within the framework of parental grief. They grieve the loss of the ideal/normal child that they expected or thought they had and deal with the reality of accepting a different child.

    1. Anxiety, crying, shock

    2. Uncertainty—This is very common when the parents "know" that something is wrong with their child (e.g., not meeting developmental milestones, not responding to parental cues) and spend time looking for a definitive diagnosis

    3. Denial

    4. Anger, blame, guilt, viewing child as punishment

    5. Doctor shopping—Trying to find another diagnosis

    6. Accept the reality of a "less than perfect child" or not accept the child and not move on

B. How to tell the parents/family

    1. Be honest and realistic.

    2. Acknowledge their stress and feelings.

    3. Discuss the diagnosis and prognosis in appropriate language.

    4. Discuss the positive and negative aspects; do not focus entirely on the negatives.

    5. Provide health, developmental, and community resources.

C. Parental responses

1. Initial reaction reflects anxiety, stress, and grief.

2. Deciding who to tell about the diagnosis: family, friends, neighbors, church.

3. Accept the reality of integrating the child into the family.

4. Seek information and resources.

5. Plan for the future of the child and family.

6. Chronic sorrow—Some parents/families experience a continued sense of loss for what might have been, particularly on the anniversary of the birth or diagnosis.

D. Role of the health care professional (Freedman & Boyer, 2000)

1. Support parents/families during the initial diagnosis or seeking a diagnosis.

2. Acknowledge their feelings (positive and negative).

3. Provide accurate, current information about the diagnosis and prognosis.

4. Provide appropriate referrals (health, developmental, community).

5. Link family with other families and/or organizations and support groups as appropriate.

6. Make referrals for family and/or genetic counseling as needed.

III. Childrearing Stage—Post-Diagnosis through Preschool

The time period after the initial diagnosis and the first few years of the child's life engender several family life changes that must be dealt with in addition to learning to manage the child's I/DD. These adaptive tasks include:

A. Accepting the diagnosis and moving on

1. Family needs to give meaning to the diagnosis within existing family philosophy

2. Deciding how family members will be informed of the diagnosis

3. Comparing their family situation upwardly (better off) or downwardly (worse off) with other families with children having the same or similar diagnoses and prognoses

B. Locating and accessing appropriate health and social services

1. Obtain accurate prognosis and information about what to expect and treatment/care.

2. Obtain appropriate referrals for health and social services (e.g., early intervention and developmental, physical therapy, etc.) (See Chapters 8 and 9.)

C. Managing the daily care of the child

1. Learning the skills to provide physical (e.g., medications, physical therapy, seizure precautions, etc.) and developmental care (e.g., stimulation activities)

2. Developing relationships with health care professionals. Families develop long-term relationships with a variety of health care professionals (doctors;

nurses; physical, speech, and occupational therapists, etc.). Thorne and Robinson (1989) have described the evolution of collaborative, effective family-health care relationships that result in good outcomes for the child with I/DD. They call this *guarded alliance*. The stages of the relationship include:

a. Hero worship—Also referred to as naïve trust, when families initially believe that health care professionals (HCP) and system will meet their child's and family needs. It is characterized as a trusting relationship in which decision making is deferred to the experts. Extended experience with HCP and health care system leads to disillusionment as needs are not met.

b. Resignation/disillusionment—The second stage is characterized by despair, hopelessness, and powerlessness to obtain health care that families perceive as needed and appropriate. This is exacerbated in health care situations when HCP have little or inaccurate knowledge (e.g., children with I/DD do not experience pain) or deny services (e.g., vision referrals for a child with profound disabilities) based on the child's lack of productive contributions to society in the future.

c. Consumerism/team player—In this stage, families develop relationships with HCP to obtain essential services. Families become well informed about the condition and treatment and the health care bureaucracy. In team playing, families have developed reciprocal, negotiated relationships with HCP in the families, HCP recognize the limitations of the health care system, and families accept responsibility and primary decision making for their child. This reciprocal trust involves families placing some trust in the HCP and the HCP acknowledging the competence of families to make valid decisions related to the care of their child. Thus, the relationship is characterized by mutual trust and collaboration.

3. Family management style (FMS)—FMS is a family approach to managing the daily care of the child and the effects of the I/DD on the family (Knafl, Breitmayer, Gallo, & Zoeller, 1996). Five FMS have emerged based upon the following factors:

a. Child's identity, view of condition, self-view, and self-care behaviors; parenting philosophy and mutuality; care-management approach; prominence of child's I/DD on family life; and family's and child's future well- being.

b. FMS styles

i. Thriving—Families accept and accommodate child; parents have positive, mutual parenting philosophy; they are proactive and confident in managing the child's condition; the I/DD does not dominate the family.

ii. Accommodating—Similar to thriving with the exception that mothers tend to be more confident in care management, with parenting philosophy and mutuality less than the thriving families.

iii. Enduring—In this style, families may view the child as a tragic figure, with parents very protective; may view care as burdensome.

iv. Struggling—In this style, the child's identity and self-view varies, sometimes positive and other times negative; mothers tend to view the care as burdensome and place the I/DD in the foreground of family life; fathers are more confident and do not place the I/DD in the foreground of family life.

v. Floundering—In this style, the child is always viewed as a tragic figure with a negative, limited future; parents do not have a mutual parenting philosophy and share discordant views of the I/DD; families react to every crisis and employ few resources in dealing with problems.

D. Meeting child's developmental needs—Parents' developmental expectations become stable over time and are primarily formed by the time the child reaches age 3; they tend to lower developmental expectations as their child matures. Parental expectations are directly influenced by the HCP who work with their child.

1. Involved in early intervention programs.

2. Engage in normal developmental activities within limits of child's abilities

3. Normalization of family life—After the family has adapted (usually within the first three years post-diagnosis), families tend to structure their family life by treating the child as normally as possible within the child's abilities. Attributes of family normalization are:

    a. Acknowledging the condition and the potential threat to lifestyle

    b. Adopting normalcy lens for defining the child and family; engaging in parenting behaviors and family routines that are consistent with a normalcy lens

    c. Engaging in parenting behaviors and family routines that are consistent with normalization

    d. Developing a treatment regimen that is consistent with normalcy

    e. Interacting with others based on a view of the child and family as normal (Deatrick, Knafl, & Murphy–Moore, 1999, pp. 211–212)

E. Dealing with stress and crises in the early years, there may be periods of ongoing as well as situational stress periods. These critical periods are often associated with health and developmental issues.

1. Hospitalization and/or surgeries—Relocation of the child to an unfamiliar environment and the associated anxiety, uncertainty, and vulnerability of the situation engenders family stress.

2. Unexpected illness of child or family members.

3. Failure to meet normal developmental milestones. Delays or limited ability to meet the usual physical and/or cognitive milestones may engender a temporary sense of grief and loss.

4. Chronic sorrow has been postulated as a response by parents to the diagnosis of an infant/child with an I/DD. It is postulated that it is the reaction to the loss of the ideal or normal child and is a "periodic recurrence of permanent, pervasive sadness or other grief associated with a significant loss" (Eakes, Burke, & Hainsworth, 1998, p. 179). This sadness is not constant, but may be triggered by certain events.

   a. Anniversary of birth and/or diagnosis of the child

   b. Missed or delayed developmental physical milestone such as delayed walking or inability to walk

   c. Inability of child to obtain advanced degrees or pursue a career

   d. Marriage and parenthood

F. Developing a social support network—Social support has been shown to reduce family stress. Families develop support at three ecological levels. The network size and density is related to the ability of families to live successfully in this abnormal situation (Kazak, 1986).

   1. Family/intimate relationships—Which family members are informed; will they be involved in care; financial support

   2. Friendships—Who is told and extent and frequency of support

   3. Neighborhood and community

G. Meeting developmental and emotional/social needs of other family members. Individual families often function differently after the diagnosis of an I/DD.

   1. Family developmental needs include:

      a. Marital relationship—A child's I/DD may either strengthen a strong marriage or cause dissolution of a weak one. Marital instability has been seen with a child with greater behavioral problems.

      b. Maternal depression, anxiety, and worry—Increased depression has been noted among these mothers, particularly Latina mothers (Monsen, 1999).

      c. Social isolation—In focusing on the child and their care, families may restrict interaction with the community.

      d. Financial restrictions—Families may have reduced resources as mothers may stay home to take care of the child; fathers may refuse promotions that necessitate relocation from a community where the family has established health care and social supports. Additional expenses related to child's condition also reduce the family's financial resources and may restrict vacations, etc.

   e. Open communication among family members about all aspects of the condition is positively related to family functioning and adaptation.

   f. Sibling needs for attention, discipline, family activities.

   g. Role flexibility.

   h. Redefine personal expectations.

   i. Share family responsibilities.

   j. Counseling and/or support groups for parents and/or siblings.

   k. Parent training programs focused on dealing with the child with an I/DD (Briskin & Liptak, 1995).

2. Parental issues—In the past, researchers focused on the negative effects of having a child with an I/DD on the parents and family; the majority of families effectively adapt to this situation. Currently, researchers are examining the positive aspects of this experience and are trying to determine what enables families to successfully adapt and manage this chronic stress situation (Clare, Garnier, & Gallimore, 1998; Miltiades & Pruchno, 2001).

   a. Uncertainty about future health, growth and development, and ultimate family of future

   b. Concerns about ability to meet child's needs including health, behavior, and emotional development (Lam & Mackenzie, 2002)

   c. Positive effects—May strengthen marriage, improve family communication, develop more ties to community, increase empathy for others, become advocate for disabled

   d. Negative effects—Lower self-esteem, depression, fewer life options, impaired family functioning, deterioration of parental physical health

3. Sibling issues—Sibling relationships are the longest relationships within families, with siblings serving as models, caregivers, teachers, friends, and defenders. As with the parental literature, more recent studies have documented the positive aspects of having a sibling with I/DD rather than the negative effects. As noted previously, the majority of siblings deal very effectively with having a sibling with an I/DD.

   a. Knowledge of I/DD—Siblings need current, accurate information, provided by parents and/or health care professionals using appropriate language and concepts for their developmental level.

   b. Involvement in care—Older sisters often serve as caregivers for the child with the I/DD. May be assigned parenting responsibilities for other siblings.

   c. Potential social isolation if sibling is ashamed of child and does not bring friends home.

d. Stigma—Normal sibling may feel stigmatized by the situation and may have lower self-esteem.

e. Parental relationship—Differential parenting with more time spent with child with I/DD and differential disciplinary practices.

f. High-risk siblings—Sibling emotional and psychological difficulties have been associated with lower socioeconomic status, differential parenting, and feelings of guilt about the sibling with an I/DD.

H. Role of health care professionals

1. Provide ongoing parental support and information

2. Develop collaborative, positive health care relationships with parents and siblings.

3. Encourage sibling involvement with the child with an I/DD within their capabilities.

4. Encourage sibling visitation when child is hospitalized.

5. Sibling support groups as needed.

IV. Childrearing Stage—School-Age and Adolescence

The school-age stage is a relatively stable developmental period with the focus on education and developing peer relationships, while adolescence, with rapid physical, hormonal, and emotional changes, often creates instability within the family.

A. Family issues with the school-age child with an I/DD

1. Education

a. Deciding upon type, either special education or mainstreaming/inclusion (see Chapter 10)

b. Consistent involvement with chosen educational approach or changes as needed and appropriate

c. Negotiating with school personnel to provide required care (e.g., medications, continence care)

d. Re-assimilation of child into school after protracted absences due to illness, hospitalization, surgery, etc.

e. Locating additional health care and social services as child's needs change

f. Encouraging social relationships with peers

g. Identifying child care resources and/or respite, dependent upon severity of condition and caregiving demands

h. Beginning to promote autonomy and self-care within child's capabilities

    i. Educating teachers, staff, and community about child and abilities (see Chapter 10)

B. Adolescence (see Chapter 11)

  1. Power struggles often occur between adolescents, parents, and other family members as they seek control. Parents may be reluctant to give up control, fearing that care routines may not be followed and subsequent negative outcomes.

  2. Dealing with issues of sexuality (see Chapter 13)

    a. Sexual expression—Parents may deny sexuality in their adolescent with I/DD or feel unable to deal with it due to lack of knowledge, how to convey appropriate information, timing, etc.

    b. Managing menses

    c. Sex education

    d. Birth control

    e. Sexually transmitted diseases/AIDS

    f. Pregnancy

    g. Sexual abuse

  3. Dating and opposite/same-sex relationships including dealing with peer rejection and isolation

  4. Continued promotion of self-care and autonomy

  5. Job/vocational training

  6. Locating health care and resources for transition to adult needs (see Chapter 13)

  7. Sibling informational needs/supports as they question continuing care responsibilities, marrying, and having children; genetic counseling as needed

V. Launching/Postparental Stage—Adult and Older Adult

In adulthood, children leave the family, may seek further education, obtain jobs, and start their own families. These options may be limited for adult children with I/DD. Some adult children lead independent lives with jobs and independent living arrangements. However, "the majority of these adult children are living with and financially dependent upon their families, are under- or unemployed, and socially isolated" (Keogh, Bernheimer, & Guthrie, 2004, p. 219).

A. Adult (see Chapter 12)

  1. Determining living arrangements—Continue living with family or independent, semi-independent, or assisted living arrangements

  2. Continuing education or training—Community college

3. Job—In community or sheltered workshop

4. Helping adult child avoid social isolation and depression

5. Marriage and parenting (Kantz, 1992; Sheerin, 1998)

    a. Supporting marriage

    b. Becoming a parent—What are family responsibilities for child care if adult child has a child; locating appropriate parenting programs; continued resources and supports

    c. Assuming parental responsibilities for child of the adult child with I/DD with health and financial implications

B. Later adulthood—Increased lifespans of adult children with I/DD have led to previously rare family issues related to additional health problems of the adult children (e.g., heart disease, cancer, osteoporosis, dementia, etc.) as well as deteriorating parental health (Pruchno & Patrick, 1999). (See Chapter 14.)

    1. Managing behavior change including increased aggression and hostility and possible loss of self-care skills.

    2. Dealing with physical effects of aging and/or the secondary effects of the I/DD on the adult child.

    3. Deteriorating health of parents, specifically mother, and inability to provide care for adult child.

    4. Ongoing family care responsibilities may devolve to the oldest female sibling. This caregiver may be providing care for parents and sibling with I/DD as well as own nuclear family.

    5. Identifying family support groups focused on family issues for this stage in family lifespan.

    6. Relief of stress for primary caregiver; if the caregiver views caregiving as a burden, they are 62% more likely to experience an early death (Schultz & Beach, 1999).

    7. Making plans for the future—The majority of families do no planning for the future.

        a. Out of home placement

            i. Living with another family member; African American families use this option most frequently as they believe family members should care for their family member with an I/DD.

            ii. Group home or assisted living arrangements; often long (years) waiting lists, so families need to plan in advance.

            iii. Nursing homes or long-term care facilities.

        b. Health and social services appropriate for needs of family member.

        c. Respite care for caregivers if family member remains in home.

    d. Power of attorney, custody, and financial arrangements—Who has legal authority for health care decisions; financial and legal affairs.

  8. Death and bereavement of parents and adult child

  9. Sibling issues

    a. Strongest bonds/relationships are between sisters.

    b. Youngest brothers in families tend to have least information about the sibling with an I/DD.

    c. Oldest sister tends to become care provider for both the adult and child and parents.

    d. Trend of smaller families with fewer children may mean fewer sibling options and support availability in the future.

VI. Role of Health Care Professionals in Working with Families

A. Support the family through various stages across the lifespan.

B. Respect the family's definition of the situation and their means of providing care for their family member.

C. Develop collaborative relationships with the family rather than an authoritarian, paternalistic relationship.

D. Acknowledge the skills, knowledge, and competence of the family in providing appropriate care.

E. Listen to the family and actively collaborate with them in health care decisions.

F. Provide anticipatory guidance for families regarding issues arising at various points in the lifespan.

VII. Summary

The comprehensive care of an individual with I/DD, of any age, often involves interaction with family members. This chapter has explored a number of family theories, relationships, and issues that must be considered by nurses and health care professionals working with this population.

References

Briskin, H., & Liptak, G. S. (1995). Helping families with children with developmental disabilities. *Pediatric Annals, 24,* 262–266.

Clare, L., Garnier, H., & Gallimore, R. (1998). Parents' developmental expectations and child characteristics: Longitudinal study of children with developmental delays and their families. *American Journal on Mental Retardation, 103,* 117–129.

Clawson, J. A. (1998). A child with chronic illness and the process of family adaptation. *Journal of Pediatric Nursing, 11,* 52–61.

Deatrick, J. A., Knafl, K. A., & Murphy-Moore, C. (1999). Clarifying the concept of normalization. *Image: Journal of Nursing Scholarship, 31,* 209–214.

Eakes, G. G., Burke, M. L., & Hainsworth, M. A. (1998). Middle-range theory of chronic sorrow. *Image: Journal of Nursing Scholarship, 30,* 179–184.

Freedman, R. I., & Boyer, N. C. (2000). The power to choose: Support for families caring for individuals with developmental disabilities. *Health and Social Work, 25,* 59–68.

Kantz, J. L. (1992). Enhancing the parenting skills of developmentally disabled parents: A nursing perspective. *Journal of Community Nursing, 9,* 209–219.

Kazak, A. E. (1986). Families with physically handicapped children: Social ecology and family systems. *Family Process, 25,* 265–281.

Keogh, B. K., Berhheimer, L. P., & Guthrie, D. (2004). Children with developmental delays twenty years later: Where are they? How are they? *American Journal on Mental Retardation, 109,* 219–230.

Knafl, K. A., Breitmayer, B., Gallo, A., & Zoeller, L. (1996). Family response to childhood chronic illness: Description of management styles. *Journal of Pediatric Nursing, 11,* 315–326.

Lam, L., & Mackenzie, A. E. (2002). Coping with a child with Down syndrome: The experiences of mothers in Hong Kong. *Qualitative Health Research, 12,* 223–227.

Miltiades, H. B., & Pruchno, R. (2001). Mothers of adults with developmental disability: Change over time. *American Journal on Mental Retardation, 106,* 548–561.

Monsen, R. B. (1999). Mothers' experiences of living worried when parenting children with spina bifida. *Journal of Pediatric Nursing, 14,* 157–163.

Pruchno, R., & Patrick, J. H. (1999). Mothers and fathers of adults with chronic disabilities. *Research on Aging, 21,* 682–713.

Schultz, G., & Beach, S. R. (1999). Caregiving as a risk factor for mortality: The caregiver health effects study. *Journal of the American Medical Association, 282,* 2215–2219.

Seligman, M., & Darling, R. (1997). *Ordinary families, special children: A systems approach to childhood disability* (2nd ed.). New York: The Guilford Press.

Sheerin, F. (1998). Parents with learning disabilities; A review of the literature. *Journal of Advanced Nursing, 28,* 126–133.

Thorne, S. E., & Robinson, C. A. (1989). Guarded alliance: Health care relationships in chronic illness. *Image: Journal of Nursing Scholarship, 21,* 153–157.

Health Care Policy Issues

VI

Cultural and Ethnic Issues

Wendy M. Nehring, RN, PhD, FAAN, FAAMR
and Sheryl White-Scott, MD, FAAMR

25

Objectives

At the completion of this chapter, the learner will be able to:

1. Distinguish among the definitions of culture, race, and ethnicity.
2. Describe cultural characteristics.
3. Discuss the factors that influence assimilation to the majority culture.
4. Discuss the implications of the census projections for percentages of ethnic groups now and in the future.
5. Synthesize the cultural influences on poverty and health.
6. Identify steps for health professionals to become more culturally sensitive and competent.
7. Analyze the statistics concerning minorities with intellectual and developmental disabilities (I/DD).
8. Discuss culturally sensitive assessment and intervention strategies for use with minority families who have a member with I/DD.

Key Points

- The United States is a multicultural society.
- Individuals from a particular ethnic background are heterogenous; they may share similar traditions, but may be assimilated to various degrees and may be influenced by other subcultures, such as socioeconomic level.
- Little information is known about growth, developmental milestones, and parenting practices for different cultures.
- More minority children than nonminority children are identified as having an I/DD.
- Care of the person with I/DD who is also a member of a minority must be culturally sensitive and involve a comprehensive assessment and intervention plan.

I.   Introduction

A. The United States is a multicultural society and it is imperative that each individual is knowledgeable and sensitive to each culture's mores and tenets.

B. Little is known and written about in regards to persons with I/DD who are also members of a minority culture.

C. Persons with I/DD belong to a subculture.

D. A third subculture, poverty, may also be an aspect of the life of a person with I/DD.

II.   Definitions

A. Culture

1. Slaughter-Defoe and colleagues (1990) defined culture as "the sum total of mores, traditions, and beliefs of how we function, and encompasses other products of human works and thoughts specific to members of an intergenerational group, community, or population" (p. 363).

2. Rehm (1999) defined culture as "a dynamic and negotiated social construction arising from interaction and resulting in shared understandings among people in contact with one another" (p. 66).

3. Lynch and Hanson (1998) emphasized that culture is dynamic with traditions, behaviors, mores, and beliefs constantly influenced by acculturation.

B. Race

1. Individuals with similar identity factors, such as social and political status (Rehm, 1999).

C. Ethnicity

1. Individuals with characteristics, such as geographic origin, religion, and/or language, in common (Rehm, 1999).

III. Cultural Characteristics (St. Clair & McKenry, 1999)

A. Communication—assess communication patterns

B. Space—assess patterns of personal space

C. Time—assess how time is measured

D. Social organization—assess whether family prefers close nuclear familial arrangements or integrated community interactions

E. Environmental controls—assess health and illness beliefs and traditions as well as whether the family is internally or externally oriented

F. Biological variations—assess genetic variations, nutritional habits, skin color, body structure, and susceptibility to disease (Giger & Davidhizar, 1999).

IV. Acculturation Is the Assimilation of the Majority Culture over Generations.

Assimilation is influenced by:

A. Socioeconomic status

B. Educational level

C. Number of generations living in the United States

D. Proximity to other cultures

E. Proximity to members of own cultural group

F. Gender

G. Age

H. Immigration experiences

I. Ability to comprehend and speak English. The Bureau of Primary Health Care of the Health, Resources, and Services Administration (HRSA) (2001) found that primary care providers often ordered fewer or more diagnostic tests due to a lack of understanding when the individual was unable to clearly describe their symptoms.

J. Sociopolitical climate and cultural stigma, if present (Lynch & Hanson, 1998)

V. Intellectual Differences

It is not important to discuss whether different cultures have innately different intellectual levels, but to learn what are the cultural learning priorities (Fagan, 2000). Individuals living in rural, agricultural societies experience life and cultural characteristics listed above differently from individuals living in urban, technological societies.

VI. History

It is very important to understand the history of the culture in order to provide culturally competent care.

VII. Census Projections

A. In 2020, the United States Census Bureau (2002b) predicts that the percentage of persons of Caucasian backgrounds in the U.S. will equal 63.8%. In 2050, the Caucasian population will drop to 52.8% and in 2100, this percentage will drop even further to 40.3%.

B. Hispanics and Asian and Pacific Islanders percentages will triple. Currently, the Hispanic population is approximately 12.1%. This percentage is projected to increase to 16% in 2020, 24.3% in 2050, and 33.3% in 2100 (U.S. Census Bureau, 2002b). Specifically, Hispanic children will comprise 20% of all children in the United States in 2100 (Federal Interagency Forum on Child and Family

Statistics, 2003). Asian and Pacific Islanders will increase from the current 4% to 12.6% in 2100 (U.S. Census Bureau, 2002b).

C. In contrast, the Black population will remain stable, increasing from 12.2% in 2001 to 13% in 2100 (U.S. Census Bureau, 2002b).

VIII. Culture and Poverty

A. More children from minority cultures live in poverty (Blackwell & Tonthat, 2003; Federal Interagency Forum on Child and Family Statistics, 2003).

B. Health status decreases as poverty increases.

C. Poverty influences intelligence (Breslau et al., 2001). This may be due to the fact that immigrants often have lower levels of education with many lacking a high school diploma (U.S. Census Bureau, 2002a).

IX. Cultural Influences on Health

A. In 2001, 24% of Hispanic children, 14% of Black children, and 7% of Caucasian children did not have health insurance nor an identified primary care provider (Federal Interagency Forum on Child and Family Statistics, 2003).

B. Uninsured adults with chronic conditions have been found to be less likely to obtain evidence-based standards of practice in the treatment of their condition than are people with insurance.

C. Children from minority cultures also had less access to private health care providers (Weinick & Krauss, 2000).

D. With increased numbers of children born to interracial and ethnic couples, diseases that have been identified as occurring more frequently in certain ethnic groups will become more diffuse and will require close assessment of an individual's ethnic background through a pedigree analysis (Lashley, 1998).

E. Researchers have found that African Americans had less trust in their primary care providers due to personal privacy issues and the fear of experimentation against their will (Boulware, Cooper, Ratner, LaVeist, & Powe, 2003).

F. Little information is available on patterns of growth, developmental milestones, and parenting practices for different cultures.

X. Cultural Competence in Nurses and Health Care Professionals

A. Campinha-Bacote's (1999) model of cultural competence includes four constructs:

1. Cultural awareness—Initial attempts to understand one's own cultural mores, traditions, and beliefs and prejudices about other cultures leading to an appreciation of one's own and other cultures.

2. Cultural knowledge—Learn about the mores, traditions, and beliefs of other cultures.

3. Cultural skill—Acquire in-depth knowledge of other cultures in order to adapt health care according to cultural values and beliefs concerning health care and specific beliefs about illness and health.

4. Cultural encounters—Competence in providing culturally sensitive care increases as care-giving experiences increase.

5. Obtaining cultural competence is a lifelong process (Roberts & Evans, 1997).

B. Specifically, culturally sensitive health care professionals are able to:

1. Discern cultural differences in family strengths, child rearing practices, and family coping methods.

2. Involve the family in the development and follow-up of the treatment plan for the child.

3. Set health goals based on the family's cultural beliefs, traditions, and mores.

4. Assist the family to negotiate and obtain needed health care and associated services in places that are culturally sensitive and, at best, of the same cultural background.

5. Respect that family's cultural values, beliefs, traditions, and mores (Rehm, 1999).

C. Health care professionals must assess their own viewpoints about persons with I/DD and learn about different cultural opinions of persons with I/DD; they must become culturally sensitive and competent in their practice (Habel, 2001; Robinson & Rathbone, 1999)

XI. Persons with I/DD from Other Cultures

A. Definition of I/DD is found in Chapter 2.

B. The prevalence of I/DD is found in Chapter 4.

C. According to the U.S. Census Bureau (2001), based on 1997 data, the percentage of minority adults with disabilities of any kind with activity limitations was 21.3% Blacks (15.7% severely disabled), 13.8% Hispanics (9.7% severely disabled), and 13% Asians and Pacific Islanders (8.5% severely disabled).

D. Pleis and Coles (2003) reported slightly higher results from their 1999 data: 35% Native American and Alaskans, 26% African American, 18% Hispanic, and 17% Asian and Pacific Islanders.

E. Data available on the numbers of children from different cultures with disabilities can be estimated from the numbers of children in special education (U.S. Department of Education, Office of Special Education Programs, 2002).

1. The number of U.S. children, ages 6 to 21 years, in the 2001–2002 academic year in special education was approximately 5.9 million children.

2. Of that number, 20.3% were Black, 15.4% Hispanic, 1.9% Asian and Pacific Islanders, and 1.3% American Indian and Alaskans.

3. The greatest percentage of children in special education in New Mexico (52.5%) and California (42.3%) were Hispanic.

4. The greatest percentage of children in special education in the District of Columbia (90.8%), Mississippi (54.5%), and Louisiana (53.2%) were Black.

5. The reported number of children, aged birth to 2 years, in early intervention programs in 2001 was 246,199 students.

6. The greatest percentage of children in early intervention in California (50.9%) and New Mexico (49.2%) were Hispanic.

7. The greatest percentage of children in early intervention in the District of Columbia (70.6%) and Mississippi (53.9%) were Black.

F. African American (Black) and Native American children have been found to be overrepresented in special education (Fujiura & Yamaki, 2000; Oswald, Coutinho, Best, & Nguyen, 2001; U.S. Department of Education, 2002). This may be a result of:

1. Language

2. Discrimination by school administrators and/or teachers

3. Discrimination by intelligence testers

4. Poverty

G. Preventive care is often lacking for persons with I/DD. Lewis and colleagues (2002) found a large percentage of adults with I/DD receiving psychotropic medications without appropriate diagnosis (see Chapters 18 and 19).

H. In recent years, many children are being internationally adopted and often have growth and developmental concerns (e.g., Judge, 2003) (see Chapter 9).

I. Families with a member with an I/DD had lower income levels and were more likely to need governmental support. Minority status resulted in lower levels of income and often dependence on welfare (Fujiura, 1998; Fujiura & Yamaki, 1997).

XII. Culturally Sensitive Assessment and Intervention Strategies for Use with Minority Families with a Member with I/DD

A. Areas of focus (McCallion, Janicki, & Grant-Griffin, 1997). Questions should be developmentally-age appropriate.

1. Perception of the I/DD (Bennett, Zhang, & Hojnar, 1998)

a. Is there an educational, health, or social emphasis?

b. What are health beliefs in relation to the I/DD?

c. Is the diagnosis and etiology understood? Who knows the diagnosis and etiology? Explore positive and negative beliefs about the etiology (e.g., bad blood, family curse, blessing from God, etc.).

d. What current supports does the family use?

e. How does the family's culture and/or religion affect this perception? Are cultural health practices used by this family? (Rogers-Dulan & Blacher, 1995; Skinner, Correa, Skinner, & Bailey, 2001; Zola & Groce, 1993)

2. Definition of the family

a. What is the family's structure? List the members of the identified family (McCubbin, Thompson, Thompson, McCubbin, & Kaston, 1993).

b. Is the family's locus of control internal or external?

c. Who is the head of the family?

d. What member of the family makes the majority of health care decisions?

e. Who is (are) the major caregiver(s) for the person with an I/DD?

f. Where does the family member with an I/DD live? If the family member with an I/DD lives away from their biological family, for example, in a group home or developmental center, what part does the biological family play in the life of the person with an I/DD?

g. Researchers have found that African Americans with an I/DD living in group homes are often segregated in homes that only have African Americans living in them. Caucasians with an I/DD live in group homes where only Caucasians reside. The group homes where African Americans lived were often less safe, less hygienic, and were located in rural settings (Howard et al., 2002).

h. Who does the person with an I/DD interact with in the family most frequently? Who do they have the closest relationships with?

i. What are the communication patterns of this family?

j. Does the family have pets?

3. Caretaker identification

a. Who is the primary caretaker, if any, of the person with an I/DD? What responsibilities do they have? How do they perceive the stress in their lives? What outlets do they have? What formal and informal supports do they use? What is the relationship of the primary caretaker to the family member with an I/DD?

b. Does this person speak English? What is their acculturation?

c. What is the cultural stigma to having a family member with an I/DD?

d. Is the caretaker's health affected?

e. If the family member with an I/DD is a child, do the parents treat the siblings differently?

f. Increased levels of depression have been found in Latino mothers caring for a child with an I/DD (Blacher, Lopez, Shapiro, & Fusco, 1997; Blacher, Shapiro, Lopez, Diaz, & Fusco, 1997) and increased levels of stress have been found in Korean mothers (Shin, 2002). These researchers compared these cultures with American, Caucasian mothers.

4. Process family uses for decision making

   a. Determine who is mainly responsible for making decisions in this family.

   b. Obtain contact information and make sure that this (these) individual(s) are present when important health decisions and/or insurance decisions are discussed.

   c. There has been no research reported on the decision-making processes used by families with a member with an I/DD.

   d. McCallion and colleagues (1997) did find that families closely considered advice and recommendations from extended family members and friends.

5. Expectations of each family member

   a. Identify the expectations that each family member has for themselves and the other members of their family. Assess for discrepancies and the influence of culture and acculturation on these opinions.

   b. What is the social role for each family member? This may influence the family's investment, including financial, in this individual.

   c. Provide recommendations for or loans of articles and books that discuss family and individual experiences with a family member, usually a child, who has an I/DD.

   d. Recommend parent and/or individual support groups in the geographical area that the family lives. May want to accompany the family or individual to their first meeting.

   e. After permission from the family, could facilitate a visit from a parent or individual with the same diagnosis.

6. Family and individual support systems

   a. Identify the family and individual informal and formal support systems. Discern whether these supports are positive and helpful. List their strengths and limitations. Identify if there are any negative supports and what steps may need to be taken to assist in the alleviation of the stress from this relationship.

   b. Assess any stigma that the family and/or individual with an I/DD may experience (Gartner, Lipsky, & Turnbull, 1991).

   c. Does the family and/or individual with an I/DD have difficulty with access to transportation? To health care?

   d. Who is (are) the primary health care provider(s) for the family member with an I/DD? Is the family and/or individual with an I/DD aware of other health care services they might receive (if applicable)? Does the individual with an I/DD see a specialist for that specific condition?

e. If needed, seek an interdisciplinary assessment for the individual with an I/DD.

7. Patterns of and reason for relocation

a. What is the reason(s) for the family to relocate to this country and/or this city? How often have they moved and why?

8. Family and cultural values

a. Identify the family's and individual's with an I/DD's cultural health values and how they influence health care decisions. What is most important?

b. Identify help-seeking styles and child-rearing practices and beliefs.

9. Initial language

a. What members of the family speak English? Do they understand and speak English well? Does the individual with an I/DD understand and speak English well? If not, who interprets for the family? Health care providers should not rely on a child, younger than 12 years, as the interpreter for the family. This is very important for purposes of informed consent.

b. Does the individual with an I/DD have language difficulties that require accommodation and/or speech equipment? Is the health care provider able to understand the person with an I/DD?

c. How many languages do the family and/or individual speak? What is the primary language spoken? (Barrera, 1993)

10. Relationships with primary health care providers

a. What is the family's opinion about sharing information and asking questions of primary health care providers? What is the family's opinion about frequency of visits with the primary care provider? Specialty care provider?

b. Build trust with the family and individual with an I/DD.

c. Identify family and individual barriers to complying with the health care management plan.

d. Provide interdisciplinary care.

e. Minority children see a primary care physician less often than Caucasian children. African Americans and Hispanics use the emergency department more frequently for primary health care than do Caucasian families (Federal Interagency Forum on Child and Family Statistics, 2003).

f. Health care assessment instruments should be culturally sensitive, age appropriate, and in the family's primary language (Center for Children with Chronic Illness and Disability, 1999).

g. Health care providers should be aware of current research and statistics regarding the health care management of persons of all ages, and from different cultures, with an I/DD.

XIII. Summary

We live in a multicultural and global society. Having an I/DD, being from a minority culture, and/or being poor, add multilayers. The nurse and other health care professionals must be knowledgeable and sensitive to cultural mores and tenets.

References

Barrera, I. (1993). Effective and appropriate instruction for all children: The challenge of cultural/linguistic diversity and young children with special needs. *Topics in Early Childhood Special Education, 13,* 461–487.

Bennett, T., Zhang, C., & Hojnar, L. (1998). Facilitating the full participation of culturally diverse families in the IFSP/IEP process. *Infant-Toddler Intervention, The Transdisciplinary Journal, 8,* 227–249.

Blacher, J., Lopez, S., Shapiro, J., & Fusco, J. (1997). Contributions to depression in Latina mothers with and without children with retardation: Implications for caregiving. *Family Relations, 46,* 325–334.

Blacher, J., Shapiro, J., Lopez, S., Diaz, L., & Fusco, J. (1997). Depression in Latina mothers of children with mental retardation: A neglected concern. *American Journal of Mental Retardation, 101,* 483–496.

Blackwell, D. L., & Tonthat, L. (2003). Summary health statistics for U.S. children: National Health Interview Survey, 1999. *Vital Health Statistics 10* (210). Hyattsville, MD: National Center for Health Statistics.

Boulware, L. E., Cooper, L. A., Ratner, L. E., LaVeist, T. A., & Powe, N. R. (2003). Race and trust in the health care system. *Public Health Reports, 118*(3, Special Issue), 358–365.

Breslau, N., Chilcoat, H. D., Susser, E. S., Matte, T., Liang, K. Y., & Peterson, E. L. (2001). Stability and change in children's intelligence quotient scores: A comparison of two socioeconomically disparate communities. *American Journal of Epidemiology, 154,* 711–717.

Bureau of Primary Health Care, Health Resources, and Services Administration. (2001). *Provider's guide to quality and culture.* Retrieved October 16, 2001 from http://erc.msh.org

Campinha-Bacote, J. (1999). A model and instrument for addressing cultural competence in health care. *Journal of Nursing Education, 38,* 203–207.

Center for Children with Chronic Illness and Disability. (1999). *Children, youth, and families: Building on cultural strengths. The second five years* (pp. 6–7). Washington, DC: Author.

Fagan, J. F. (2000). A theory of intelligence as processing: Implications for society. *Psychology, Public Policy, and Law, 6,* 168–179.

Federal Interagency Forum on Child and Family Statistics. (2003). *America's children: Key national indicators of well-being 2003.* Vienna, VA: National Maternal and Child Health Clearinghouse.

Fujiura, G. T. (1998). Demography of family households. *American Journal of Mental Retardation, 103,* 225–235.

Fujiura, G. T., & Yamaki, K. (1997). Analysis of ethnic variations in developmental disability prevalence and household economic status. *Mental Retardation, 35,* 286–294.

Fujiura, G. T., & Yamaki, K. (2000). Trends in demography of childhood poverty and disability. *Exceptional Children, 66,* 187–199.

Gartner, A., Lipsky, D. K., & Turnbull, A. P. (1991). *Supporting families with a child with a disability: An international outlook.* Baltimore: Paul H. Brookes.

Giger, J. N., & Davidhizar, R. E. (1999). *Transcultural nursing: Assessment and intervention* (3rd ed.). St. Louis, MO: Mosby.

Habel, M. (January 15, 2001). Caring for people of many cultures: The challenge for nursing. *NurseWeek*, 21–22.

Howard, D. L., Sloane, P. D., Zimmerman, S., Eckert, K., Walsh, J. F., & Buie, V. C. (2002). Distribution of African Americans in residential care/assisted living and nursing homes: More evidence of racial disparity? *American Journal of Public Health, 92*, 1272–1277.

Judge, S. (2003). Developmental recovery and deficit in children adopted from Eastern European orphanages. *Child Psychiatry and Human Development, 34*, 49–62.

Lashley, F. R. (1998). *Clinical genetics in nursing practice* (2nd ed.). New York: Springer.

Lewis, M. A., Lewis, C. E., Leake, B., King, B. H., & Lindemann, R. (2002). The quality of health care for adults with developmental disabilities. *Public Health Reports, 117*, 174–184.

Lynch, E. W., & Hanson, M. J. (Eds.). (1998). *A guide for working with children and their families: Developing cross-cultural competence* (2nd ed.). Baltimore: Paul H. Brookes.

McCallion, P., Janicki, M., & Grant-Griffin, L. (1997). Exploring the impact of culture and acculturation on older families caregiving for persons with developmental disabilities. *Family Relations, 46*, 347–357.

McCubbin, H. I., Thompson, E. A., Thompson, A. I., McCubbin, M. A., & Kaston, A. J. (1993). Culture, ethnicity, and the family: Critical factors in childhood chronic illnesses and disabilities. *Pediatrics, 91*, 1063–1070.

Oswald, D. P., Coutinho, M. J., Best, A. M., & Nguyen, N. (2001). Impact of sociodemographic characteristics on the identification rates of minority students as having mental retardation. *Mental Retardation, 39*, 351–367.

Pleis, J. R., & Coles, R. (2003). *Summary health statistics for U.S. adults: National Health Interview Survey, 1999.* Vital Health Statistics 10 (212). Hyattsville, MD: National Center for Health Statistics.

Rehm, R. S. (1999). Family culture and chronic conditions. In P. L. Jackson & J. A. Vessey (Eds.). *Primary care of the child with a chronic condition* (3rd ed., pp. 66–82). St. Louis, MO: Mosby.

Roberts, R. N., & Evans, J. E. (1997). Cultural competency. In H. M. Wallace, R. F. Biehl, J. C. MacQueen, & J. A. Blackman (Eds.). *Mosby's resource guide to children with disabilities and chronic illness* (pp. 117–136). St. Louis, MO: Mosby.

Robinson, E. G., & Rathbone, G. N. (1999). Impact of race, poverty, and ethnicity on services for persons with mental disabilities: Call for cultural competence. *Mental Retardation, 37*, 333–338.

Rogers-Dulan, J., & Blacher, J. (1995). African American families, religion, and disability: A conceptual framework. *Mental Retardation, 33*, 226–238.

Shin, J. Y. (2002). Social support for families of children with mental retardation: Comparison between Korea and the United States. *Mental Retardation, 40*, 103–118.

Skinner, D. G., Correa, V., Skinner, M., & Bailey, D. B. Jr. (2001). Role of religion in the lives of Latino families of young children with developmental delays. *American Journal on Mental Retardation, 106*, 297–313.

Slaughter-Defoe, D. T., Nakagwa, K., Takanishi, R., & Johnson, D. J. (1990). Toward cultural/ecological perspectives on schooling and achievement in African- and Asian-American children. *Child Development, 61*, 363–383.

St. Clair, A., & McKenry, L. (1999). Preparing culturally competent practitioners. *Journal of Nursing Education, 38*, 228–234.

U.S. Census Bureau. (2001). *Americans with disabilities: 1997—Table 1.* Retrieved September 1, 2003 from http://www.census.gov/hhes/www/disable/sipp/disab97/ds97t1.html

U.S. Census Bureau. (2002a). *Population profile of the United States: 2000 (Internet release).* Retrieved September 1, 2003 from http://www.census.gov/population/pop-profile/2000/

U.S. Census Bureau. (2002b). *Projections of the resident population by race, Hispanic origin, and nativity: Middle series.* Retrieved August 31, 2003 from http://www.census.gov/population/projections/nation/summary/

U.S. Department of Education, Office of Special Education Programs. (2002). *Racial/ethnic composition (number) of students ages 6–21 served under IDEA, Part B by disability, during the 2001–2002 school year—All disabilities.* Retrieved August 31, 2003 from http://www.ideadata.org/tables25th/ar_aa15.htm

Weinick, R. M., & Krauss, N. A. (2000). Racial/ethnic differences in children's access to care. *American Journal of Public Health, 90,* 1771–1774.

Zola, I. K., & Groce, N. E. (1993). Multiculturalism, chronic illness, and disability: Some issues are universal. *Children's Health Issues, 2*(1), 4–5.

Ethical and Legal Issues

Teresa A. Savage, RN, PhD

26

Objectives

At the completion of this chapter, the learner will be able to:

1. Articulate ethical and legal issues using the appropriate terminology.
2. Describe ethical principles underlying the care for people with intellectual and developmental disabilities (I/DD).
3. Identify legal issues in the care of people with I/DD.

Key Points

- The self-determination of people with I/DD should be respected and facilitated unless there is evidence they do not have the capacity to make certain decisions.
- Autonomy can be exercised by a surrogate, but only if all efforts to maximize the person's decision-making capacity have failed.
- Guardianship, whether plenary or limited, should be sought only if it is in the best interests of the person with I/DD.

I.   Overview

Ethical issues surrounding persons with I/DD focus on the support needed for self-determination. All people need some degree of support and often people with I/DD need more than average. Especially in health care, people with I/DD may need support in accessing health care and making health care decisions. The law provides mechanisms for identifying others to make health care decisions for people with I/DD who may lack the capacity for making a specific decision. The law offers a dichotomy, however, of determining whether a person is competent or incompetent. Often the capacity to make decisions is not a dichotomy but a gradation of skills and abilities dependent upon the decision to be made, the context, and the available support.

The self-advocacy movement is shifting from paternalism to a "dignity of risk" approach. It can be argued, however, that paternalism is still appropriate in some circumstances. Children under 18 years require supervision and guidance whether or not they have a diagnosis of I/DD. Those with the diagnosis may require more supervision if their skills in judgment and reasoning are immature. Over the age of 18 years, some adults may require more supervision that will enable them to live and work in the least restrictive environment. Usually the greater the degree of I/DD, the more support, supervision, and assistive care needed.

II.   Issues of Autonomy

A. Autonomy is enacted by respect for persons regardless of cognitive and/or motoric abilities; decisional capacity is presumed for all adults unless evidence is to the contrary.

B. Decisional capacity is the "ability to comprehend information, weigh the potential benefits and risks of the choices, appreciate the implications of the information to one's situation, and to make a choice" (Grisso & Appelbaum, 1998, p. 31). Competence is the legal term; one is competent until adjudicated to be incompetent.

C. Persons unable to make their own health care decisions should have decisions made by a surrogate using substituted judgment.

  1. Substituted judgment standard—A surrogate decides based on what that person would have decided if capable; the person, when previously capable of deciding, expressed wishes pertaining to this or a similar situation and the surrogate's decisions reflect those wishes (President's Commission for the Study of Ethical Problems in Medicine and Biomedical and Behavioral Research, 1983).

  2. Ideally, the person will have support to make his or her own decisions; lacking that, however, a surrogate should be identified. For health care decisions, state statutes may describe a process to follow to identify a surrogate decision maker.

3. For people who are nonverbal, augmentative communication may be employed to learn their wishes (check specific state laws or use augmentative communication, if present).

D. Parents are the legal guardians of children age 17 years and younger and make their health care decisions.

1. Older children and adolescents with I/DD should be included in decision making according to their abilities and the import of the decisions.

2. Parents are expected to use the best-interests standard for decision making, rather than the substituted judgment standard.

3. Best-interests standard—A surrogate decides what is the best decision for the person with I/DD without input from that person (President's Commission, 1983).

4. For children who cannot communicate, persons closest to the child such as a parent or caregiver can interpret their responses, e.g., what behaviors indicate pain, discomfort, pleasure, or satisfaction (McGrath, Rosmus, Canfield, Campbell, & Hennigar, 1998).

E. Persons 18 years and older with I/DD are presumed to be competent unless they have been declared incompetent. They may not always have the capacity to make health care decisions. Their capacity to decide should be assessed in light of the decision(s) to be made.

1. In the past, health care providers may have allowed parents of the adult with I/DD to make decisions although they had not sought legal guardianship when the child reached 18 years. Each state should have statutes indicating under what circumstances next-of-kin can provide consent for health care.

2. For those persons who do not have decisional capacity, a surrogate can be chosen according to state statutes, or a legal guardian can be appointed.

3. Physiologic and environmental factors can affect decisional capacity.

    a. Medication can cause conditions that can interfere with attention and concentration.

    b. Disruption of the routine and clinic atmospheres can cause stress for the person with I/DD and interfere with attention and concentration.

    c. Health care providers should attempt to structure the environment in such a way as to optimize the person's ability to attend to and concentrate on information.

F. Informed consent is "a product of the relationship between person and consent context" (Fisher, 2003, p. 29).

1. Although intended for consent related to research participation, Fisher's goodness-of-fit ethic can be useful for consent related to treatment.

2. Suggestions for enhancing informed consent ability are:

    a. Using understandable language and multiple modalities (pictures, videos, demonstrations)

    b. Repeating information

    c. Paying attention to context that can be stress producing (e.g., wearing white lab coats)

    d. Providing opportunities for decision making

    e. Being aware of acquiescence

G. Situations requiring health care decisions

    1. General health decisions—The person's decisional capacity should be assessed and the person, if capable, should give or refuse consent for medical treatment. The person should be made aware of mandatory testing/treatment required by the state for participation in specific programs. Health care providers should plan the examination, test, or treatment to minimize distress to the person and others. Ideally, health care providers should be selected based on their experience with persons with I/DD.

        a. Primary care—routine examinations, immunizations, screening, preventative treatment (e.g., mammograms, Pap smears, dental examinations)

        b. Secondary care—habilitation, treatment to prevent complications related to underlying disability (e.g., bracing to reduce deformity from spasticity)

        c. Tertiary care—rehabilitation, treatment of complications resulting from underlying disabilities (e.g., scoliosis surgery, gastrostomy tube for dysphagia and aspirations)

    2. Life-sustaining treatment

        a. Application of technologies such as tracheostomy, tube feedings, dialysis, mechanical ventilation, shunt for hydrocephalus, or any life-prolonging medical intervention.

        b. Project BRIDGE methodology consists of inviting persons with I/DD to tell their stories so that their wishes can be known for current decisions, or future decisions if they are unable to participate in decision making (Reynolds, 1999). Having a Values History, in lieu of an advance directive, may also be helpful (Freedman, 1998).

        c. For persons who are unable and have never been able to participate in decision making, family members (according to state statute) or a legally appointed guardian makes decisions. Assistance from the health care facility's ethics committee may be helpful.

        d. End-of-life decisions may need to be made whether or not the person has a terminal illness. Historically, treatment has been withheld or withdrawn from people with severe I/DD based on the belief that the person has a poor quality of life *because* of the I/DD. This assumption is erroneous and reflects a bias against people with I/DD. However, because a person has an I/DD and his or her preferences are not known, the person should not be forced to endure medical treatment that could be burdensome and increase the person's suffering.

e. Palliative care for people with I/DD and a terminal illness may be very similar to care for people without I/DD, but there may be distinct differences. The decision to withhold treatment and provide palliative care in otherwise nonterminal illness may be appropriate for persons with I/DD. Treatment may be more burdensome; for example, it may be necessary to sedate someone who needs hemodialysis for end-stage renal disease or chemotherapy and frequent blood draws for cancer treatment. In some circumstances, if the prognosis for cure is good, the benefit of treatment may outweigh the burdens. If treatment is unlikely to be curative, or the burden outweighs the benefit, it is ethical to forgo treatment. In those cases, palliative care should be provided in the least restrictive setting (Douglas et al., 2000; Lin, 2003; Lohiya, Tan-Figueroa, & Crinella, 2003; Nelson, 2003; Tuffrey-Wijne, 2002, 2003).

3. Special considerations in health care decisions—Laws vary from state to state, so health care providers should check with their legal affairs department

a. Reproductive issues—Sexual expression should be addressed within the social, cultural, and moral perspectives of the person's family and community.

   i. Contraception—Education regarding sexuality and appropriate social behavior should occur appropriate to the person's developmental level; contraceptive choice should be customized for the person. Methods requiring infrequent dosing, such as Norplant, may be more effective than reliance on barrier methods. Decisions about child-bearing, as with all major life decisions, should be carefully considered.

   ii. Sterilization—Given the history of forced sterilization, many state laws were changed to outlaw involuntary sterilization; however, as recently as 1994, Pennsylvania authorized the involuntary sterilization of a 26-year-old woman (Block, 2000). Should the woman with I/DD request sterilization, as with all major health decisions, her capacity to make this decision should be assessed and her decision-making process facilitated by people of her choosing.

   iii. Pregnancy and abortion—If the pregnancy was desired, then the woman should receive prenatal care and plan for labor and delivery, ideally with a practitioner experienced in caring for women with I/DD. If the pregnant woman is incapable of making decisions regarding the pregnancy, then the surrogate decision maker, or legal guardian, should make decisions in the woman's best interests. This may include continuing the pregnancy and adopting the child, placing the child with an adoption agency, or terminating the pregnancy. (There may also be criminal charges of rape since the woman is unable to consent to sexual intercourse.) In some states, a guardian has been appointed for the fetus, so health care providers should be aware of their state's law and proclivities.

b. Electroshock treatment and psychotropic medication—Again, historical abuses have practitioners cautious in the application of ECT and psychotropic medication use in people with both I/DD and mental illness. However, there are data to support the use of ECT in people with I/DD (Aziz, Maixner, DeQuardo, Aldridge, & Tandon, 2001; Cutajar & Wilson, 1999; Little, McFarlane, & Ducharme, 2002). If the standard of care is ECT or psychotropic medication, then the ethical focus becomes the consent process where a guardian or a committee may be involved. State laws provide a method for obtaining consent when the person is unable to consent (O'Sullivan & Borcherding, 2002).

c. Organ transplantation—Donation—Living donation: If consent can be obtained from the person with I/DD to donate, and all other criteria for organ donation is met, then a person with I/DD is not specifically excluded from donating part or all of an organ (United Network for Organ Sharing, 2004). It may be useful to consult the ethics committee at the transplant center when donation is contemplated. Donation after death: If the person with I/DD could give informed consent regarding organ donation upon death, then organs can be retrieved. If the wishes of the person are unknown, the next of kin may be able to donate organs after death, depending upon state statute.

d. Organ transplantation—Recipient: There is a dearth of literature on organ transplantation for people with I/DD. Transplant centers set their criteria for transplantation. Because of the risks and the need for strict adherence to post-transplant care, some people with I/DD (and many without I/DD) may not be candidates for transplants. U.K., Australian, Canadian, and U.S. transplant centers have performed kidney transplants in people with I/DD (Baqi, Tejani, & Sullivan, 1998; Benedetti et al., 1998), but it is suspected that many people with I/DD who would be eligible for organs are not listed (Leonard, Eastham, & Dark, 2000). In addition to issues of consent, there is concern about the immune system and the effect of long-term immunosuppression on someone with a predisposition to malignancies.

e. Participation in medical research—Abuses such as the Willowbrook Hepatitis study and polio vaccine studies represent a disregard for the rights and personhood of people with I/DD. In order to protect people with I/DD from exploitation in research, they were systematically excluded. The value of determining efficacy of treatments with certain groups would be denied to people with I/DD if they are excluded from research. The National Institutes of Health require justification for excluding certain vulnerable groups from research. The National Bioethics Advisory Commission (1998) issued a report on research with persons lacking decision-making capacity and made a number of recommendations for change that would permit inclusion of people with I/DD in research. Recognizing the challenges, some authors propose methods of obtaining consent from people with I/DD (Fisher, 2003; Freedman, 2001), while another opposes including people with I/DD in research (Edwards, 2000).

   i.   Have the person identify a trusted family member or friend to be present during the consent discussions.

   ii.   Alter the consent environment to reduce stress and enhance the person's welfare.

   iii.   Alter the research design, if needed, to reduce the person's vulnerability to harm.

   iv.   Be aware of the tendency of the person to acquiesce to authority.

   v.   Use understandable language, repeat information, and use multiple modalities to convey information.

   vi.   If the research is likely to be beneficial to the person, but the person lacks capacity to consent, a surrogate may provide permission authorizing the person's inclusion in research; assent, the affirmative agreement to participate, must be obtained from the person. The lack of objection is not adequate to presume assent.

   vii.   If the research is nontherapeutic and poses more than minimal risk of harm, a surrogate may not authorize a person's inclusion in research.

H. Ethics concerns/questions

  1. A person's right to self-determination must be weighed with others' obligation to protect; how paternalism is balanced with autonomy is individual to each situation.

  2. Paternalism has a role in protecting society's most vulnerable people, but it can be oppressive, and therefore must be justified.

  3. Persons with I/DD should be permitted to make choices that could result in harm if they are exercising their autonomy. They should have the dignity of risk, as do others without I/DD (Millar, 1998).

  4. Health care providers have a role in fostering the autonomy of persons who may lack decisional capacity. Through familiarity with resources for assessing decisional capacity, deliberating ethical issues, and determining legal status for informed consent, the health care providers can make appropriate referrals, assist in the assessment process and ethical deliberations, and thereby protect and advocate for the rights of persons with I/DD.

III. Issues of Beneficence

A. Beneficence is the ethical principle of doing or bringing about good.

B. Advocacy

1. Health care providers advocate for persons with I/DD by fostering their autonomy through informed decision making. If a surrogate is the decision maker, the health care provider can assist in the decision-making process by participating in team conferences to determine the wishes and best interests of the person with I/DD.

2. Integration into the community should occur with accommodations to special needs and vigilance in preventing exploitation or abuse.

C. Self-determination

1. Persons should have access to services that would maximize their potential for pursuit of those objectives that fulfill their lives.

2. Persons without I/DD are expected to make choices determining the course of their lives; persons with I/DD may not have the same choices. They may not desire to pursue educational, therapeutic, or employment activities. Because of their disability, they are expected to work in an environment appropriate to their functional social level. Should the person with I/DD be "forced" to go to school, therapy, or work as part of life, or be allowed to refuse? Should a person upon reaching age 65 be allowed to retire and stop attending workshop or day programs?

IV. Issues of Nonmaleficence

A. Nonmaleficence is the principle of preventing harm.

B. Prevention of exploitation

1. Persons with I/DD may require supervision in living arrangements, educational and therapy programs, employment, and social activities. The degree and type of supervision will vary, but should be aimed at the least restrictive required to protect the person from harm. If appropriate, and as a last resort, guardianship may be necessary.

   a. Plenary guardianship means that the guardian makes all decisions related to the person and the person's property.

   b. Limited guardianship means that the guardian makes decisions only pertaining to a limited area, specified by the court, such as health care decisions or managing the person's money.

2. There is ethical tension between respecting the person's autonomy and wishing to protect the person from possible harm when that person may not be able to self-protect. Limited guardianship may offer a compromise between autonomy and paternalism.

C. Prevention of abuse

    1. Appropriate supervision during all activities, including traveling to and from home, work, school, and other places, is imperative.

    2. Again the tension between autonomy and the person's right to privacy must be weighed against the risk of abuse.

V.   Issues of Justice

A. Justice represents fairness and equity; a just distribution of the goods and burdens of society.

B. Liberty

    1. Living arrangements should reflect the least restrictive environment that can be secured.

    2. The person should be offered a choice in vocation/employment that is consistent with skills, aptitude, social skills, and personal preferences.

    3. The person should have access to leisure activities appropriate for developmental and maturational level, skills, and personal preferences.

C. Criminal justice

    1. People with I/DD may not have access to necessary supports when they interact with the criminal justice system, either as victims, potential witnesses, defendants, or prisoners, so that they can receive fair treatment (American Association on Mental Retardation (AAMR), 2003).

    2. Health care providers may be asked to assess capacity or otherwise assist persons with I/DD to exercise their rights.

    3. It is the position of the American Association on Mental Retardation that "individuals whose capabilities are greater than those of people whose disabilities require either extensive or pervasive supports must be held responsible by some form of incarceration, even to potentially drastic levels, inclusive of life imprisonment. Still, the U.S. Supreme Court has consistently held that mental retardation and mental disabilities constitute mitigating circumstances, and evidence of its existence must be included in jury deliberations, both in the guilt/innocence phase and the sentencing phase" (American Association on Mental Retardation, 2001, p. 1).

D. Distributive justice

    1. Nondiscrimination in health care (see also Chapter 5)

       a. Access to life-saving technologies if desired, or intensive care and emergency care—There may be a presumption that life-saving technologies, ICU treatment, and/or resuscitation is not desired by the person with I/DD or surrogate because of the underlying belief I/DD cannot be cured. There may also be a presumption that use of high technology resources for persons with I/DD is inappropriate allocation. Some institutions have established futility policies, prohibiting admission of some categories of patients, such as those in persistent vegetative state, into their ICU. Health care providers should provide information to the person with I/DD and/or surrogate so they may weigh the benefits and burdens of the proposed treatment. There should not be a unilateral decision to withhold treatment. Ethics consultation may be necessary to resolve conflict between health care providers and the person or surrogate.

b. Access to rehabilitative and habilitative services—Persons with I/DD may benefit from rehabilitative and/or habilitative services although the person may not reach a certain level of recovery or attain a prescribed level of functioning. Their participation in rehabilitation and/or habilitation should be based on their choice to participate, their progress towards goals, and their potential for progress.

2. Testing to identify I/DD for prenatal decision making

   a. Risk identification

      i. Carrier status

      ii. Genetic counseling regarding probabilities of having an affected child

   b. Pre-implantation genetic diagnosis (PGD)

      i. With in vitro fertilization, a single cell can be tested for specific genetic conditions.

      ii. The President's Council on Bioethics (2004) promotes equitable access to the benefits of genetic technologies and urges tolerance of and respect for genetic differences.

3. Prenatal testing

   a. The "triple screen" is a screening test that measures three pregnancy hormones: alpha-fetoprotein, human chorionic gonadotropin, and unconjugated estriol. The "quadruple screen" also includes inhibin A. Abnormalities in hormone levels may indicate the fetus has a neural tube defect or Down syndrome. Further testing is warranted if the screening is abnormal.

   b. Testing is usually predicated on the belief that the woman would desire pregnancy termination if a genetic condition is detected in the fetus. Prenatal testing should be available to gain information about the fetus when the risks of the testing outweigh the knowledge to be gained. Informed consent should be secured before testing, and conducting the test should not be conditional on the woman's agreement to terminate the pregnancy if an abnormality is found.

     c. A disability rights approach on prenatal testing is to provide education regarding the purpose of screening and the disabilities being screened prior to testing, rather than afterward, if an abnormality is detected (Parens & Asch, 2003).

     d. Asch (1999, p. e14) says "If the child with a disability is not a problem for the world, and the world is not a problem for the child, perhaps we can diminish our desire for prenatal testing and selective abortion and can comfortably welcome and support children of all characteristics."

4. Newborn screening

     a. Blood test to identify inborn errors of metabolism, which can be treated to prevent I/DD.

     b. Mandatory tests vary from state to state; most states do not require parental consent, but parents may refuse the testing.

5. Health care provider's role in prevention

     a. Health care providers can facilitate informed decision making through assessing the patient's level of understanding and providing education on the specific health care issue requiring a decision.

     b. Health care providers should participate in policy and procedure development and revision in their agencies to ensure that patients' rights are respected regarding diagnostic testing and treatment in the prevention of I/DD.

VI. Legislation

A. Federal laws

1. Americans with Disabilities Act of 1990 (ADA)—An antidiscrimination law for people with disabilities. The law uses "civil rights remedies to eliminate the marginalization of people with disabilities" (Herr, 2003, p. 206). The goals of the ADA are to provide equal opportunity through accommodations if needed, accessibility, reasonable modifications to procedures or policies, integration, and full involvement of citizens with disabilities into public policy.

2. Olmstead decision—U.S. Supreme Court decision requiring federal, state, and local governments to provide funds for integrating people with disabilities into community-based services in the least restrictive settings (http://www.cms.hhs.gov/olmstead).

3. Rehabilitation Act of 1973—Prohibits discrimination based on handicapping condition; promotes independent living through community supports, personal assistance services, and vocational rehabilitation services.

4. Developmental Disabilities Assistance and Bill of Rights Act of 2000 (Public Law 106-402)—The purpose of the law is to ensure and assist states and

localities in providing free, least-restrictive education for children with I/DD, to ensure their rights are protected, and to assess effectiveness of this support; to provide and evaluate early intervention services for children birth–3 years of age; and to provide scholarship assistance to educate special education personnel in exchange for service obligation.

5. Medicaid Home and Community-Based Waiver Program (Public Law 97-35)—Allows states to use federal Medicaid funds for home health care, homemaker services, respite, case management, and residential and employment services for Medicaid recipients. This URL has an overview of state home and community-based services waivers: http://www.cms.hhs.gov/medicaid/1915c/mrddadult.pdf (Omnibus Budget Reconciliation Act of 1981).

6. Federal Crime Bill of 1994—Prohibits execution of people with mental retardation, but does not define it nor stipulate when in the criminal proceedings a person would undergo assessment to determine mental retardation. The U.S. Supreme Court, in the ruling of *Atkins v. Virginia*, found that execution of people with mental retardation is "cruel and unusual" and therefore prohibited by the Eighth Amendment to the Constitution (Legal Information Institute, 2002).

B. State statutes

1. Health care providers should consult the legal affairs department in their agencies to ascertain relevant law for persons with I/DD.

2. Health care providers should be familiar with state laws pertaining to the protection of the rights of persons with I/DD.

3. Health care providers can impact public policy as registered voters and as professionals who provide testimony at public hearings when legislators need input on issues pertaining to the lives of persons with I/DD. Health care providers may also serve on local, regional, or statewide committees, such as IDEA partnerships, or with self-advocacy organizations such as People First. Such positions may provide an opportunity for health care providers to educate the public on the abilities and needs of persons with I/DD and their families.

4. Twenty-six of the 40 states with the death penalty now prohibit execution of people with mental retardation (Death Penalty Information Center, 1997).

VII. Summary

The care of persons with I/DD, of any age, involves a variety of ethical and legal issues. Nurses and other health care professionals must be cognizant of these issues, continue to be informed, and hold discussions as needed so that the individual with I/DD's rights are not compromised.

References

American Association on Mental Retardation. (2001) *Fact sheet: The death penalty.* Retrieved April 30, 2004 from: www.aamr.org/Policies/faq_death_penalty.shtml

American Association on Mental Retardation. (2003). *ARC position statement on criminal justice.* Retrieved April 30, 2004 from: www.aamr.org/Policies/pos_criminal_justice.shtml

Americans with Disabilities Act and the Olmstead decision. Retrieved April 27, 2004 from http://www.cms.hhs.gov/olmstead

Asch, A. (1999). Prenatal diagnosis and selective abortion: A challenge to practice and policy. *American Journal of Public Health, 89,* 1649–1657.

Aziz, M., Maixner, D. F., DeQuardo, J., Aldridge, A., & Tandon, R. (2001). ECT and mental retardation: A review and case reports. *Journal of ECT, 17*(2), 149–152.

Baqi, N., Tejani, A., & Sullivan, E. K. (1998). Renal transplantation in Down syndrome: A report of the North American Pediatric Renal Transplant Cooperative. *Pediatric Transplantation, 2,* 211–215.

Benedetti, E., Asolati, M., Dunn, T., Walczak, D. A., Papp, P., Bartholomew, A. M. et al. (1998). Kidney transplants in recipients with mental retardation: Clinical results in a single-center experience. *American Journal of Kidney Diseases, 31,* 509–512.

Block, P. (2000). Sexuality, fertility, and danger: Twentieth-century images of women with cognitive disabilities. *Sexuality and Disability, 18,* 239–254.

Cutajar, P., & Wilson, D. (1999). The use of ECT in intellectual disability. *Journal of Intellectual Disability Research, 43*(Pt 5), 421–427.

Death Penalty Information Center. (1997). *State statutes prohibiting the death penalty for people with mental retardation.* Retrieved April 30, 2004 from: http://www.deathpenaltyinfo.org/article.php?scid=28&did=138

Developmental Disabilities Assistance and Bill of Rights Act of 2000. Public Law 106–402, 114 Stat. 1677 (2000).

Douglas, S. P., Crook, E. D., Kujdych, N., Lowe, D. A., Sparks, J., & Dottes, A. (2000). Dignity or denial? Decisions regarding initiation of dialysis and medical therapy in the institutionalized severely mentally retarded. *The American Journal of Medical Sciences, 320,* 374–378.

Edwards, S. D. (2000). An argument against research on people with intellectual disabilities. *Medicine, Health Care and Philosophy, 3,* 69–73.

Fisher, C. B. (2003). Goodness-of-fit ethic for informed consent to research involving adults with mental retardation and developmental disabilities. *Mental Retardation and Developmental Disabilities Research Reviews, 9,* 27–31.

Freedman, R. I. (2001). Ethical challenges in the conduct of research involving persons with mental retardation. *Mental Retardation, 39,* 130–141.

Freedman, R. I. (1998). Use of advance directives: Facilitating health care decisions by adults with mental retardation and their families. *Mental Retardation, 36,* 444–456.

Grisso, T., & Appelbaum, P. S. (1998). *Assessing competence to consent to treatment: A guide for physicians and other health professionals.* New York: Oxford University Press.

Herr, S. S. (2003). The potential of disability nondiscrimination laws. In S. S. Herr, L. O. Gostin, & Koh, H. H. (Eds.). *The human rights of persons with intellectual disabilities: Different but equal.* New York: Oxford University Press.

Legal Information Institute. (2002). *Atkins v. Virginia.* Retrieved April 30, 2004 from: http://supct.law.cornell.edu/supct/html/00-8452.ZS.html

Leonard, H., Eastham, K., & Dark, J. (2000). Heart and heart-lung transplantation in Down's syndrome: The lack of supportive evidence means each case must be carefully assessed. *British Medical Journal, 320,* 816–817.

Lin, R. J. (2003). Withdrawing life-sustaining medical treatment—A physician's personal reflection. *Mental Retardation and Developmental Disabilities Research Reviews, 9*, 10–15.

Little, J. D., McFarlane, J., & Ducharme, H. (2002). ECT use delayed in the presence of comorbid mental retardation: A review of clinical and ethical issues. *Journal of ECT, 18*, 218–222.

Lohiya, G-S, Tan-Figueroa, L., & Crinella, F. M. (2003). End-of-life care for a man with developmental disabilities. *Journal of the American Board of Family Practice, 16*(1), 58–62.

McGrath, P. J., Rosmus, C., Canfield, C., Campbell, M. A., & Hennigar, A. (1998). Behaviours caregivers use to determine pain in nonverbal, cognitively impaired individuals. *Developmental Medicine & Child Neurology, 40*, 340–343.

Millar, B. (1998). The dignity of risk and the right to failure: A lesson from patient-focused care. *Journal of Clinical Nursing, 7*, 295–296.

National Bioethics Advisory Commission. (1998). *Research involving persons with mental disorders that may affect decisionmaking capacity.* (Vol. I & II). Washington, DC: U.S. Government Printing Office.

Nelson, L. J. (2003). Respect for the developmentally disabled and forgoing life-sustaining treatment. *Mental Retardation and Developmental Disabilities Research Reviews, 9*, 3–9.

Omnibus Budget Reconciliation Act of 1981. Pub. L. No. 97-35, §§501, 95 Stat. 818 (1981).

O'Sullivan, J. L., & Borcherding, B. G. (2002). Informed consent for medication in persons with mental retardation and mental illness. *Health Matrix, 12*, 63–92.

Parens, E., & Asch, A. (2003). Disability rights critique of prenatal genetic testing: Reflections and recommendations. *Mental Retardation and Developmental Disabilities Research Reviews, 9*, 40–47.

President's Commission for the Study of Ethical Problems in Medicine and Biomedical and Behavioral Research. (1983). *Deciding to forego life-sustaining treatment: Ethical, medical, and legal issues in treatment decisions.* Washington, DC: U.S. Government Printing Office.

President's Council on Bioethics. (2004). *Reproduction and responsibility: The regulation of new biotechnologies.* Washington, DC: U.S. Government Printing Office.

Rehabiliation Act of 1973, Pub. L. No. 93-112, 87 Stat. 355 (1973).

Reynolds, D. F. (1999). Project BRIDGE—People with disabilities participate in their health care decisions. *Bioethics Forum, 15*(2), 36–45.

Tuffrey-Wijne, I. (2002). The palliative care needs of people with intellectual disabilities: A case study. *International Journal of Palliative Nursing, 8*, 222–232.

Tuffrey-Wijne, I. (2003). The palliative care needs of people with intellectual disabilities: A literature review. *Palliative Medicine, 17*, 55–62.

United Network for Organ Sharing. (2004). *Living donation facts.* Retrieved April 26, 2004 from: www.unos.org/ContentDocuments/Living_Donation_Facts.pdf

Economic and Policy Issues

Theodore A. Kastner, MD, MS and Kevin K. Walsh, PhD

27

Objectives

At the completion of this chapter, the learner will be able to:

1. Understand how government programs, both federal and state, fund health care services.

2. Identify the primary economic programs that fund primary care and acute care services, and understand trends in health care financing (e.g., managed care) and how they have affected individuals with intellectual and developmental disabilities (I/DD).

3. Understand how specialized health care for people with I/DD can best be provided and funded; identify various models of health care services for this population.

4. Identify the primary funding arrangements for long-term care and how they interact with primary care and acute care systems.

Key Points

- Health care needs in adults and children with I/DD pose additional challenges in access, clinical care, and funding when compared to the general population.

- Government agencies play a major role in the provision and funding of health care services in this population.

- Government-funded health care services require several partnerships: federal and state, public and private, payers and providers.

- Workable specialized community-based health care services for individuals with I/DD exist but have not yet demonstrated complete efficacy.

I. Populations and the Need

A. Populations of interest

 1. Health care for adults and children with I/DD requires specialized skills and systems (Crocker, 2000; DeJong, Palsbo, & Beatty, 2002).

 a. The definition of developmental disabilities usually defines eligibility and linkage to services; typically, federal definitions are incorporated into state policies.

 b. Size of the population—Prevalence of I/DD in the general population is between 2.5% and 3%; by 2002 over 393,000 individuals received residential services in settings with 15 or fewer residents (Prouty, Smith, & Lakin, 2003).

 2. Health care for children with special health care needs (CSHCN) is closely related to health care in I/DD and is often included in this latter group during childhood (American Academy of Pediatrics, Committee on Child Health Financing, 1995; American Academy of Pediatrics, Committee on Children with Disabilities, 1998).

 3. Clinical characteristics of the populations

 a. Children with special health care needs differ from adults in that the dynamics of child development present different stages over time; additionally, the causes of disease often differ (e.g., in children there are more rare or low-incidence conditions and fewer common ones, differing from adult care in which there are few rare conditions and a preponderance of common ones) (American Academy of Pediatrics, Committee on Children with Disabilities, 1998).

 b. Adults with I/DD range in disability from very mild and not dissimilar from the general population to profoundly disabled with many complex and multiple disabilities.

 4. Within the general population of individuals with I/DD, there are subgroups with specialized needs (e.g., Down syndrome, autism, dual diagnosis, seizure management, aging issues, multiply handicapped, and technology-dependent).

 5. Over the last half of the 20th century, and especially over the past 25–30 years, a significant shift in care has taken place from institutional settings to community-based settings, giving rise to increased challenges in the consistent provision of *quality* health care (Lewis, Lewis, Leake, King, & Lindemann, 2002; Schalock, Baker, & Croser, 2002; Walsh & Kastner, 1999).

B. Needs of the population

 1. Access to quality primary health care and dental care in community settings with knowledgeable and experienced practitioners

2. Access to specialty care, tertiary care, ancillary care, and other services including durable medical equipment (DME), pharmacy, home health services, rehabilitation, and other services

3. Care coordination services to assure appropriate, effective, and efficient health care delivery (American Academy of Pediatrics Committee on Children with Disabilities, 1999; Crocker, 2000; Walsh, Kastner & Criscione, 1997)

   a. Definition and description of care coordination activities and elements.

   b. Benefits and outcomes of care coordination

      i.   fiscal benefits and outcomes

      ii. clinical benefits and outcomes

      iii. system integration

      iv. quality and satisfaction (Lewis et al., 2002; Walsh & Kastner, 1999)

II. Historical Background on Relevant Health Care Policy

A. Children with special health care needs

   1. In 1912 the Marine Hospital Service became the U.S. Public Health Service and, in the same year, the Children's Bureau was established.

   2. The Social Security Act of 1935 provided for Aid to Dependent Children and the Maternal and Child Health Grants program under Title V, which was later expanded to include other areas. In 1954, the Children's Bureau became part of the U.S. Department of Health Education and Welfare and began a limited focus on children with mental retardation.

   3. In 1956, the Social Security Act Amendments authorized payments for Adults Disabled in Childhood, about 30% of which were provided to individuals with mental retardation.

   4. Maternal and Child Health funds have been used to develop university-based research and training centers under the Leadership Education in Neurodevelopmental and Related Disabilities (LEND) programs, which provide long-term, graduate-level interdisciplinary training to health professionals.

   5. As part of these LEND programs and service centers, Maternal and Child Health–sponsored residency training and fellowship training programs have flourished, typically in university-based tertiary treatment settings.

   6. Recently, specialty boards in Neurodevelopmental Disabilities (American Board of Psychiatry and Neurology) and Developmental and Behavioral Pediatrics (American Board of Pediatrics) have been created.

B. Individuals with mental retardation and related developmental disabilities

1. Earliest formal health care systems existed in institutional settings, which were funded by state funds until Medicaid ICF/MR funding for these facilities became available during the Kennedy administration (Crocker, 2000; Kasten & Coury, 1991; Tarjan, Eyman, & Miller, 1969).

2. The President's Panel on Mental Retardation was created in 1961, which led to many programmatic developments such as the establishment of general health programs (e.g., the WIC—Women, Infants, and Children program—to promote normal growth of children and prenatal health of mothers) and programs specifically designed to affect individuals with I/DD (e.g., the University Affiliated Facilities—UAF, later changed to University Affiliated Programs—UAP, and now known as University Centers for Excellence in Developmental Disabilities Education, Research, and Service—UCEDD).

3. Programs and services specifically for individuals with mental retardation and related developmental disabilities were developed within Medicaid, under Title XIX of the Social Security Act to support ICF/MR settings and, in 1981, the Home and Community-Based Services (HCBS) waiver program.

III. Current Health Care Policy Environment

A. Fee-for-Service vs. managed care—States are increasingly turning to managed care to provide basic primary care services, while "carving out" certain services to remain in the Medicaid fee-for-service model (American Academy of Pediatrics, Committee on Child Health Financing, 1995; Kastner, Walsh, & Criscione, 1997a, 1997b).

B. Medicaid eligibility vs. Medicaid *and* Medicare eligibility ("dually eligible")— These two federal program impose rules and requirements for services that must be included in state plans. For example, Medicaid includes a minimum set of services; Medicare eligibility precludes a state from mandating membership of individuals with I/DD in Medicaid managed care.

C. Mental health care poses challenges in both the general population in managed care and in individuals with I/DD (Beasley & Hurley, 2003).

D. Other influences

1. Surgeon General's Conference—Increased recognition of the need to formally address health care in individuals with mental retardation and related developmental disabilities (U.S. Public Health Service, 2002) (see Chapter 7).

2. President Bush's New Freedom Initiative—This initiative for people with disabilities has given rise to the creation of the Aging and Disability Resource Center Grant Program (http://www.whitehouse.gov/infocus/newfreedom/).

3. Nongovernmental health-related organizations

    a. American Academy of Pediatrics (AAP)—A traditional health care providers' association, composed mostly of pediatricians, committed to the attainment of optimal physical, mental, and social health of infants, children, adolescents, and young adults. Disabilities issues are generally addressed by work groups or specialized committees. The AAP forms the primary professional group (e.g., pediatricians) of those providing health care for individuals with I/DD. AAP has championed the concept of the "medical home" in health care.

    b. Society for Developmental and Behavioral Pediatrics (SDBP)—An international, interdisciplinary organization seeking to improve care and knowledge in developmental and behavioral pediatric areas.

    c. American Academy of Developmental Medicine and Dentistry (AADMD)—A recently formed professional group dedicated to improving the health status of individuals with disabilities through teaching, research, and advocacy.

    d. Family Voices—A national advocacy organization devoted to improving health care for children and youth with special health care needs.

IV. Financing of Health Care in I/DD

A. Federal programs

1. Overview

    a. Health care is funded under two major federal programs—Medicaid and Medicare. Medicaid programs are administered by each state whereas Medicare is administered by the federal government through the Centers for Medicare and Medicaid Services (CMS).

    b. Medicaid is a program for individuals who meet criteria based on poverty. Medicaid benefits differ across the states. Medicaid services in states include mandatory services and elective services. Medicaid covers long-term care.

    c. Medicare is a program for older adults that pays for a complex array of services under several programs. It includes physicians' visits, hospitalization, and, to a limited extent, prescriptions but does not include long-term care. Many individuals with I/DD are eligible for Medicare benefits either by virtue of their age or the age of their parents.

    d. Many individuals are eligible for both Medicare and Medicaid benefits ("dually eligible").

2. Medicaid

    a. Created in 1965 under Title XIX of the Social Security Act to pay for medical assistance for low-income individuals and families, Medicaid is jointly funded by the federal and state governments to provide health care and medical long-term care assistance. It is the nation's largest source of funding for medical and health-related services for people with limited income. Medicaid requires states to provide, at a minimum, a specific set of services (e.g., physician services, hospitalizations, laboratory services). Additional optional services, often of high importance to persons with I/DD, include dental coverage, pharmacy services, and the like. Coverage of these optional services is often subject to change as state budgets may be unable to fund them.

    b. Medicaid programs of importance to individuals with I/DD:

        i. Aged, Blind, and Disabled (ABD)—designation leading to specific benefits based on eligibility; many eligibility provisions specifically include individuals who are aged, blind, or disabled.

        ii. Early and Periodic Screening, Diagnosis, and Treatment (EPSDT)—Created by the Omnibus Budget Reconciliation Act of 1989 (OBRA 89) this program provides comprehensive and preventive child health diagnosis, screening, and treatment services. Available to Medicaid recipients under the age of 21.

        iii. Intermediate Care Facilities/Mental Retardation (ICFs/MR)—The original Medicaid legislation provided coverage for intermediate care facilities—nursing facilities for elderly and disabled persons. An optional Medicaid benefit was created by Section 1905(d) of the Social Security Act to fund "institutions" (four or more beds) specifically for people with mental retardation (ICFs/MR). In order to promote habilitation, these facilities must provide "active treatment." Although the federal government considers any facility with four or more beds to be an institution, ICFs/MR can vary in size from small community-based homes to large congregate care centers with hundreds of beds.

        iv. Medicaid waivers—A Medicaid waiver may be granted when a cost-neutral application is submitted by a state to the federal government (Centers for Medicare and Medicaid Services—CMS) to "waive" certain Medicaid rules and regulations in order to expand the number of persons who are served or to expand the range of services covered. Waivers address clinical conditions such as developmental disability, traumatic brain injury, HIV/AIDS, or serious and persistent mental illness. All states operate Home and

Community Based Services (HCBS) waiver programs, which provide community services in lieu of ICFs/MR-institutional settings. For children with special health care needs, a popular option is the Katie Beckett Waiver, which provides home-based care as an alternative to institutionalization.

    v.   State Children's Health Insurance Plan (SCHIP)—Created by the Balanced Budget Act of 1997, this program gives states the option of offering health insurance for children, up to age 19, who are not already insured under Medicaid. Approximately one-half of states used SCHIP to expand access to the full range of Medicaid benefits including EPSDT. The other half created a new benefit package that may not offer the same range of services covered under Medicaid.

3. Medicare: Policy basis and relevance to I/DD

    a.   Created in 1965 under Title XIX of the Social Security Act, Medicare extended health coverage to almost all Americans aged 65 or older.

    b.   Social Security Amendments in 1972 expanded Medicare to provide coverage to two additional high risk groups—disabled persons receiving cash benefits for 24 months under the social security program and persons suffering from end-stage renal disease.

    c.   Pharmacy benefits were added in 2003. This controversial expansion of benefits included copays and deductibles for all Medicare recipients, including those individuals with Medicaid who were previously not responsible for a financial contribution.

4. Combined federal and state roles

    a.   All levels of government share responsibility for funding and providing health care services for most individuals with I/DD; linkage and coordination among governmental agencies, practitioners, health facilities/providers, and other nongovernmental groups is essential to quality.

B. State programs

1. States structure and administer Medicaid programs at the state level under the auspices of the federal Centers for Medicare and Medicaid Services (CMS), formerly known as HCFA (Health Care Financing Administration).

2. Medicaid-funded health care for people with I/DD is generally provided through either "fee-for-service" programs in which practitioners submit claims and are paid by their state (often through a fiscal intermediary), or in "Medicaid managed care" in which practitioners are paid through arrangements with managed care organizations (typically, HMOs). Implementation of Medicaid managed care requires approval of a waiver by CMS.

3. Service availability in managed care

   a. Medicaid managed care represents an opportunity for states to modify the range of services and payment mechanisms offered to support people with I/DD in the community. New services may include care management, quality improvement initiatives, or integration of acute and long-term care. The concept of managed care is believed to include financial risk for the contractor (such as the HMO) or health care provider, although this is not always the case.

   b. Payment mechanisms to HMOs are typically based upon capitation and may include capitation, capitation with risk corridors, full-risk capitation, or capitation with some preserved fee-for-service elements. Payment mechanisms used by HMOs when contracting with health care providers generally rely upon fee-for-service, but can include forms of capitation if these are mutually agreeable (Kastner, Walsh & Criscione, 1997a, 1997b).

   c. The range of services covered under Medicaid managed care is generally equal to or greater than those covered under fee-for-service. However, medical management structures (utilization management/quality improvement) may limit access to some services.

   d. States and HMOs rely upon the concept of "medical necessity" in determining what services are to be provided to a specific individual. In many cases, coverage for habilitative services such as physical therapy, occupational therapy, and speech therapy may be limited due to restrictive definitions of "medical necessity."

4. "Carving in" and "carving out"

   a. When implementing a Medicaid waiver, such as one for Medicaid managed care, a state must decide what services to provide through HMOs and what services to provide under the existing fee-for-service program.

   b. A "carve-out" is a service that a state Medicaid administration excludes from managed care and leaves in the fee-for-service system. For example, a state may elect to pay for durable medical equipment or certain high-cost medications under fee-for-service arrangements and will "carve them out" of the Medicaid managed care contract.

   c. A "carve-in" is a service that is specifically *included* in the state's Medicaid plan for a particular group. For example, a state Medicaid program may carve in mental health benefits for its aged, blind, and disabled population.

5. Privatized service systems

   a. Some states elect to "privatize" the service delivery system using private organizations called contracted system administrators (CSAs), administrative service organizations (ASOs), or similar terms. These organizations manage systems issues such as network development, credentialing, and claims processing. In addition, they may subcontract to various provider groups or other organizations for care management, direct services, support services, and so forth.

    b. Specialty clinical settings often exist and provide services to individuals with I/DD including funded clinics, specialized practices or practice groups, or clinics attached to federally funded settings (such as University Affiliated Centers of Excellence in Developmental Disabilities—UCEDDs).

C. Families and commercial health insurance

    1. Families often share in paying for health care, especially for children with special health care needs, through *co-pays* and other *out of pocket* expenses (Altman, Cooper, & Cunningham, 1999; Fujiura, 1998).

    2. Insurance for children with special health care needs is often obtained through the parents' employers and provided through commercial health plans. Most adults with I/DD lack private insurance as they are unemployed. The majority of health services for adults with I/DD are funded by Medicaid or Medicare or both.

    3. Health savings accounts are a new benefit authorized under revisions to the federal Medicare program (in 2003) but available in the commercial market. This program builds upon the former medical savings account program and allows employers to offer a high deductible insurance coverage in conjunction with the employee making tax-exempt deposits to a health savings account. Concerns relate to the effects of healthy persons choosing to leave the insurance pool and creating stratification in the marketplace. Persons with I/DD could eventually pay higher premiums as a result of being in a high-risk pool.

V. Models of Health Care Services Delivery

A. Acute care services—Include all preventive, primary, secondary, and tertiary services offered in the community; they can be delivered under various models (Pulcini & Howard, 1997).

    1. Medicaid fee-for-service—Practitioners provide services to eligible individuals, billing Medicaid directly.

    2. Medicaid managed care—Practitioners are in one of several relationships with a managed care organization, typically a health maintenance organizations (HMO). Payment for services rendered comes from the HMO either in a fee-for-service arrangement or on a *capitated* basis, that is a set *per person per month* (PMPM) fee for all health care services (Crocker, 2000; Kastner, Walsh, & Criscione, 1997a).

3.   In many states, children with I/DD and children with special health care needs receive expanded health benefits and care coordination under specific programs such as SCHIP, EPSDT, specific waiver programs, or other state programs.

B. The Medical Home–American Academy of Pediatrics—The medical home denotes a practice setting in which people with I/DD and their families receive care from a pediatrician or physician whom they know and trust (American Academy of Pediatrics, Medical Home Web site: http://www.medicalhomeinfo.org).

C. Medicaid and state DD authority efforts

1.   Initiatives for children—SCHIP's

2.   ESPDT initiatives

3.   Structural efforts—Establishment and funding of specialty clinics and program interventions in states (e.g., Down syndrome (Chicoine, McGuire, Hebein, & Gilly, 1994); primary care (Ziring et al., 1988); dual diagnosis and crisis intervention (Davidson et al., 1995)).

4.   University Centers of Excellence in Developmental Disabilities (UCEDDs, formerly UAPs)

D. Market-based and other model efforts—Part IV, Appendix D of the Surgeon General's report (2001) outlines several creative health care system strategies including:

1.   Comprehensive health care integrated with social services funded by Medicaid health care funds by using fee-for-service or capitated payments through managed care organizations.

2.   Inclusive health services that provide care to specialized populations in community settings (e.g., rural initiatives or mother and infant care); often grant funded.

3.   Specialty outreach services that encompass either regional or statewide initiatives.

4.   As managed care penetrates the aged, blind, and disabled marketplace, additional opportunities will arise for entrepreneurial care providers to work through managed care organizations in regional or statewide efforts.

E. Practitioner issues

1.   Nurse practitioners and other advanced practice nurses—There are increasing opportunities, in both primary care and specialty settings, to employ nurse practitioners and other advanced practice nurses into care systems for individuals with I/DD; therefore, basic baccalaureate and advanced practice education at the graduate level will become critical (Brown & Grimes, 1993; Richer, Jorden, & Taylor, 2001; Walsh, Hammerman, Josephson, & Krupka, 2000).

2.   Credentials—Traditional health care credentials have not included the care of I/DD, although recently certifications have been developed (Palmer,

Percey, Tivnan, Tunnessen, & Scheiber, 2003); for example, the American Board of Pediatrics offers certification in developmental-behavioral pediatrics and, in conjunction with the American Board of Psychiatry and Neurology, offers a certificate in neurodevelopmental disabilities (see http://www.abp.org/certinfo/SUBSPEC/ssproc.htm).

3. New health care professional groups are forming around the population of individuals with I/DD, such as the American Academy of Developmental Medicine and Dentistry (http://www.aadmd.org).

F. Health care in out-of-home placements and other settings

1. Secondary/tertiary care settings (hospitals, ancillary and specialized services such as rehabilitation).

2. Long-term care

a. Individuals with I/DD may receive health care through traditional long-term care placements (e.g., ICFs/MR and nursing homes).

b. Medicare does not cover long-term care services, but they can be covered by Medicaid in nursing homes.

c. Long-term care for individuals with I/DD can be provided in public or private (ICFs/MR) facilities.

d. States can "waive" the requirement for ICFs/MR level and provide long-term care under the HCBS waiver; when enrolled in waivers, those with I/DD typically seek health care in community settings.

VI. Related Topics

A. Cost burden of illness in I/DD (Braddock, 2002; Burke et al., 1999; Glidden & Floyd, 1997)

B. Cost comparisons of institutional vs. community care (Felce, Lowe, Beecham, & Hallam, 2000; Rhoades & Altman, 2001; Walsh, Kastner, & Green, 2003)

C. Obesity reduction and achieving fitness (Dykens, Rosner, & Butterbaugh, 1998; Fujiura, Fitzsimons, Marks, & Chicoine, 1997; Lancioni & O'Reilly, 1998)

D. The role of health services research (Brown, Lakin, & Burwell, 1997; Jette & Keysor, 2002; Perrin, 2002)

VII. Summary

Economic and policy issues are often complicated and difficult to understand. In this chapter, the major economic and policy issues of this time have been plainly addressed. Nurses and health care professionals caring for individuals with I/DD need to be cognizant and concerned about these issues and active in their solutions.

References

Altman, B. M., Cooper, P. F., & Cunningham, P. J. (1999). The case of disability in the family: Impact on health care utilization and expenditures for nondisabled members. *The Milbank Quarterly, 77,* 39–75.

American Academy of Pediatrics, Committee on Child Health Financing. (1995). Guiding principles for managed care arrangements for the health care of infants, children, adolescents, and young adults. *Pediatrics, 95,* 613–615.

American Academy of Pediatrics, Committee on Children with Disabilities. (1999). Care coordination: Integrating health and related systems of care for children with special health care needs. *Pediatrics, 104*(4 Pt 1), 978–981.

American Academy of Pediatrics, Committee on Children with Disabilities. (1998). Managed care and children with special health care needs: A subject review. *Pediatrics, 102,* 657–660.

Beasley, J. B., & Hurley, A. D. (2003). The design of community supports for individuals with developmental disabilities and mental health needs. *Mental Health Aspects of Developmental Disabilities, 6,* 81–84.

Braddock, D. (2002). Public financial support for disability at the dawn of the 21st century. *American Journal on Mental Retardation, 107,* 478–489.

Brown, S. A., & Grimes, D. E. (1993). *Nurse practitioners and certified nurse-midwives: A meta-analysis of studies on nurses in primary care roles.* Silver Spring, MD: American Nurses Association.

Brown, S. L., Lakin, K. C., & Burwell, B. O. (1997). Beneficiary centered care in services to persons with developmental disabilities. *Health Care Financing Review, 19,* 23–46.

Burke, T. A., McKee, J. R., Pathak, D. S., Donahue, R. M. J., Parasuraman, T. V., & Batenhorst, A. S. (1999). Costs of epilepsy in an intermediate care facility for persons with mental retardation. *American Journal on Mental Retardation, 104,* 148–157.

Chicoine, B., McGuire, D., Hebein, S., & Gilly, D. (1994). Development of a clinic for adults with Down syndrome. *Mental Retardation, 32,* 100–106.

Crocker, A. C. (2000). Community-based and managed health care. In M. L. Wehmeyer & J. R. Patton (Eds.). *Mental retardation in the 21st century.* Austin, TX: Pro-Ed.

Davidson, P. W., Cain, N. N., Sloan-Reeves, J. E., Giesow, V. E., Quijano, L. E., & Van Heyningen, J. (1995). Crisis intervention for community-based individuals with developmental disabilities and psychiatric disorders. *Mental Retardation, 33,* 21–30.

DeJong, G., Palsbo, S. E., & Beatty, P. W. (2002). The organization and financing of health services for persons with disabilities. *The Milbank Quarterly, 80,* 261–301.

Dykens, E. M., Rosner, B. A., & Butterbaugh, G. (1998). Exercise and sports in children and adolescents with developmental disabilities: Positive physical and psychosocial effects. *Child & Adolescent Psychiatric Clinics of North America, 7,* 757–771.

Felce, D., Lowe, K., Beecham, J., & Hallam, A. (2000). Exploring the relationships between costs and quality of services for adults with severe intellectual disabilities and the most severe challenging behaviors: A multivariate regression analysis. *Journal of Intellectual & Developmental Disability, 4,* 307–326.

Fujiura, G. T. (1998). Demography of family households. *American Journal on Mental Retardation, 103,* 225–235.

Fujiura, G. T., Fitzsimons, N., Marks, B., & Chicoine, B. (1997). Predictors of BMI among adults with Down syndrome: The social context of health promotion. *Research in Developmental Disabilities, 18,* 261–273.

Glidden, L. M., & Floyd, F. J. (1997). Disaggregating parental depression and family stress in assessing families with developmental disabilities: A multisample analysis. *American Journal on Mental Retardation, 102,* 250–266.

Jette, A. M., & Keysor, J. J. (2002). Uses of evidence in disability outcomes and effectiveness research. *The Milbank Quarterly, 80,* 325–345.

Kasten, E. F., & Coury, D. L. (1991). Health policy and prevention of mental retardation. In J. L. Matson & J. A. Mulick (Eds.). *Handbook of mental retardation* (2nd ed., pp. 336–344). New York: Pergamon Press.

Kastner, T., Walsh, K. K., & Criscione, T. (1997a). Overview and implications of Medicaid managed care for people with developmental disabilities. *Mental Retardation, 35,* 257–269.

Kastner, T., Walsh, K. K., & Criscione, T. (1997b). Technical elements, demonstration projects, and fiscal models in Medicaid managed care for people with developmental disabilities. *Mental Retardation, 35,* 270–285.

Lancioni, G. E., & O'Reilly, M. E. (1998). A review of research on physical exercise with people with severe and profound developmental disabilities. *Research in Developmental Disabilities, 19,* 477–492.

Lewis, M. A., Lewis, C. E., Leake, B., King, B. H., & Lindemann, R. (2002). The quality of health care for adults with developmental disabilities. *Public Health Reports, 117,* 174–184.

Palmer, F. B., Percey, A. K., Tivnan, P., Tunnessen, J. D., & Scheiber, S. C. (2003). Certification in neurodevelopmental disabilities: The development of a new subspecialty and results of the initial examinations. *Mental Retardation & Developmental Disabilities Research Reviews, 9*(2), 128–131.

Perrin, J. M. (2002). Health services research for children with disabilities. *The Milbank Quarterly, 80,* 303–324.

Prouty, R. W., Smith, G., & Lakin, K. C. (Eds.). (2003). *Residential services for persons with developmental disabilities: Status and trends through 2002.* Minneapolis: University of Minnesota, Research and Training Center on Community Living, Institute on Community Integration.

Pulcini, J., & Howard, A. M. (1997). Framework for analyzing health care models serving adults with mental retardation and other developmental disabilities. *Mental Retardation, 35,* 209–217.

Rhoades, J. A., & Altman, B. M. (2001). Personal characteristics and contextual factors associated with residential expenditures for individuals with mental retardation. *Mental Retardation, 39,* 114–129.

Richer, E. R., Jorden, M. E., & Taylor, C. J. (2001). Assessing successful entry into nurse practitioner practice: A literature review. *Journal of the New York State Nurses Association, 32*(2), 14–18.

Schalock, R. L., Baker, P. C., & Croser, M. D. (2002). *Embarking on a new century: Mental retardation at the end of the twentieth century.* Washington, DC: American Association on Mental Retardation.

Tarjan, G., Eyman, R. K., & Miller, C. R. (1969). Natural history of mental retardation in a state hospital. *American Journal of Diseases of Children, 117,* 609–620.

U.S. Public Health Service. (2002). *Closing the gap: A national blueprint to improve the health of persons with mental retardation. Report of the Surgeon General's conference on health disparities and mental retardation.* Washington, DC: Author.

Walsh, K. K., Hammerman, S., Josephson, F., & Krupka, P. (2000). Caring for people with developmental disabilities: Survey of nurses about their education and experience. *Mental Retardation, 38,* 33–41.

Walsh, K. K., & Kastner, T. A. (1999). Quality of health care for people with developmental disabilities: The challenge of managed care. *Mental Retardation, 37,* 1–15.

Walsh, K. K., Kastner, T., & Criscione, T. (1997). Characteristics of hospitalizations for people with developmental disabilities: Utilization, costs, and the impact of care coordination. *American Journal on Mental Retardation, 101,* 505–520.

Walsh, K. K., Kastner, T. A., & Green, R. G. (2003). Cost comparisons of community and institutional residential settings: Historical review of selected research. *Mental Retardation, 41,* 103–122.

Ziring, P. R., Kastner, T., Friedman, D. L., Pond, W. S., Barnett M. L., Sonnenberg, E. M., et al. (1988). Provision of health care for persons with developmental disabilities living in the community: The Morristown Model. *Journal of the American Medical Association, 260,* 1439–1444.

Index